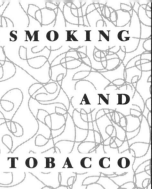

SMOKING

AND

TOBACCO

CONTROL

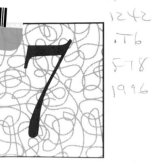
MONOGRAPH

7

The FTC Cigarette Test Method for Determining Tar, Nicotine, and Carbon Monoxide Yields of U.S. Cigarettes

Report of the NCI Expert Committee

U.S. DEPARTMENT OF HEALTH AND HUMAN SERVICES
Public Health Service
National Institutes of Health

Foreword

In response to the emerging scientific evidence that cigarette smoking posed a significant health risk to the user, in the early 1950's the major cigarette manufacturers began widespread promotion of filtered cigarettes to reassure smokers that, regardless of whatever unhealthy constituents were in cigarette smoke, filters were a "scientific" breakthrough.

Advertisements for Viceroy's "health guard filter" stated, "DENTISTS ADVISE—Smoke VICEROYS—The Nicotine and Tars Trapped by The Viceroy Filter CAN NEVER STAIN YOUR TEETH!" and "Leading N.Y. Doctor Tells His Patients What to Smoke—Filtered Cigarette Smoke Is Better For Health. The Nicotine and Tars Trapped . . . Cannot Reach Mouth, Throat Or Lungs." Chesterfield was "Best for you—*low* in nicotine, highest in quality," while L&M's were "Just What the Doctor Ordered." Lorillard Tobacco Company stressed its science-based Kent micronite filter (the original micronite filter was made of asbestos) and claimed it removed seven times more tar and nicotine than any other cigarette, which "put Kent in a class all by itself where health protection is concerned." Of course, we know today that not only were these claims patently false, but the cigarette companies knew it.

In the early 1950's the Federal Trade Commission (FTC) challenged a variety of health claims made for cigarettes in their advertising, including claims about tar and nicotine. In 1955 FTC published advertising guidelines that, among other things, prohibited claims by cigarette manufacturers that a particular brand of cigarettes was low in tar and nicotine or lower than other brands, when it had not been established by competent scientific proof that the claim was true and the difference was significant. Cigarette manufactures, however, continued to advertise tar numbers. In the absence of a standardized test methodology, this resulted in what is referred to as a "tar derby"—a multitude of inconsistent, noncomparable claims that did not give consumers a meaningful opportunity to assess the relative tar delivery of competing brands. The tar derby ended in 1960 when discussions with FTC culminated in an industry agreement to refrain from tar and nicotine advertising.

In 1966, however, the U.S. Public Health Service (PHS) prepared a technical report on "tar" and nicotine that concluded, "The preponderance of scientific evidence strongly suggests that the lower the 'tar' and nicotine content of cigarette smoke, the less harmful would be the effect." In reaching this conclusion, the report noted the clear relationship between dose of cigarette smoke received by the smoker and disease risk. Regardless of how dose was calculated—by number of cigarettes smoked per day, age of initiation, total number of years one smoked, or depth of inhalation, mortality rates among smokers increased. When smokers quit smoking, their risk was reduced in proportion to the length of time off cigarettes.

Subsequent to the PHS statement, FTC reversed its decision banning tar and nicotine claims in advertising and established a standardized testing protocol for assessing tar and nicotine yields. Today that protocol is widely known as the FTC test method. In 1980 the protocol was broadened to include measurement of the carbon monoxide yields of cigarettes as well.

The initial protocol adopted by FTC was largely based on the work of U.S. Department of Agriculture chemist C.L. Ogg, as published in the *Journal of the Association of Official Agricultural Chemists* in 1964. It appears, however, that this protocol was based on one person's observations about how people smoked.

Much the same protocol had been proposed by American Tobacco Company researchers in 1936. Writing in the July issue of *Industrial and Engineering Chemistry*, J.A. Bradford and colleagues noted, "The present writer's arbitrarily selected rate is a 35-cc puff of 2-second duration taken once a minute."

However, cigarettes consumed at that time were vastly different from those manufactured and marketed later. In fact, tar and nicotine levels began to decline during the 1950's, concurrent with the mass marketing of filter cigarettes. Market share of filter cigarettes increased from almost zero in 1950 (0.6 percent of the market) to 50 percent by decade's end. Total cigarette sales, which had begun to decline after the first public statements about the hazards of smoking in the early 1950's, rebounded to new highs.

Although filter efficiency may have contributed to some of the reduction in tar/nicotine yields in the 1950's, the decline resulted mostly from less tobacco being used to make filtered as opposed to unfiltered cigarettes. However, during the 1960's and 1970's major cigarette design changes resulted in significantly lower machine-measured cigarette yields. The changes included increased use of ventilated tobacco rods and filters, use of more porous cigarette papers, and increased use of expanded and reconstituted tobacco. Concurrent with these modifications in cigarette design, cigarette manufacturers increasingly made use of additives in manufacturing. Today about 600 different compounds are routinely added to domestic cigarette brands, yet no routine testing is performed to determine whether these compounds pose any additional health risk to the smoker when they are burned in a cigarette.

U.S. market share of cigarettes yielding 15 mg tar or less went from 3.6 percent in 1970 to 44.8 percent by 1980. The sales-weighted average tar and nicotine yields of all U.S. cigarettes are now approximately 12 mg tar and 0.9 mg nicotine. By comparison, sales-weighted yields in the early 1950's were 35 mg tar and 2.5 mg nicotine.

As consumption of low-yield cigarettes began to proliferate, the public health community became concerned that these products were not what they seemed. Increasingly, scientific studies documented that smokers who switched to these low-yield products smoked them differently, thus negating the reason many of them changed in the first place—to lower their health risk.

The U.S. Congress also voiced its concern in 1978 when it enacted the Health Services and Centers Act. Section 403 of that legislation directed the U.S. Department of Health and Human Services (DHHS) to conduct a "study or studies of (1) the relative health risks associated with smoking cigarettes of varying levels of tar, nicotine, and carbon monoxide; and (2) the health risks associated with smoking cigarettes containing any substances commonly added to commercially manufactured cigarettes." The Secretary of the Department of Health and Human Services addressed this issue as part of the 1981 Surgeon General's report, *The Health Consequences of Smoking: The Changing Cigarette.* The overall conclusion of that report was clear: "There is no safe cigarette and no safe level of consumption." Although the report did note that smoking cigarettes with lower yields of tar and nicotine reduces the risk of lung cancer to some extent, the benefits are minimal in comparison with giving up cigarettes entirely. Evidence relating to heart disease, other cancers, or chronic obstructive lung disease was not sufficient to permit conclusions to be drawn. As to the accuracy of the FTC test method, the report stated: "The 'tar' and nicotine yields obtained by present testing methods do not correspond to the dosages that the individual smokers receive: In some cases they may seriously underestimate these dosages."

Growing numbers of questions were raised about the accuracy of the FTC test protocol to measure tar, nicotine, and carbon monoxide levels from low-yield cigarettes—questions raised not just by the public health community but also within the tobacco industry. Competitors complained to FTC that Brown and Williamson's (B&W) Barclay brand cigarette did not test accurately with the FTC test method. They argued that the brand was designed with unique air ventilation channels that caused it to test low on the FTC method. The ventilation channels, which remained open when Barclays were smoked on the FTC machine, were rendered inoperable when a human being smoked the cigarettes. In April 1983 FTC announced that its testing method understated values for constituents in Barclay cigarettes, and as a result, until new testing methods were developed, FTC would no longer report an official rating for Barclay cigarettes. Later, FTC took similar steps with respect to other B&W cigarette varieties that used a filter design similar to Barclay's.

Eventually FTC closed its cigarette testing laboratory, in part because of insufficient expertise within the agency to carry out an increasingly complex and costly testing program. Since 1987, constituent levels for domestic cigarette brands have been determined for the manufacturers by the Tobacco Institute Testing Laboratory with oversight by FTC. The Tobacco Institute serves as a trade organization as well as the information and lobbying arm of the tobacco industry.

In June 1994 the Chairman of the House Subcommittee on Health and the Environment wrote the Director of the National Cancer Institute (NCI), asking him to convene a meeting of experts to ". . . review and make recommendations on the accuracy and appropriateness of the Federal Trade Commission's method for determining the relative 'tar' and nicotine content of cigarettes." A similar request was received from the FTC Chairman asking that NCI convene a consensus conference on the topic and outlining several areas it wished to be considered.

On December 5 and 6, 1994, a meeting of the NCI ad hoc expert committee was convened under the aegis of the President's Cancer Panel to examine this issue. The committee consisted of 11 individuals from diverse scientific backgrounds and experience. The committee had the benefit of excellent presentations from 14 experts whose professional careers were not only involved in research on smoking, but who have been active contributors to this field of scientific inquiry. Two of the individual participants were cigarette industry scientists, who participated in all discussions.

From the outset of the committee's deliberations, it was clear that the intent of the meeting was not to redesign the FTC testing protocol but, rather, to examine the protocol and make suggestions for improvement, if warranted. To provide a framework for discussion, the committee was asked to consider three basic questions:

1. **Does the evidence presented clearly demonstrate that changes are needed in the current FTC protocol for measuring tar, nicotine, and carbon monoxide? If yes, what changes are required?**

2. **Should constituents other than tar, nicotine, and carbon monoxide be added to the protocol?**

3. **Does the FTC protocol provide information useful to smokers in making decisions about their health?**

I. The committee reached the following conclusions with respect to the first question.

   A. The smoking of cigarettes with lower *machine-measured* yields has a small effect in reducing the risk of cancer caused by smoking, no effect on the risk of cardiovascular diseases, and an uncertain effect on the risk of pulmonary disease. A reduction in *machine-measured* tar yield from 15 mg tar to 1 mg tar does not reduce relative risk from 15 to 1.

   B. The FTC test protocol was based on cursory observations of human smoking behavior. Actual human smoking behavior is characterized by wide variations in smoking patterns, which result in wide variations in tar and nicotine exposure. Smokers who switch to lower tar and nicotine cigarettes frequently change their smoking behavior, which may negate potential health benefits.

   C. Accordingly, the committee recommends the following changes to the FTC protocol:

1. This system should also measure and publish information on the range of tar, nicotine, and carbon monoxide yields that most smokers should expect from each cigarette sold in the United States.

2. This information should be clearly communicated to smokers.

3. A simple graphic representation should be provided with each pack of cigarettes sold in the United States and in all advertisements. The representation should not imply a one-to-one relationship between measurements and disease risk.

4. The system must be accompanied by public education to make smokers aware that individual exposure depends on how the cigarette is smoked and that the benefits of switching to lower yield cigarettes are small compared with quitting.

D. There should be Federal oversight of cigarette testing, but such testing should continue to be performed by the tobacco industry and at industry expense.

E. The questions involved in the purpose, methodology, and utility of the FTC protocol are complex medical and scientific issues that require ongoing involvement of Federal health agencies, including the National Institutes of Health, the Food and Drug Administration, and the Centers for Disease Control and Prevention.

F. The system should be reexamined at least every 5 years to evaluate whether the protocol is maintaining its utility to the smoker.

G. When a cigarette manufacturer makes significant changes in cigarette design that affect yields, it should notify the appropriate Federal agency.

II. With regard to the second question, the committee recommends that to avoid confusing smokers, no smoke constituents other than tar, nicotine, and carbon monoxide be measured and published at the present time. Smokers should be informed of the presence of other hazardous smoke constituents with each package and with all advertisements. These constituents should be classified by toxic effects.

III. In considering the third question, the committee reached the following conclusions:

A. Information from the testing system is useless to smokers unless they have ready access to it. The information from the testing system should be made available to all smokers, including those who smoke generic brands and other brands not widely advertised.

B. Brand names and brand classifications such as "light" and "ultralight" represent health claims and should be regulated and accompanied, in fair balance, with an appropriate disclaimer.

C. The available data suggest that smokers misunderstand the FTC test data. This underscores the need for an extensive public education effort.

As Chairman of the President's Cancer Panel under whose aegis this meeting was convened, I would like to express here my admiration and deep appreciation to the members of the NCI ad hoc committee and its expert consultants for a job well done. In transmitting this report to both the U.S. Congress and the Federal Trade Commission, it is my sincere hope that the recommendations contained herein will receive the serious and thoughtful consideration they deserve.

Harold P. Freeman, M.D.
Chairman, President's Cancer Panel

Acknowledgments

The FTC Cigarette Test Method for Determining Tar, Nicotine, and Carbon Monoxide Yields of U.S. Cigarettes: Report of the NCI Expert Committee was developed under the general editorship of the Smoking and Tobacco Control Program (STCP), National Cancer Institute (NCI), **Donald R. Shopland**, Coordinator.

In organizing the December 5-6, 1994, meeting of the NCI Ad Hoc Committee of the President's Cancer Panel on the FTC Test Method for Determining Tar, Nicotine, and Carbon Monoxide Levels in Cigarettes, NCI had the expert advice and assistance of many individuals both in and out of Government service. In particular, the Coordinator and STCP staff members would like to acknowledge the following individuals who served as part of an informal planning group for the conference:

Judith Wilkenfeld, Esq.
Food and Drug Administration
Rockville, MD

Jack E. Henningfield, Ph.D.
Addiction Research Center
National Institute on Drug Abuse
Baltimore, MD

Michael P. Eriksen, Sc.D.
Centers for Disease Control and Prevention
Atlanta, GA

Shira D. Modell, Esq.
Federal Trade Commission
Washington, DC

Special recognition is due **John M. Pinney** and **Joseph G. Gitchell**, Pinney Associates, Bethesda, MD, for their help with overall conference organization and planning. Mr. Pinney also served as facilitator for all consensus deliberations by the expert panel.

We would like to express our sincere appreciation to the following members of the NCI Ad Hoc Committee of the President's Cancer Panel.

Chairman, President's Cancer Panel

Harold P. Freeman, M.D.
Director of Surgery
Harlem Hospital Center
New York, NY

Executive Secretary, President's Cancer Panel

Maureen O. Wilson, Ph.D.
National Cancer Institute
Bethesda, MD

Panelists

Fred Bock, Ph.D.
Miami, FL

Dorothy K. Hatsukami, Ph.D.
Associate Professor of Psychiatry
University of Minnesota
Minneapolis, MN

Sandra Headen, Ph.D.
Social/Community Psychologist
University of North Carolina School of
    Public Health
Chapel Hill, NC

Dietrich Hoffmann, Ph.D.
Associate Director and Chief
Division of Environmental Carcinogenesis
American Health Foundation
Valhalla, NY

John R. Hughes, M.D.
Professor
Departments of Psychiatry, Psychology,
    and Family Practice
University of Vermont
Burlington, VT

Diana Petitti, M.D., M.P.H.
Director
Division of Research and Evaluation
Kaiser Permanente
Pasadena, CA

William S. Rickert, Ph.D.
President
Labstat, Inc.
Kitchener, Ontario
CANADA

Saul Shiffman, Ph.D.
Professor
Department of Psychology
University of Pittsburgh
Pittsburgh, PA

Maxine L. Stitzer, Ph.D.
Professor
Department of Psychiatry and Behavioral
    Sciences
Johns Hopkins University School of Medicine
Francis Scott Key Medical Center
Baltimore, MD

Ray Woosley, M.D., Ph.D.
Chair
Department of Clinical Pharmacology
Georgetown University
Washington, DC

Invited Speakers

Neal L. Benowitz, M.D.
Professor of Medicine and Chief
Division of Clinical Pharmacology and
    Experimental Therapeutics
University of California, San Francisco
San Francisco, CA

Joel B. Cohen, Ph.D.
Distinguished Service Professor and Director
Center for Consumer Research
University of Florida
Gainesville, FL

Gary A. Giovino, Ph.D., M.S.
Chief
Epidemiology Branch
Centers for Disease Control and Prevention
Atlanta, GA

Michael R. Guerin, Ph.D.
Section Head, Organic Chemistry
Oak Ridge National Laboratory
Oak Ridge, TN

Jeffrey E. Harris, M.D., Ph.D
Massachusetts General Hospital
Associate Professor
Department of Economics
Massachusetts Institute of Technology
Cambridge, MA

Jack E. Henningfield, Ph.D.
Chief
Clinical Pharmacology Branch
Addiction Research Center
National Institute on Drug Abuse
Baltimore, MD

Dietrich Hoffmann, Ph.D.
Associate Director and Chief
Division of Environmental Carcinogenesis
American Health Foundation
Valhalla, NY

Lynn T. Kozlowski, Ph.D.
Professor and Head
Department of Biobehavioral Health
Pennsylvania State University
University Park, PA

C. Lee Peeler, Esq.
Associate Director
Division of Advertising Practices
Federal Trade Commission
Washington, DC

Harold C. Pillsbury, Jr.
Rockville, MD

Jonathan M. Samet, M.D., M.S.
Chairman
Department of Epidemiology
Johns Hopkins University
    School of Hygiene and Public Health
Baltimore, MD

James P. Zacny, Ph.D.
Assistant Professor
Department of Anesthesia and Critical Care
University of Chicago
Chicago, IL

**Tobacco Industry
Representatives**

J. Donald deBethizy, Ph.D.
Vice President, Product Evaluation
R.J. Reynolds Tobacco Company
Bowman Gray Technical Center
Winston-Salem, NC

David E. Townsend, Ph.D.
Principal Scientist
R.J. Reynolds Tobacco Company
Bowman Gray Technical Center
Winston-Salem, NC

The Coordinator and STCP staff members also gratefully acknowledge the authors who made this monograph possible. Attributions for those chapters with authors follow.

Chapter 1. **Cigarette Testing and the Federal Trade Commission: A Historical Overview**   C. Lee Peeler, Esq.
Federal Trade Commission
Washington, DC

Chapter 2. **Review of the Federal Trade Commission Method for Determining Cigarette Tar and Nicotine Yield**

Harold C. Pillsbury, Jr.
Rockville, MD

Chapter 3. **Changes in Cigarette Design and Composition Over Time and How They Influence the Yields of Smoke Constituents**

Dietrich Hoffmann, Ph.D.
American Health Foundation
Valhalla, NY

Mirjana V. Djordjevic, Ph.D.
American Health Foundation
Valhalla, NY

Klaus D. Brunnemann, M.S.
American Health Foundation
Valhalla, NY

Chapter 4. **Attitudes, Knowledge, and Beliefs About Low-Yield Cigarettes Among Adolescents and Adults**

Gary A. Giovino, Ph.D., M.S.
Centers for Disease Control and
   Prevention
Atlanta, GA

Scott L. Tomar, D.M.D., Dr.P.H.
Centers for Disease Control and
   Prevention
Atlanta, GA

Murli N. Reddy, M.S.
Centers for Disease Control and
   Prevention
Atlanta, GA

John P. Peddicord, M.S.
Centers for Disease Control and
   Prevention
Atlanta, GA

Bao-Ping Zhu, Ph.D., M.B.B.S., M.S.
Centers for Disease Control and
   Prevention
Atlanta, GA

Luis G. Escobedo, M.D., M.P.H.
Centers for Disease Control and
   Prevention
Atlanta, GA

Michael P. Eriksen, Sc.D.
Centers for Disease Control and
   Prevention
Atlanta, GA

Chapter 13.	**Cigarette Design Technologies Reduce Smoke Yield and Expand Consumer Choices: The Role and Utility of the FTC Test Method**	David E. Townsend, Ph.D. R.J. Reynolds Tobacco Company Bowman Gray Technical Center Winston-Salem, NC
SECTION IV.	**Overview of 1980 to 1994 Research Related to the Standard Federal Trade Commission Test Method for Cigarettes**	Michael D. Mueller, M.S.P.H. R.O.W. Sciences, Inc. Rockville, MD

Finally, the Coordinator and STCP staff members would like to acknowledge the significant contributions of the following staff members of R.O.W. Sciences, Inc., Rockville, MD, and MasiMax Resources, Inc., Rockville, MD, who provided technical and editorial assistance in the preparation of this monograph. In particular, we would like to acknowledge the contribution of *Richard H. Amacher*, M.S., who served as Project Manager from September 1989 through August 1995 for the contract under which this publication was produced. We would also like to thank *Marilyn M. Massey*, M.P.H., MasiMax Resources, and *Jacqueline M. Tressler*, R.O.W. Sciences, who currently serve as Project Manager and Subcontract Manager, respectively, for the contract under which this publication was produced, for their valuable contribution during the final phases of the mongraph's development. Special recognition is also due to *James R. Libbey*, M.P.I.A., who served as Managing Editor for this publication, and *Traci Cherrier*, who served as Senior Conference Specialist for the NCI ad hoc committee meeting that resulted in this monograph.

R.O.W. Sciences, Inc.

Douglas Bishop, Art Director

Catherine W. Chapman, Executive Assistant

Rebecca A. Charton, Senior Librarian

Ruth E. Clark, Word Processing Specialist

Daria T. Donaldson, Proofreader

Catherine Hageman, Word Processing Supervisor

Stephen P. Luckabaugh, Information Specialist

Frances Nebesky, Senior Copyeditor

Sheila Proudman, Technical Writer/Resource Coordinator

Esther M. Roberts, Administrative Assistant

Donna Selig, Copyeditor/Proofreader

Keith W. Stanger, Graphics Services Coordinator

Donna Cay Tharpe, Quality Control Proofreader

Sonia Van Putten, Word Processing Specialist

MasiMax Resources, Inc.

Rebecca H. Razavi, Copyeditor/Proofreader

Aida M. Teymouri, Administrative Secretary

ABOUT THE MONOGRAPH

This volume is the seventh in the series of Smoking and Tobacco Control monographs published by the National Cancer Institute since 1991. The monographs were specifically established by NCI to provide an authoritative source of information about issues important to those individuals and institutions involved in smoking and tobacco use control.

This report was compiled in response to a request to the National Cancer Institute by the then Chairman of the Subcommittee on Health and the Environment, U.S. House of Representatives, asking that a scientific panel of experts be convened to review and make recommendations on the accuracy and appropriateness of the Federal Trade Commission's test method for assessing constituent yields for cigarettes on the U.S. market. The NCI received a similar but more detailed letter from the Chairman of the Federal Trade Commission in which the Commission outlined several areas for the NCI ad hoc committee to consider (see page xix).

The Coordinator of NCI's Smoking and Tobacco Control Program, who was given overall responsibility for the project, established a small informal advisory group consisting of individuals from the FTC and various PHS agencies to help organize the conference, suggest committee members, and plan the agenda.

The NCI Ad Hoc Committee of the President's Cancer Panel on the FTC Test Method for Determining Tar, Nicotine, and Carbon Monoxide Levels in Cigarettes was convened December 5-6, 1994, in Bethesda, MD. Harold P. Freeman, M.D., Chairman of the President's Cancer Panel, also chaired these proceedings.

However, prior to the December conference the 11 members of the NCI ad hoc committee (these individuals are identified in the "Acknowledgments" to the monograph) were provided several resource materials in support of their deliberations. These resources included copies of the 1981 Surgeon General's report *The Health Consequences of Smoking: The Changing Cigarette. A Report of the Surgeon General*, a detailed bibliography of the relevant worldwide scientific literature, and a copy of an NCI-commissioned White Paper titled "Overview of 1980 to 1994 Research Related to the Standard Federal Trade Commission Test Method for Cigarettes." The White Paper, which is published as Section IV of this monograph, represents a noncritical summary of those research findings published since the 1981 Surgeon General's report. Full copies of all articles were made available on demand to members of the NCI ad hoc committee by NCI's information science contractor, R.O.W. Sciences, Inc., of Rockville, MD.

The December 5-6, 1994, conference was organized similar to a consensus conference. Prior to the formal opening of the conference, the committee was asked to consider the three questions laid out on page vi of the "Foreword."

On the first day, subject matter experts were invited to make formal, structured presentations before the NCI ad hoc committee. (See "Acknowledgments" for list of speakers.) The 13 individual chapters published in Section I of this monograph are based on these presentations. Each presentation was approximately 30 minutes in length, followed by a question-and-answer session. Both members of the NCI ad hoc committee and invited speakers fully participated in these discussions. During the second day of deliberations, committee members and invited speakers participated in a more open-ended discussion, with the goal of reaching consensus on the three questions.

Open discussions ended midday December 6. Members of the NCI ad hoc committee then met to finalize their recommendations and findings; these were presented to the public during a press conference midafternoon December 6. *The FTC Cigarette Test Method for Determining Tar, Nicotine, and Carbon Monoxide Yields of U.S. Cigarettes: Report of the NCI Ad Hoc Committee* is the culmination of that effort.

Individuals wishing to receive a copy of the audiotapes of the December meeting may order these directly from Caset Associates at (703) 352-0091. The cost per set is $75. Those individuals interested in receiving a copy of the written transcript should contact Mr. Donald R. Shopland, National Cancer Institute, Executive Plaza North, Room 241, 6130 Executive Boulevard, Bethesda, MD 20892-7337.

U.S. HOUSE OF REPRESENTATIVES

COMMITTEE ON ENERGY AND COMMERCE

SUBCOMMITTEE ON HEALTH AND THE ENVIRONMENT

2415 RAYBURN HOUSE OFFICE BUILDING
WASHINGTON, DC 20515-6118
PHONE (202) 225-4952

June 7, 1994

Dr. Samuel Broder
Director
National Cancer Institute
National Institutes of Health
Building 31
Room 11A48
9000 Rockville Pike
Bethesda, Maryland 20892

Dear Dr. Broder:

I am writing to request that the National Cancer Institute sponsor a scientific conference which would review and make recommendations on the accuracy and appropriateness of the Federal Trade Commission's method for determining the relative "tar" and nicotine content of cigarettes. As you know, there is growing concern over the current testing method because many public health and addiction experts believe it may mislead smokers about the relative safety of a low tar, low nicotine product.

It has been suggested that a major reason for reliance upon the FTC test procedure is to allow consumers the option of reducing their risk of disease by smoking a brand deemed low in "tar" and nicotine. Consumer preference for low tar and nicotine rated cigarettes accelerated during the 1970's when NCI supported research strongly suggested that such cigarettes offered the consumer a reduced risk of lung cancer. The shift in consumer demand to these newer low yield cigarettes was quite rapid. In 1972 less than 2 percent of all cigarettes sold in the U.S. had a tar yield of less than 15 mg. However, the major cigarette manufacturers were quick to use the FTC tar and nicotine numbers in their advertising and by the end of the decade 40 percent of all cigarettes sold were under 15 mg. During the 1980's considerable doubt was expressed by many public health officials as to whether the tar and nicotine yields of cigarettes based on a protocol developed in the 1950's accurately reflect actual exposure and health risk levels when smoking today's cigarettes. Today approximately 60 percent of all brands are considered low-tar.

The NCI can provide an invaluable public service in sponsoring a scientific forum to address these issues and formulate alternative recommendations. It would be particularly helpful if a conference on this matter, perhaps in collaboration with the National Institute on Drug Abuse and the Federal Trade Commission, could be convened by October 1994.

Your consideration of this request is greatly appreciated. Please do not hesitate to contact me or Ripley Forbes of the Subcommittee staff if we can answer any questions or provide assistance in developing a conference agenda. I look forward to hearing from you.

With every good wish, I am

Sincerely,

HENRY A. WAXMAN
Chairman, Subcommittee on
Health and the Environment

Contents

Cigarette Testing and the Federal Trade Commission: A Historical Overview[1]

C. Lee Peeler

Cigarette manufacturers began advertising their products' tar and nicotine content before there was a standardized procedure for testing cigarette output. In 1955, after a series of cases challenging a variety of claims made for cigarettes (including tar and nicotine claims),[2] the Federal Trade Commission (Commission or FTC) published cigarette advertising guides. Among other things, the guides prohibited claims that a particular brand of cigarettes was low in tar and nicotine or lower than other brands "when it has not been established by competent scientific proof . . . that the claim is true, and if true, that such difference or differences are significant" (Federal Trade Commission, 1988a).

However, cigarette manufacturers continued to advertise tar numbers. In the absence of a standardized testing methodology, their claims resulted in what is often referred to as the "tar derby"—a multitude of inconsistent, noncomparable claims that did not give consumers a meaningful opportunity to assess the relative tar delivery of competing brands. The tar derby ended in 1960, when discussions with the Commission culminated in an agreement by the industry to refrain from tar and nicotine advertising (Federal Trade Commission, 1988b).

In 1964 the first Surgeon General's report on the health risks of smoking concluded that cigarette smoking was a cause of lung cancer in men (U.S. Department of Health and Human Services, 1964). In 1966 the Public Health Service stated that "The preponderance of scientific evidence strongly suggests that the lower the tar and nicotine content of cigarette smoke, the less harmful would be the effect" (U.S. Department of Health and Human Services, 1981, p. v).

It was in this environment that the Commission initiated two major steps in 1966 to encourage cigarette manufacturers to provide consumers with comparative information about their products' tar and nicotine yields.

---

[1] These remarks are the views of the staff of the Bureau of Consumer Protection. They do not necessarily represent the view of the Commission or any individual commissioner.

[2] *See, e.g., R.J. Reynolds Tobacco Co. v. FTC*, 192 F.2d 535 7th Cir. (1951) (claims that Camel does not impair the physical condition of athletes and aids digestion); *American Tobacco Co.*, 47 F.T.C. 1393 (1951) (Lucky Strike cigarettes advertised as less irritating to the throat than competing brands and containing less tar than four other leading brands); *P. Lorillard Co.*, 46 F.T.C. 735 (1950) (Old Gold cigarettes advertised as lowest of seven leading brands in nicotine and throat irritating tars, and Beech-Nut cigarettes as providing "definite defense against throat irritation"). *See also, e.g., Leighton Tobacco Co.*, 46 F.T.C. 1230 (1950) (Phantom cigarettes represented as causing no irritation of any kind).

First, it ended the ban on tar and nicotine advertising by announcing that factual statements of the tar and nicotine content of mainstream cigarette smoke could be made if they were supported by tests conducted in accordance with the so-called "Cambridge Filter method" and if they were not accompanied by claims about reduced health hazards (Federal Trade Commission, 1988a). Second, it authorized establishment of a laboratory to analyze cigarette smoke and invited public comment on what modifications, if any, should be made to the Cambridge Filter method for purposes of the laboratory's procedures and how the test results should be expressed (*Federal Register*, 1966). The modified Cambridge Filter method ultimately adopted by the Commission is often referred to as the "FTC method."

By mid-1967 the laboratory was ready to begin testing cigarettes (*Federal Register*, 1967).[3] The Commission agreed, pursuant to Senator Warren Magnuson's request,[4] to report the test results to Congress periodically, a process that continues today.

From the outset, the testing was intended to obtain uniform, standardized data about the tar and nicotine yield of mainstream cigarette smoke, *not* to replicate actual human smoking. The Commission recognized that individual smoking behavior was just that—too individual to gauge what a hypothetical "average" smoker would get from any particular cigarette: "No two human smokers smoke in the same way. No individual smoker always smokes in the same fashion" (Federal Trade Commission, 1967). The purpose of the testing was "not to determine the amount of 'tar' and nicotine inhaled by any human smoker, but rather to determine the amount of tar and nicotine generated when a cigarette is smoked by machine in accordance with the prescribed method" (Federal Trade Commission, 1967). Indeed, the Cambridge Filter method did not attempt to duplicate an "average" smoker but was "an amalgam of many choices" (Federal Trade Commission, 1967). Because no test could accurately duplicate human smoking, the Commission believed that the most important thing was to make certain the results presented to the public were based on a reasonable, standardized method and could be presented to consumers in an understandable manner.

The Commission next attempted to increase consumer awareness of the ratings produced by its laboratory. In 1970 it proposed a trade regulation rule that would have required disclosure of tar and nicotine ratings in all cigarette

---

[3] For the first dozen years of its existence, the laboratory tested only for tar and nicotine. In 1980 the protocol was modified to add testing for carbon monoxide.

[4] Expressing the opinion held at that time by many people in the Federal Government, Senator Magnuson stated that "By encouraging smokers to switch to low tar/nicotine cigarettes, we can contribute meaningfully to the physical health of our nation. Publication of the Commission's testing results is one important facet

The Commission expressed its views concerning dissemination of tar and nicotine figures in an October 1967 letter to the National Association of Broadcasters: "The Commission favors giving smokers as much information about the risks involved in smoking as is possible and to that end favors mandatory disclosure of tar and nicotine content, as measured by a standard test."

advertising (*Federal Register*, 1970). The rulemaking was suspended indefinitely a short time later, when five of the major cigarette manufacturers and three small companies agreed voluntarily among themselves to include the ratings produced by the Commission's protocol in their advertisements. That agreement, modified to reflect the discontinuance of the Commission's laboratory, remains in effect today.[5]

There are a number of ways to lower a cigarette's tar and nicotine rating, including adding filters that literally trap some of the constituents of the tobacco smoke before they reach the machine, wrapping the tobacco plug in paper that burns relatively quickly, and placing ventilation holes around the circumference of the filter so that when a smoker or smoking machine puffs on the cigarette, air is drawn into the filter and the resulting diluted mixture of air and smoke yields lower tar and nicotine ratings than an undiluted puff of smoke would yield. The last technique is often referred to as "aeration."

These types of changes in cigarette technology have focused the Commission's attention on its protocol on two separate occasions since 1970. In both cases, the Commission solicited public comments on certain aspects of the FTC method. However, in neither instance did the information received by the Commission form a sufficient basis for changing the protocol, even though the limitations on the predictiveness of the FTC method caused by compensatory smoking were clearly recognized by the mid-1980's. ("Compensatory behavior" is the tendency of consumers to offset the benefits of a positive change in their behavior by making a second, negative change. For example, a smoker who switches to a brand with lower tar and nicotine ratings might smoke more cigarettes each day or smoke each one more intensively, that is, inhale more deeply and/or take more puffs per cigarette.) Following is a review of the two events referred to above.

Aeration first became an issue for the Commission in 1977, when Lorillard, Inc., suggested that the depth to which cigarettes were inserted in the Commission's smoking machine be decreased when the standard depth would block some of a cigarette's ventilation holes, thereby impairing its filtration system and resulting in higher ratings than if the holes were open. The Commission solicited public comments on this question and also on whether the insertion depth should be decreased beyond the point where consumers cover the cigarette with their fingers or lips (*Federal Register*, 1977).

Of the seven cigarette companies that commented, only Lorillard supported varying the standard insertion depth. However, none of the responders addressed the question of whether the new insertion depth would be more consistent with actual smoking practices. After reviewing

---

[5] The American Tobacco Company did not sign the voluntary agreement, but similar disclosures have been contained in its advertisements, pursuant to a 1971 consent agreement with the Commission. [*In re American Brands, Inc.*, 79 F.T.C. 255 (1971).]

the comments, the Commission noted that the development of cigarettes with ventilation holes near the tip had complicated the comparability of its tar and nicotine ratings,[6] but "that a change in the insertion depth would cause a lack of continuity with previous test results" (*Federal Register*, 1978, pp. 11856, 11857). The Commission decided not to modify the protocol "in the absence of information indicating that a new insertion depth would be more consistent with the manner in which smokers insert cigarettes in actual use" (*Federal Register*, 1978, p. 11857).

Another controversy concerning the test method arose in the early 1980's and involved the Brown & Williamson Tobacco Corporation's (B&W) Barclay cigarette, which was designed with a channel ventilation system rather than air holes.[7] Competitors claimed that Barclay, which had received an official FTC rating of 1 mg tar in 1981, did not test accurately on the FTC smoking machine because the channels remained open during testing but were rendered inoperable in practice. After careful consideration, the Commission determined that its present test method did not accurately measure Barclay's tar, nicotine, and carbon monoxide. It revoked the 1-mg rating, estimating that Barclay should be rated between 3 and 7 mg of tar (based on testing by independent consultants) and invited comments on a number of issues relating to possible modification of its testing method, including using new cigarette holders on the smoking machine that would simulate the reduction in ventilation that occurred when people smoked Barclay (*Federal Register*, 1983). The Commission asked which modifications would yield the most appropriate results for all cigarettes and whether modification of the cigarette testing method would result in unintended consequences and affect possible innovation in cigarettes design (*Federal Register*, 1983).

The Commission also took this opportunity to reiterate that its ratings were relative; that the amount of tar, nicotine, and carbon monoxide any particular cigarette delivered depended on how it was smoked; and that in the case of ventilated filter cigarettes, delivery would be increased if ventilation holes were blocked (*Federal Register*, 1983). It then invited

---

[6] Quoting its 1967 statement that the purpose of testing was not to determine the amount of constituents inhaled by a human smoker but to determine the amount generated when a cigarette was smoked by a machine in accordance with a prescribed protocol (see above), the Commission noted that:

> The point of this statement was that the FTC's "tar" and nicotine values represented valid standards for making comparisons among different cigarettes. Thus, if the consumer smoked each different cigarette the same way, he would inhale "tar" and nicotine in amounts proportional to the relative values of the FTC figures. A person who smoked a 10 mg "tar" cigarette would ingest half the "tar" he would by smoking a 20 mg "tar" cigarette providing he smoked the same way. The development of cigarettes with ventilation areas within 11 mm of the tip has complicated this simple relationship. (*Federal Register*, 1978, p. 11856)

[7] In conventional aerated cigarettes, air and smoke mixed together as they passed through the filter. Outside air drawn into Barclay's channels, however, went directly into the smoker's mouth before first mixing with any smoke; dilution was supposed to occur in the mouth, not in the filter. Competitors alleged that because the exit holes for the channels were close to the smoker's lips, they were crushed or covered by lips, thus reducing dilution.

comments on a wide range of issues concerning compensatory smoking behavior:

> Should the Commission further examine the implications for its testing program of the issues raised by compensatory smoking behavior, including hole blocking, when consumers smoke lower "tar" cigarettes? What is the evidence that smokers use higher "tar" cigarettes differently than lower "tar" cigarettes? What is the evidence regarding the extent of hole blocking by smokers of different ventilated filter cigarettes? Are there problems regarding compensatory smoking behavior which are significant enough to warrant further exploration of changes in the method, beyond those necessitated by the Commission's findings concerning Barclay? What lines of inquiry would generate the most useful information if such an examination is undertaken? For example, should the Commission explore a system of categories or "bands" of "tar" content rather than specific numerical estimates? Also, should consumers be advised that the cigarettes' actual "tar" delivery depends on how it is smoked? (*Federal Register*, 1983)

Shortly after the initial comment period closed,[8] a Federal district court issued an opinion in the Commission's action against B&W over advertisements that continued to describe Barclay as a 1-mg tar cigarette, despite the Commission's revocation of Barclay's 1-mg rating [*FTC v. Brown & Williamson Tobacco Corp.*, 580 F. Supp. 981 (D.D.C. 1983), *aff'd in part, remanded in part*, 778 F.2d 35 (D.C. Cir. 1985)]. During that litigation, B&W contended that "recent scientific evidence demonstrates that the FTC system is so flawed that it is itself deceptive" [580 F. Supp. at 984].[9] The court recognized that compensatory smoking behavior complicated the ratings question but rejected B&W's contention that the system provided no benefit to consumers:

> The FTC system attempts only to determine how much relative tar and nicotine a smoker would get in his mouth were he to smoke two cigarettes in the same manner. B&W has utterly failed to show that the system does not do this. Nor has it shown that a better method for determining the relative health

---

[8] Comments responsive to the April 13, 1983, *Federal Register* notice were originally due by June 30, 1983. On June 4, 1984, however, the Commission reopened the comment period because certain information that was relevant to the questions addressed in that notice, but had been previously under a court-ordered seal, was now publicly available (*Federal Register*, 1984).

[9] B&W argued that all cigarettes were subject to compensatory smoking behavior and thus all tar numbers were "soft." The Commission acknowledged that low-yield cigarettes were subject to substantial variations in actual smoker intake but contended that Barclay tested differently on the machine from other cigarettes. The Commission's position was that the tar ratings provided a rough comparative scale; that is, a 1-mg cigarette should be comparable to all other 1-mg cigarettes, if all are smoked in an identical manner.

hazards of the many different varieties of cigarettes on the
market is currently feasible [580 F. Supp. at 985].

The comments ultimately submitted in response to the Commission's
questions about compensatory smoking reflected sharply disparate views.
On the one hand, the American Heart Association (AHA), American Lung
Association (ALA), and American Cancer Society (ACS) identified problems
with the existing methodology, expressed concern over the impact of
compensatory smoking behavior, and suggested extensive research to
improve the current testing and reporting procedures.[10]

On the other hand, Philip Morris, R.J. Reynolds Tobacco Company,
and American Brands asserted that compensatory smoking behavior was
not relevant to the testing methodology and that devising a protocol that
accounted for compensatory smoking would require establishing a profile of
the average smoker, something the Commission had previously declined to
do because of the impossibility of accounting for all the relevant variables.
Lorillard stated that data on compensatory smoking were very limited and
therefore recommended that the existing system be kept intact. Liggett &
Myers suggested that perhaps all cigarette testing should be abolished because
smoking behavior could seriously affect tar and nicotine yields and smokers
could not be taught to change their behavior.

In response to the Commission's question about possible implementation
of a "banding" system for its tar and nicotine ratings, B&W (which had
just had Barclay's rating revoked) argued that the current system caused
manufacturers to emphasize small differences that might not exist, given
the realities of compensatory smoking, and that it should be replaced with
a system that would group products into high-tar, medium-tar, low-tar, and
ultralow-tar "bands." Philip Morris and American Brands argued that banding
would lead to a concentration of brands at the upper limit of each category
(in contrast to the existing system, which encouraged reductions across the
board). American Brands also contended that banding would confuse
consumers, whereas Philip Morris noted that it would substitute the
Government's judgment about the significance of differences in tar ratings
for that of the individual consumer.

---

[10] The ALA stated that given the reality of compensatory smoking, low-tar cigarettes might not be as safe as
some consumers were being led to believe and that the Commission's testing and reporting procedures were
contributing to questionable advertisements for "safe" cigarettes. The ACS stated that the Commission's test
method should be modified to reflect current understanding of compensatory smoking behavior. The AHA
expressed its view that the Commission's testing and reporting procedures fostered the belief among
consumers that low-tar cigarettes were safer than high-tar brands. However, epidemiological evidence
showing a correlation between the risk of coronary heart disease and the number of cigarettes smoked
per day, but not a reduced rate of such disease among low-tar smokers, suggested that smokers of those
cigarettes might be engaging in compensatory smoking.

The ALA and ACS recommended that research be conducted to determine how actual intake of tar and
other smoke constituents by smokers related to the FTC's ratings; following completion of this research,
the Commission should test each cigarette under a range of conditions replicating actual smoking behavior
and report those results with a warning that individual yield depends on individual smoking patterns.

In short, there was no clear consensus as to specific action the Commission could (or should) take to eliminate the limitations of the test method. At the same time, abandoning the testing system without instituting another method of tar testing would have been premature because then-current epidemiological evidence suggested that there had been a reduction in lung cancer deaths that might be attributable to declines in average tar levels that had occurred since the 1950's (U.S. Department of Health and Human Services, 1981).[11] Accordingly, at that time the Commission made no changes to its cigarette test method to address compensatory smoking.

In early 1987 the Commission decided to close its cigarette testing laboratory. The Commission found that closing the laboratory was necessary for several reasons, chiefly because the cost of the laboratory was significant and the Commission would have had to commit significant additional funds to continue its operation. The Commission also was persuaded that the same information could be obtained from other sources and that other means were available to verify the accuracy of industry testing results. In fact, the Commission's operation of a testing system for the industry at taxpayer expense was highly unusual. The common scenario is for the industry to conduct its own testing under Government-specified testing protocols.

Since 1987 the Tobacco Institute Testing Laboratory (TITL) has continued to test most cigarettes, using the Commission's approved methodology; the companies report the results to the Commission pursuant to a compulsory request, and the Commission publishes the results. TITL keeps the Commission informed of proposed changes in the testing procedure and solicits Commission approval for all significant changes. TITL's work is regularly monitored by the Commission's contractor, Harold Pillsbury, Jr. (this volume), who has virtually unrestricted access to the laboratory and makes unannounced visits to inspect it and check the testing process. Mr. Pillsbury also checks the data for consistency from run to run and from year to year. Most industry members also have testing facilities; however, the numbers published by the Commission are primarily TITL numbers. (Generic and private label brands, as well as new cigarettes and cigarettes that are not widely available, are not tested by TITL.)

Since the closing of its laboratory, the Commission has continued to review advertising for today's low- and ultralow-yield cigarettes for deceptive claims. In January 1995 the Commission approved a consent agreement with the American Tobacco Company, settling charges over advertisements that allegedly misused the Commission's tar and nicotine ratings by stating that consumers would get less tar by smoking 10 packs of Carlton brand cigarettes

---

[11] In 1954 the tar yield of the sales-weighted average cigarette was 37 mg (U.S. Department of Health and Human Services, 1981). By 1981 cigarettes yielding 15 mg of tar or less had 56 percent of the domestic market (Federal Trade Commission, 1984).

(which are rated as having 1 mg of tar per cigarette) than by smoking a single pack of certain other brands of cigarettes (rated as having more than 10 mg of tar per cigarette).

The Commission's desire to ensure that smokers have accurate and useful information about their cigarettes led to its request for the conference, whose reports are contained in this monograph.

QUESTION-AND-ANSWER SESSION

Mr. Peeler conducted a question-and-answer session simultaneously with Mr. Pillsbury; see page 12.

REFERENCES

Federal Register. 31(215): 14278, November 4, 1966.

Federal Register. 32(147): 11178, August 1, 1967.

Federal Register. 35(154): 12671, August 8, 1970.

Federal Register. 42(79): 21155, April 25, 1977.

Federal Register. 43(56): 11856 and 11857, March 22, 1978.

Federal Register. 48(72): 15953-15955, April 13, 1983.

Federal Register. 49(108): 23120-23121, June 4, 1984.

Federal Trade Commission. "Statement of Considerations." Press release. August 1, 1967, p. 2.

Federal Trade Commission. *Report to Congress for 1981 Pursuant to the Federal Cigarette Labeling and Advertising Act.* Washington, DC: Federal Trade Commission, 1984, p. 30 (Table 11).

Federal Trade Commission. *Trade Regulation Reporter.* Vol. 6. Chicago: Commerce Clearing House, Inc., 1988a, ¶ 39,012.70.

Federal Trade Commission. *Trade Regulation Reporter.* Vol. 3. Chicago: Commerce Clearing House, Inc., 1988b, ¶ 7853.51 at 11730.

U.S. Department of Health, Education, and Welfare. *Smoking and Health, Report of the Advisory Committee to the Surgeon General of the Public Health Service.* PHS Publication No. 1103. Rockville, MD: U.S. Department of Health and Human Services, Public Health Service, 1964.

U.S. Department of Health and Human Services. *The Health Consequences of Smoking: The Changing Cigarette. A Report of the Surgeon General.* DHHS Publication No. (PHS) 81-50156. Rockville, MD: U.S. Department of Health and Human Services, Public Health Service, Office on Smoking and Health, 1981.

Review of the Federal Trade Commission Method for Determining Cigarette Tar and Nicotine Yield

Harold C. Pillsbury, Jr.[1]

The "Federal Trade Commission (Commission or FTC) method" is the methodology that the Commission adopted almost 30 years ago for testing cigarettes. This methodology is still used today by the Tobacco Institute Testing Laboratory (TITL), with some minor modifications. The FTC method determines the relative yield of individual cigarettes by smoking them in a standardized fashion, according to a predetermined protocol, on a smoking machine. The FTC test method was based on the "Cambridge Filter method" developed by Ogg (1964), which called for 2-second, 35-mL puffs to be taken until a 23-mm butt length remained on the cigarette. More about how these parameters were selected is presented below.

For the testing procedure, as implemented initially by the FTC's cigarette testing laboratory and currently by TITL, cigarettes are collected by an independent firm that purchases two packages of each cigarette variety[2] in each of 50 locations throughout the United States. (If some varieties or brands are not available in certain locations, additional packs will be purchased in locations where they are available.) They are mailed to the testing laboratory; the postmark serves as verification that they were purchased in different locations. Individual cigarettes to be tested are selected on a random basis, two from each pack. Before being smoked, the cigarettes are "conditioned" by being placed on storage trays in a room maintained at 75 °F and 60 percent relative humidity for not less than 24 hours.

The machine used in the Commission's laboratory had 20 "ports" (openings); the smoking machine currently used by TITL also has 20 ports. Each opening is fitted with a filter holder, into which a cigarette is inserted for smoking, and a filter pad, on which particulate matter from the cigarette smoke is collected. Gases pass through the pad and are collected in specially designed plastic bags.

---

[1] These remarks are the views of the staff of the Bureau of Consumer Protection. They do not necessarily represent the view of the Commission or any individual commissioner.

[2] A particular brand of cigarettes may have more than a dozen varieties, depending on whether it is available in different lengths, in regular and menthol flavors, in hard and soft packaging, and in regular, light, and ultralight versions. For example, the Commission's 1994 tar and nicotine report lists 20 varieties of Marlboro.

The machines are calibrated to take one puff of 2-second duration and 35-mL volume every minute. Cigarettes are smoked to a butt length of 23 mm or the length of the overwrap plus 3 mm, whichever is longer. When the cigarette has been smoked down to the prescribed length, it burns through a string that has been placed on that mark; this causes a microswitch to be flipped, which in turn disconnects that particular port of the smoking machine. (Although this seems like a fairly unsophisticated way of terminating the test, more sophisticated methods—such as infrared detectors and thermal sensors—have been tried and rejected over the years.)

Five cigarettes of each variety are smoked, one at a time, using the same filter holder.[3] (A total of 100 cigarettes of each variety are smoked to get the official tar, nicotine, and carbon monoxide ratings.) After the smoke from those five cigarettes has been filtered through each filter pad, the holder is removed and weighed. The difference between the weight of the holder before and after the smoking process divided by the number of cigarettes smoked is the total particulate matter collected from the cigarette smoke.

The filter pad is then extracted with a solvent,[4] and the moisture content is determined by injecting a measured amount of the extract into a gas chromatograph and comparing the resulting peak against the standard curve. Ratings for the three constituents reported by the Commission are then determined as follows:

- Nicotine: As with moisture, a specified amount of the extract from the filter pad is injected into a gas chromatograph, and the resulting peak is compared against the standard curve.[5]

- Carbon monoxide: The gas collected in the plastic bag is passed through an infrared detector to determine carbon monoxide levels.

- Tar: Tar level is determined by subtracting water and nicotine levels from total particulate matter.

Tar and carbon monoxide figures are rounded up or down to the nearest milligram, while nicotine figures are rounded to the nearest 10th of a milligram. Varieties with tar and carbon monoxide results below 0.5 mg per cigarette or nicotine results below 0.05 mg are reported as <0.5 mg or <0.05 mg, respectively, because the FTC test method is not sensitive enough to report these components at lower levels.

Although the ratings are based on 100 cigarettes, at least 150 (and preferably 200) cigarettes of each variety are needed for the test to ensure

---

[3] To make certain that the machine is working properly, at least 4 of the 20 ports are reserved on each run for "monitor" cigarettes—cigarettes with known yields for tar, nicotine, and carbon monoxide.

[4] The solution contains extractant and internal standards: 2-propanol containing 1 mg anethole per mL as an internal standard for nicotine and 20 mg ethanol per mL as an internal standard for water.

[5] Ultraviolet spectroscopy was used to determine nicotine until 1980, when it was replaced by gas chromatography.

that 100 are successfully smoked. Common technical problems that can cause a filter pad to be discarded include lighting failures and port leaks. During the last year of the FTC laboratory's operation, fewer than 300 varieties of cigarettes were tested, and the testing cycle (which included curing, marking, and smoking the cigarettes, etc.) lasted approximately 12 months. There were 933 cigarette varieties rated by the TITL in the Commission's 1994 report.

The author once had the opportunity to ask Dr. Ogg (who worked as a tobacco chemist for the U.S. Department of Agriculture) how he came up with the specific parameters of his protocol. He said that he had based them on observations of how people smoke under different conditions. He had spent a lot of time watching people smoke (at the office, on the street, etc.), sometimes timing them with a stopwatch. His observations told him that people smoked differently under different conditions. For example, someone deep in thought might take only one or two puffs before the cigarette burned out, whereas someone who seemed extremely nervous might puff constantly. In short, there was no such thing as an "average" smoker and no way to derive a set of testing parameters that would replicate actual human smoking, so Dr. Ogg had to select parameters that seemed reasonable in light of his observations.[6] Dr. Ogg also collected cigarette butts from ash trays in hotels, restaurants, and offices and measured how long they were; the resulting average length became the butt length called for by his protocol.

When the Commission adopted a slightly modified version of the Cambridge Filter method in 1967 for use in its newly opened cigarette testing laboratory, it was the author's opinion that the Commission's procedures (as implemented on the 20-port smoking machine selected by the Commission) were clearly superior to all other methods currently in use at that time. The FTC method had its limitations, most significantly that the information it generated would not tell any individual smoker how much tar and nicotine he or she would get from a particular brand of cigarette. However, there was simply no way to get that information, and the FTC method did provide a smoker with accurate comparative information about the relative amounts of tar and nicotine delivered by various cigarettes when they were smoked in precisely the same manner. In addition, it provided a uniform analytical procedure that could be replicated in different laboratories simultaneously and in the same laboratory over time; therefore, not only could many brands of cigarettes be compared with each other at any time, but long-term pictures of tar and nicotine levels over the years also were possible.

---

[6] During the December 5-6, 1994, National Cancer Institute conference, it was learned that a protocol using the same parameters for the testing of cigarettes had been proposed by The American Tobacco Company researchers many years before Dr. Ogg published his article (Bradford et al., 1936) ("arbitrarily" selecting a 2-second, 35-mL puff once a minute, although another researcher who had studied human smoking habits used a 40-mL puff).

QUESTION-AND-ANSWER SESSION

DR. HARRIS: I was curious about the very last statement on the tape: The results are sent to the cigarette manufacturers who, in turn, report the numbers to the Federal Trade Commission?

MR. PILLSBURY: Yes. We get the tar and nicotine data directly from the cigarette manufacturers so that we can hold them responsible if there is anything wrong with the numbers.

DR. HARRIS: To your knowledge, do the numbers reported under the compulsory process by the manufacturers ever deviate from those that are measured in the Tobacco Institute laboratory?

MR. PILLSBURY: The only thing I can tell you is that they are checked.

DR. STITZER: Could you remind us how the original Cambridge Filter method was altered when the FTC method was developed?

MR. PILLSBURY: The original smoking machine was a four-port smoker that used a column of water to draw from the cigarettes. When this new machine came out, the filter pads and the holders were pretty much the same. The only thing that has been changed is that the machine has been modified so that carbon monoxide can be analyzed at the same time that the cigarettes are being smoked.

DR. STITZER: So, there wasn't a puffing protocol that went along with the original method?

MR. PEELER: We published, at the time that we adopted the method, a fairly detailed protocol for how the test was supposed to be done. I suppose the question is, did that protocol that we published differ from the original method in the parameters that were required?

MR. PILLSBURY: No. They were pretty much the same as in the original method.

DR. RICKERT: How much of a difference would you have to have in tar yields between two brands before they would be considered to be different in the statistical sense?

MR. PEELER: We publish the numbers and try to have a large enough sample so that there are differences in those numbers. But the question of whether there is a significant difference in those numbers is what we need to know from you.

DR. RICKERT: What I am referring to is that on the tables in the UK there is a footnote that reads, "Ignore differences in 2 mg in tar and CO," and I was wondering whether that is the same sort of position that we have here?

MR. PILLSBURY: The only thing that is done is they are rounded. Five and above are rounded up; four and down are rounded down. We make no criteria as to whether one with 14 mg is better for you than one with 15 mg. We are just publishing the ratings of the cigarettes as they fall.

MS. WILKENFELD: I think the answer is that, at least originally, we used to publish the table with a standard deviation and that therefore there was a significance between each degree of tar yield. We do not have confidence in yields below .5, and that is announced in the report.

DR. PETITTI: About how long does it take to finish puffing one cigarette, and what is the difference in the time that it might take to puff a cigarette that is a very-high-tar cigarette vs. a cigarette that is very low tar?

MR. PILLSBURY: The difference in the length of time it takes to smoke a cigarette is primarily a factor of how long the cigarette is, how tight the tobacco is packed, how hard it is, and how much gas flows through the cigarettes. Most of the cigarettes take approximately 10 minutes to smoke. We have had longer cigarettes that have gone up to 12 to 13 minutes.

DR. PETITTI: Could you give me a range of the shortest vs. the longest? Is it 5 minutes vs. 15, or is it 9 minutes vs. 12?

MR. PILLSBURY: Any range I would have to give you right now would be a guess, because I haven't followed the range that closely. But I believe that probably the shortest cigarette we have ever had is probably around 6 or 7 puffs per cigarette, and the longest one ran almost 15 puffs, but that was a very long cigarette.

DR. BENOWITZ: Could you explain the rationale for the parameters that are used in the current method? How did you arrive at the present protocol?

MR. PEELER: Let me ask Mr. Pillsbury to address what Dr. Ogg's rationale was in the documents because he actually had an opportunity to discuss that with Dr. Ogg. I think that if you look at the documents that the Commission published at the time of the adoption of the testing methodology in 1967, the Commission is fairly clear that, whatever Dr. Ogg's rationales were, it did not believe it could replicate average smoking conditions. And so it was picking parameters that were essentially fairly arbitrary.

MR. PILLSBURY: When we first started the lab, I talked to Dr. Ogg to quite some extent on this topic. He had actually gone out there with a stopwatch in his pocket and ridden the trains, and watched people in meetings and so forth, and tried to get some feeling for how they were smoking. He came back rather confused, because it seemed as though everybody smoked differently: from the fellow who got on the train and looked at his newspaper and lit his cigarette and never took another puff on it until it burned down to the man who was sitting down arguing with somebody, smoking like mad. So, he came up with what he considered a fairly average way of smoking, so that you didn't get a big long firebox on the end of the cigarette and you kept it burning.

As far as the butt length is concerned, they went out and picked up cigarettes from ash trays in hotels and restaurants and so forth and did actual measurements on those. And the best butt length that they could come up with was 23, or the overwrap plus 3.

MR. PEELER: Again, by the time the Commission adopted the methodology in 1967, the Commission was very clear that it was not trying to establish average smoking parameters.

DR. BOCK: I think that it goes back to the 1938 paper by the American Tobacco Company group. I talked with Bradford and Harlan in Richmond in 1953, and they, again, had gone to parties and watched what their friends were doing. They were the same parameters, I believe, and it was based on a group of probably upper-middle-income-level Richmondites.

DR. SHIFFMAN: You mentioned that the original FTC action on this was under the FTC's general authority to prevent deceptive advertising. Now, at the moment, you are also reporting the results of these tests to Congress. Has there been any evolution in the FTC's authority in this area, or is it still under this broad mandate?

MR. PEELER: No. The FTC's involvement in this issue continues to be under its authority to regulate deceptive or unsubstantiated claims in advertising. And, in the case of tar and nicotine testing in particular, there are two variations: (1) We do have a voluntary agreement from the industry to include this information in their advertising, and (2) we have had this longstanding practice of sending the reports of this testing to Congress, which was originally established in response to requests from the Commerce Committee. But the only legal authority that we have in this area is our authority to require claims in advertising to be truthful and to be substantiated.

DR. COHEN: I want to return to the point of the statistical significance of the yields. I think that is a very central question for the record. I would just like to point out that there are three different sources of variance here that ought to be considered: (1) variance due to product characteristics, such as product design features; (2) variance due to individual smoking characteristics; and (3) variance due to testing methodology.

Each of those sources of variance can be estimated separately, and it may be very important later on, as the panel does its work, to consider the implications of variance in each of those three separately.

REFERENCES

Bradford, J.A., Harlan, W.R., Hanmer, H.R. Nature of cigarette smoke. Technique of experimental smoking. *Industrial and Engineering Chemistry* 28(7): 836-839, 1936.

Ogg, C.L. Determination of particulate matter and alkaloids (as nicotine) in cigarette smoke. *Journal of the Association of Official Agricultural Chemists* 47: 356, 1964.

Changes in Cigarette Design and Composition Over Time and How They Influence the Yields of Smoke Constituents

Dietrich Hoffmann, Mirjana V. Djordjevic, and Klaus D. Brunnemann

INTRODUCTION   Since the first epidemiological reports on the association of cigarette smoking with lung cancer, the composition of tobacco blends and the makeup of commercial cigarettes in the United States as well as in Western Europe have undergone major changes. Measured on the basis of standardized machine smoking conditions, the sales-weighted average tar and nicotine deliveries in U.S. cigarette smoke have decreased from 38 mg and 2.7 mg, respectively, in 1954 to 12 mg and 0.95 mg, respectively, in 1993. The lower emissions have been primarily accomplished by using efficient filter tips and highly porous cigarette paper and by changing the composition of the tobacco blend. The latter includes the incorporation of reconstituted and expanded tobaccos into the blend. Concurrent with the reduction of tar and nicotine in the smokestream, there also occurred a reduction of carbon monoxide, phenols, and carcinogenic polynuclear aromatic hydrocarbons (PAHs). These reductions were partially tied to an increase in the nitrate content of the tobacco blend used for U.S. cigarettes. The addition of nitrate was initially targeted at decreasing the smoke yields of PAHs; however, that this also would cause a gradual increase of the carcinogenic, tobacco-specific N-nitrosamines (TSNAs) was not recognized until there was awareness of those compounds as smoke constituents in the 1970's.

These observations were based on measurements of yields from cigarettes that were smoked under standardized laboratory conditions, initially established in 1936, and adopted by the U.S. Federal Trade Commission (FTC) in 1969. These conditions do not reflect the smoking patterns of the smokers of filter cigarettes, who currently account for the consumption of 97 percent of all cigarettes produced in the United States. The current filter cigarette smoker tends to smoke more intensely and to inhale more deeply. Thus, the actual exposure to toxic and tumorigenic agents in the inhaled smoke of filter cigarettes is not necessarily in line with the machine smoking data.

BACKGROUND   In 1950 epidemiological studies reported that lung cancer was particularly prevalent among cigarette smokers (Wynder and Graham, 1950; Doll and Hill, 1950). These observations in the United States and the United Kingdom were confirmed by the Royal College of Physicians (1962) and by the U.S. Surgeon General in 1964 (U.S. Department of Health, Education, and Welfare, 1964). These reports and the emerging knowledge of the presence of carcinogens and tumor promoters in cigarette smoke led to a gradual change in the design and composition of commercial cigarettes in North America, Western Europe, and other developed countries (Hoffmann and Hoffmann, 1994a; Jarvis and Russell, 1985). The modifications were intended to reduce both the toxicity and the carcinogenic potential of the cigarette smoke. Although research on the changing cigarette was pursued in several countries, this chapter deals primarily with the developments relating to U.S. cigarettes between 1954 and 1993.

At the basis of all analytical assessments of smoke composition lies the standardization of machine smoking methods, first suggested for empirical cigarette smoking in Europe (Pfyl, 1933; Pyriki, 1934). In the United States, Bradford and colleagues (1936) developed a procedure for cigarette smoking on the basis of "arbitrarily selected" parameters of a 35-mL puff volume, a 2-second puff duration, and one puff per minute. The only goal of this method was to offer a means for comparing the smoke yields of various types of cigarettes; there was no intent to simulate human smoking patterns. The influences on smoke yields and composition that are exerted by the overall physical characteristics of a cigarette—including its length and the butt length to which it is smoked, its circumference, whether it is filtered or nonfiltered, and the effects of the puff volume, puff frequency, and puff duration; the type and cut of tobacco used as a filler; the properties of the wrapper; and the mode of precipitation of the condensate—were described in many research papers during the 1960's (Wynder and Hoffmann, 1967). For regulatory purposes, Pillsbury and colleagues (1969) adapted in principle the method of Bradford and coworkers (1936) and made some refinements to establish what became known as the FTC method; the smoking parameters were still a 35-mL puff volume, a 2-second puff duration, and a 1-puff-per-minute frequency. What was new was the definition of the butt length to which a cigarette was to be smoked. Butt lengths were set to be 23 mm for plain cigarettes and length of the filter plus overwrap with an additional 3 mm for filter cigarettes. CORESTA, the International Organization for Research on Tobacco, developed a comparable method that is widely used in most of the developed countries (CORESTA, 1991-1993).

This chapter describes the analytical data obtained with the FTC method, although many studies (Russell, 1980; Herning et al., 1981; Kozlowski et al., 1982; Fagerström, 1982; Haley et al., 1985; Byrd et al., 1994) have shown that the standardized machine smoking method does not reflect the smoking habits of consumers of filter cigarettes. This is especially so for filter cigarettes with low and ultralow smoke yields, because smokers of such cigarettes tend to inhale more deeply and draw puffs more frequently to satisfy a physiologically conditioned need for nicotine (U.S. Department of Health and Human Services, 1988).

Figure 1 presents the sales-weighted average tar and nicotine deliveries of all U.S. domestic brands for the years 1954 through 1993 (Hoffmann and Hoffmann, 1994a). This figure also shows the major changes in the makeup of U.S. cigarettes, such as the introduction of filter tips, porous cigarette

Figure 1
Sales-weighted average tar and nicotine deliveries, 1954-1993

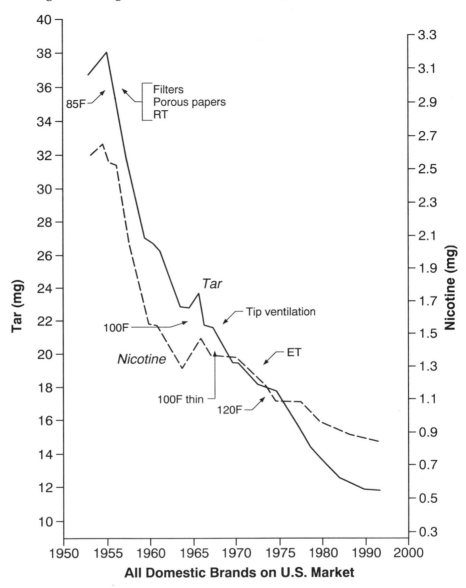

Key: RT = reconstituted tobacco; F = filter; ET = expanded tobacco.

Source: Hoffmann and Hoffmann, 1994a.

paper, reconstituted tobacco, filter tip ventilation, and use of expanded tobacco. Similar developments occurred in most industrialized countries, albeit at a somewhat slower pace and about 5 to 10 years after the introduction of these changes in the United States (Hoffmann and Hoffmann, 1994b; Jarvis and Russell, 1985; U.S. Department of Health and Human Services, 1988). Jarvis and Russell (1985) first observed for English cigarettes that the smoke delivery of nicotine was not reduced to the same extent as that of the tar. During the past 10 to 15 years, the same observation was made for U.S. cigarettes. Figure 1 does not reflect the gradual change in the tobacco blend of U.S. cigarettes with regard to an increase of the burley tobacco share from about 35.9 percent in 1950 to 46.5 percent in 1982; the remainder of the tobacco blend consists primarily of bright tobacco with about 5 to 8 percent oriental tobacco and 1 percent Maryland tobacco (Grise, 1984).

CHANGES IN CIGARETTE DESIGN AND COMPOSITION

Cigarettes With Filter Tips

Since 1955 the U.S. sales-weighted average smoke yields have declined from 38 mg tar and 2.7 mg nicotine to 12 mg and 0.95 mg, respectively (Figure 1). A major reason for the decrease in smoke yields is the wide acceptance of filter cigarettes. Their use steadily increased in America from 0.56 percent of all cigarettes smoked in 1950 to 19 percent in 1955, 51 percent in 1960, 82 percent in 1970, 92 percent in 1980, and more than 97 percent since 1993 (Figure 2) (Hoffmann and Hoffmann, 1994b; U.S. Department of Agriculture, 1993). Most filter tips (15 to 35 mm) are made of cellulose acetate; only a low percentage of cigarettes are made with composite filters of cellulose acetate with charcoal. Since about 1968, increasing proportions of the cellulose acetate filter tips are perforated with one or more lines of tiny holes placed near the middle of the filter tow. Today up to 50 percent of all cigarette filter tips in the United States have various degrees of perforations. The conventional filter cigarettes are acceptable to consumers with a maximal draw resistance of up to about 130 mm water column (Kiefer and Touey, 1967). The filters reduce primarily the smoke yields of particulate matter and thus the nonvolatile smoke constituents. The efficiency of cellulose acetate filters for total particulate matter (TPM) removal can be increased by reducing the diameter of the filaments without increasing the draw resistance (Table 1a) or by using a longer filter tip (Table 1b). In the mainstream smoke of the U.S. blended cigarette with a pH below 6.3 to 6.5, more than 90 percent of the nicotine is present in the particulate matter as a salt with organic acids (Kiefer and Touey, 1967; Brunnemann and Hoffmann, 1974).

Conventional cellulose acetate has the capability to selectively reduce some of the volatile and semivolatile compounds in the smokestream, especially when the filter is treated with certain plasticizers, such as glycerol triacetate. Some of the volatile smoke constituents that are ciliatoxic agents, such as acrolein, are removed selectively, even beyond the reduction of TPM, by retention on such treated filter tips. Phenols and cresols, a group of semivolatiles, also are removed selectively up to 80 to 85 percent, as are the highly carcinogenic dialkylnitrosamines, of which up to 75 percent can be retained on cellulose acetate filters (George and Keith, 1967; Brunnemann and Hoffmann, 1977).

Filter tips with perforations allow dilution of the smoke with air. Moreover, drawing puffs through perforated filter cigarettes reduces the velocity of the air drawn through the burning cone. As a result, less of the

Figure 2
Percentage of all U.S. cigarettes with filter tips

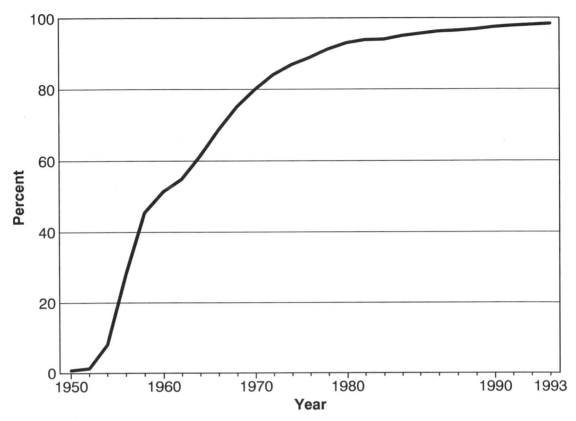

Source: U.S. Department of Agriculture, 1994.

inner core of the burning cone is depleted of oxygen, and thus the levels of carbon monoxide, hydrogen cyanide, and some other volatiles are selectively reduced in the smoke of cigarettes with perforated filter tips (Figure 3) (National Cancer Institute, 1977). Furthermore, the lower velocity of the generated smoke increases the efficiency of the filter. However, the tumorigenicity of the resulting tar does not change compared with that of the tar of a conventional, nonperforated cellulose acetate filter cigarette (National Cancer Institute, 1977). In principle, the smoke of a cigarette can be diluted to an unlimited degree by air; however, the consumers' nonacceptance of these cigarettes is the limiting factor.

The use of charcoal particles in one of two or three sections of a filter tip, or sprayed onto the cellulose acetate, also offers the opportunity to selectively reduce certain volatile smoke constituents, such as the ciliatoxic hydrogen cyanide, acetaldehyde, and acrolein (National Cancer Institute, 1977; Tiggelbeck, 1968). However, replacing one section of the filter tip with charcoal also leads to less reduction of TPM than can be achieved with

Table 1a
Effect of filament diameter on filter efficiency[a]

Approximate Filament Diameter (μ)	Pressure Drop (mm of H_2O)	Tar Removed (percent)
22	55.7	30
20	55.7	33
17	53.1	36
14	55.7	38
12.6	53.1	43

Table 1b
Effect of filter length on efficiency[b]

Filter Length (mm)	Pressure Drop (mm of H_2O)	Tar Removed (percent)
15	42	26.2
20	57	33.3
25	71	39.7
30	85	45.5
35	99	50.8

[a] *Cellulose acetate, 17 mm in length, 25-mm circumference.*
[b] *Cellulose acetate, 24.6-mm circumference.*

Key: μ = micron (10^{-6} meter); H_2O = water.

Source: Kiefer and Touey, 1967.

a filter tip of the same length but made entirely of cellulose acetate (Figure 4) (Brunnemann et al., 1990). Charcoal-containing filter tips are efficient in selectively reducing certain volatile aromatic hydrocarbons, such as benzene and toluene, from the smoke of the early puffs; yet, they release these hydrocarbons during the later puffs (Brunnemann et al., 1990).

Today, more than 70 percent of all cigarettes sold in Japan have charcoal-containing filter tips (Wynder and Hoffmann, 1994). Only a few percent of the cigarettes sold in the United States have such filters. Although more Japanese men smoke comparable numbers of cigarettes per day than American men do and the smoke yields per cigarette in Japan are similar to those in the United States, Japanese men have a significantly lower lung cancer incidence rate (Wynder and Hoffmann, 1994; Wynder et al., 1992). Among other factors, the lower yields of ciliatoxins, such as acrolein and hydrogen cyanide, in the smoke of cigarettes with charcoal filter tips may be partly responsible for the lower lung cancer rate in Japan.

Figure 3
Regression lines for all the investigated smoke components

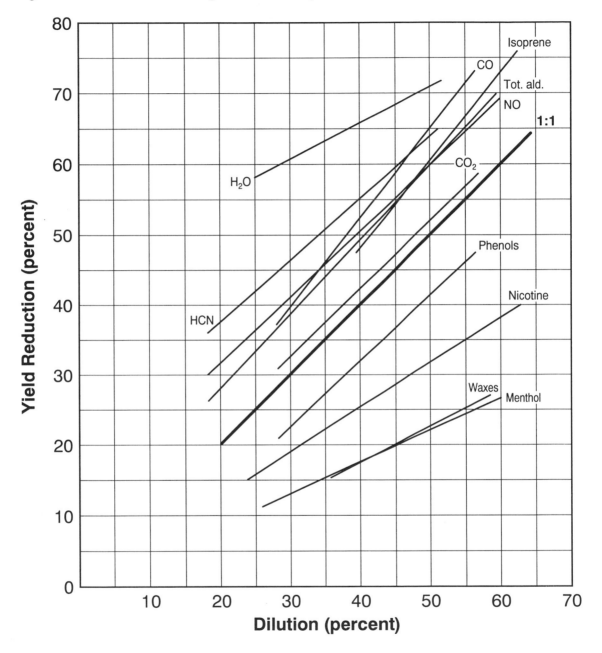

Key: *CO = carbon monoxide; tot. ald. = total volatile aldehydes; NO = nitrogen oxide; H₂O = water;*
      CO₂ = carbon dioxide; HCN = hydrogen cyanide.

Source: Norman, 1974.

Figure 4
Filtration of smoke constituents

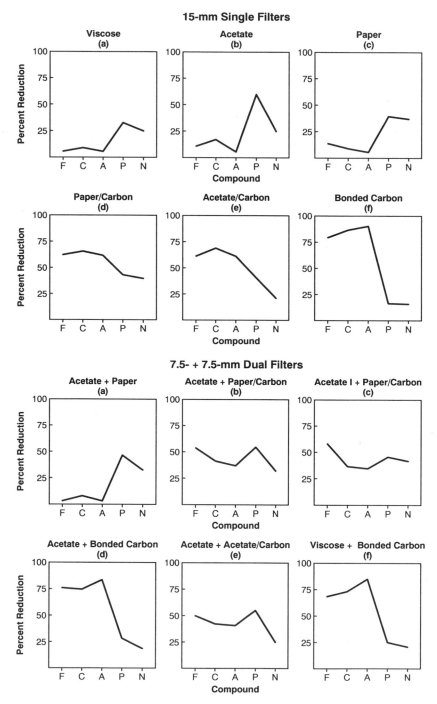

Key: *F = formaldehyde; C = hydrogen cyanide; A = acrolein; P = total phenols; N = nicotine.*

Source: Williamson et al., 1965.

Cigarette Paper With increasing permeability, porous cigarette papers significantly reduce tar, carbon monoxide, and nitrogen oxides but not low-molecular-weight gas phase components in the smokestream. Perforated cigarette paper also significantly reduces hydrogen cyanide, whereas nicotine reduction is less (National Cancer Institute, 1977) (Figure 5). In a recent study it was found that porous cigarette paper reduces not only smoke yields of carbon monoxide and tar but also of volatile nitrosamines, TSNAs, and benzo(*a*)pyrene (BaP) (Brunnemann et al., 1994). However, the reduction

Figure 5
Percentage change in smoke yield and composition with perforated, 0.5 percent citrate paper

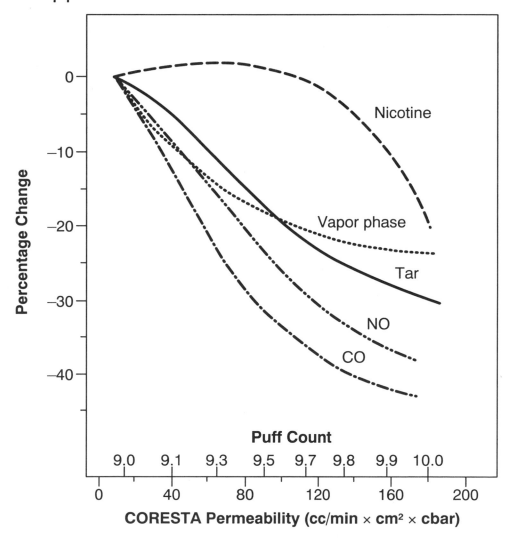

Key: *NO = nitrogen oxide; CO = carbon monoxide.*
Source: Owens, 1978.

of TSNAs and BaP is not selective. On a gram-to-gram basis, the tars obtained from cigarettes with high-porosity paper still have the same tumorigenic activity as does the tar from control cigarettes that have conventional cigarette paper (National Cancer Institute, 1977).

Reconstituted Tobacco
Reconstituted tobacco (RT) was first used after World War II as a binder for cigars and until the beginning of the 1960's on a limited scale for cigarettes (Halter and Ito, 1979). The interest in RT grew with the observation that cigarettes made exclusively from RT delivered lower smoke yields of tar, phenols, and BaP. On a gram-to-gram basis, this tar had significantly lower tumorigenicity on mouse skin and in the respiratory tract of hamsters (Wynder and Hoffmann, 1965). In 1974 the Research Institute of the German Cigarette Industry reported that forced exposure of Syrian golden hamsters to the smoke of cigarettes filled exclusively with RT gave significantly lower tumor incidence in the upper respiratory tract of the animals than treatment with the smoke of a blended cigarette containing only lamina of bright, burley, and oriental tobacco (Dontenwill, 1974).

Reconstituted tobacco, or homogenized sheet tobacco as it is sometimes called, is a paperlike sheet approaching the thickness of tobacco laminae. RT is made from tobacco dust, fines, and particles from ribs and stems; various additives may be incorporated. The process for making RT can be divided into four general classes. The first two relate to the papermaking process; the third involves a slurry; and the fourth is based on the preparation of a tobacco paste with rollers using water or low-boiling solvents. For the papermaking process, a mixture of fines, midribs, and sometimes tobacco stems is broken up and extracted with water. The extract is concentrated by evaporation. The insoluble residue is macerated further, and the resulting material is formed into a paperlike web on a papermaking machine. The web is dried and then impregnated with the concentrated extract; this web is then further dried and cut. The shredded material is added to the tobacco blend. Because the water extract of the tobacco contains nicotine and this extract is added in concentrated form to the tobacco web, this process has been considered a "nicotine-enriching process." In one papermaking process, cellulose fiber is added to increase the filling power and stability of the resulting RT.

In making RT by the slurry process, dry tobacco materials are finely divided and often mixed with small amounts of adhesive, then suspended in water. The resulting slurry is placed on a metallic band on which it is dried. The resulting sheet is shredded and added to the tobacco blend. In the rolling process, only small amounts of water are added to the mixture of tobacco fines, dust, and finely powdered ribs; this paste is placed onto rollers with different speeds, resulting in a sheet with limited filling power and tensile strength.

The potential to produce RT in various forms with different densities and filling powers and thereby to modify the tumorigenicity of tars and whole smoke encouraged the National Cancer Institute (NCI) in the 1970's to explore the use of various types of RT for recommendations of a less hazardous cigarette. The results documented that RT, especially RT resulting from the paper process with cellulose fiber as an additive, offered an opportunity to significantly reduce the cigarette smoke yields of tar, nicotine, phenols, and PAHs, as well as the tumorigenicity of the resulting tar. The most encouraging results were achieved with RT resulting from the paper process using only tobacco stems (Table 2).

Today, most blended U.S. cigarettes contain 20 to 30 percent RT, which is also now widely used in Europe, Canada, and Japan.

Puffed, Expanded, and Freeze-Dried Tobaccos   In the early 1970's a new tobacco preparation was introduced for the blended cigarette, that of "puffed," "expanded," or "freeze-dried" tobacco. Using these materials, less tobacco is required to fill a cigarette. The principle is to expand the tobacco cell walls by quick evaporation of water and other vaporizable agents. This causes a rapid pressure increase in the cells by heat and/or the reduction of external pressure.

Table 3 summarizes the smoke yields of experimental cigarettes made exclusively from puffed, expanded, or freeze-dried tobaccos. The smoke data are compared with those from the smoke of the control cigarette. The tars from the smoke of cigarettes made from expanded and freeze-dried tobaccos were significantly less tumorigenic than tar from the control cigarettes (National Cancer Institute, 1980).

Table 2
Smoke yields of cigarettes made from reconstituted tobacco (RT) by paper processes and from control cigarettes

Components	RT Stems Only	RT Blend	Control
Weight (mg)	1,011.0	1,060.0	1,226.0
Tar (mg)	11.3	11.7	25.9
Nicotine (mg)	0.2	0.7	1.7
Carbon Monoxide (mg)	11.9	11.8	16.1
NO_x (μg)	586.0	343.0	367.0
Hydrocyanic acid (μg)	73.5	81.9	201.0
Acetaldehyde (μg)	1,027.0	948.0	1,065.0
Acrolein (μg)	99.0	105.0	109.0
Benz(*a*)anthracene (ng)	13.1	9.8	46.3
Benzo(*a*)pyrene (ng)	8.9	7.4	27.8

Key: $NO_x = N$ (>95 percent) + NO_2 (<5 percent).

Source: National Cancer Institute, 1976a and 1976b.

Table 3
**Smoke analysis of cigarettes made from puffed, expanded, and freeze-dried tobaccos
and from control cigarettes**

Smoke Component	Puffed Tobacco	Expanded Tobacco	Freeze-Dried Tobacco	Control
Carbon Monoxide (mg)	9.33	11.80	12.30	18.00
Nitrogen Oxides (μg)	247.00	293.00	235.00	269.00
Hydrogen Cyanide (μg)	199.00	287.00	234.00	413.00
Formaldehyde (μg)	20.70	21.70	33.40	31.70
Acetaldehyde (μg)	814.00	720.00	968.00	986.00
Acrolein (μg)	105.00	87.70	92.40	128.00
Tar (mg)	15.60	18.20	16.30	36.70
Nicotine (mg)	0.78	0.74	0.82	2.61
Benz(*a*)anthracene (ng)	13.70	11.80	15.30	37.10
Benzo(*a*)pyrene (ng)	11.80	8.20	9.20	28.70

Source: National Cancer Institute, 1976b.

The use of puffed, expanded, or freeze-dried tobacco, together with the use of filter tips and reconstituted tobaccos, has had a major impact on the amounts of leaf tobacco needed per average U.S. cigarette. In about 1950 1,230 mg of leaf tobacco were required for one cigarette, whereas only 785 mg were needed in 1982 (Grise, 1984).

Physical Parameters of Cigarettes

Length

As the length of a cigarette increases, there is more opportunity for air to enter through the paper and for certain gaseous components, for example, carbon monoxide and hydrogen cyanide, to diffuse out of the paper into the environment. Assuming that all other factors remain the same and only the length of the cigarette increases, there will be a higher smoke yield of tar and nicotine because more tobacco is burned (Moore and Bock, 1968). In the past, it was claimed that tobacco absorbs only slightly less of the smoke particulates than a cellulose acetate filter tip (Dobrowsky, 1960). This may have been true in the early 1960's, but modern cellulose acetate filter tips are more efficient in retaining smoke particulates than the tobacco column of a cigarette.

Circumference

With the packing density remaining constant, a decrease in circumference of a cigarette reduces the amount of tobacco available for burning. As a result, tar and nicotine yields in the smokestream are reduced (Table 4) as are the yields of carbon monoxide and several other volatile smoke constituents (DeBardeleben et al., 1978).

Table 4
Effect of cigarette circumference on tar and nicotine in mainstream smoke

Circumference (mm)	Delivery (mg)	
	Tar	Nicotine
26	23.3	1.56
25	21.5	1.46
24	19.9	1.35
23	18.2	1.21

Source: DeBardeleben et al., 1978.

Tobacco Cut   Studies have shown that modifying tobacco from fine to coarse cut causes the number of puffs per cigarette to increase (DeBardeleben et al., 1978). In general, cigarettes that are filled with a more coarsely cut tobacco burn less efficiently than those made with fine-cut tobacco. One report, comparing the smoke of cigarettes filled with coarse-cut tobacco (1.27 mm) with smoke from cigarettes made with fine-cut tobacco (0.42 mm), showed only slight differences in smoke yields (Spears, 1974). However, a comparison of tars from cigarettes with given tobacco cut at rates of 20, 30, or 50 cuts per inch (1.27, 0.85, and 0.51 mm, respectively) showed in a bioassay that the finer the cut of the tobacco, the lower the tumorigenicity of the resulting tar (Wynder and Hoffmann, 1965).

Packing Density   Increasing the mass of the tobacco in a cigarette—increasing the packing density—causes yields of tar and nicotine in the smoke to rise. However, packing more than 1.0 g of tobacco into an 85-mm cigarette causes the yields of tar and nicotine in the smoke to decrease, most likely because of increased retention by the tobacco acting as a filter (Figure 6).

Tobacco Pesticides   Since 1969 the use of chlorinated pesticides has been banned in the cultivation of tobacco in the United States. As a result, 1,1,1-trichloro-2-(4,4'-dichlorodiphenyl)ethane (DDT) and 1,1,-dichloro-2-2(4,4'-dichlorodiphenyl)ethane (DDD) in tobacco and in cigarette smoke have drastically decreased. In the tobacco of a cigarette made in 1965, 13.4 ppm DDT and 20.2 ppm DDD were measured, and in the tobacco of the leading cigarette brand made in 1993, only 0.02 ppm DDT and 0.013 ppm DDD were detected, a decrease of more than 98 percent (Djordjevic et al., 1995). The small amounts of residual DDT and DDD in more recently produced cigarettes appear to originate from imported tobaccos used for blended cigarettes.

It was reported in 1981 that U.S. tobacco contains 250 ppb of the carcinogenic N-nitrosodiethanolamine (NDELA). This nitrosamine is formed by N-nitrosation of the secondary amine diethanolamine during tobacco

Figure 6
Effect of cigarette weight/packing density on particulate matter

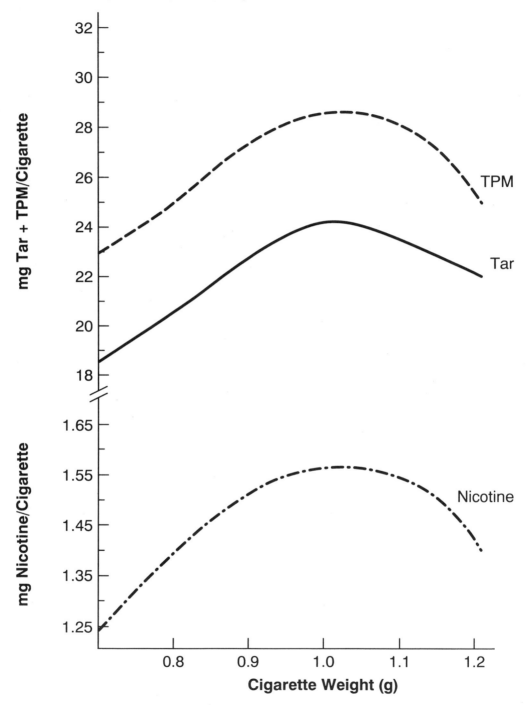

Key: TPM = total particulate matter.
Source: DeBardeleben et al., 1978.

processing. The major source of diethanolamine in tobacco in 1981 was the sucker growth inhibitor MH-30, which is the diethanolamine salt of maleic hydrazide (Brunnemann and Hoffmann, 1981). Because of the ban on MH-30 for tobacco treatment, NDELA levels have decreased to less than 100 ppb in cigarette tobacco (Brunnemann and Hoffmann, 1991). The remaining NDELA may be at least partially due to the contamination with diethanolamine from packaging materials.

Several pesticides are still being used on tobacco; these include insecticides, fumigants, and insect growth regulators (Benezet, 1989). There is only limited knowledge about the residues of these agents on cigarette tobacco and about their role during smoking.

Additives   In April 1994, the major U.S. cigarette companies released a list of 599 additives used in the manufacture of cigarettes (Tobacco Reporter Staff, 1994). Little is known about the fate of such additives during the smoking of cigarettes. An exception is menthol, which amounts to less than 2.5 mg in U.S. mentholated cigarettes (Perfetti and Gordin, 1985). Menthol is not carcinogenic in rodents (National Cancer Institute, 1979), nor does this readily volatilized compound give rise to measurable amounts of carcinogenic hydrocarbons, including BaP, during the smoking of cigarettes (Jenkins et al., 1970).

The list of additives also contains inorganic salts, such as ammonium and potassium carbonates, and bicarbonates. These additives possibly increase the pH of cigarette smoke. Beyond pH 6.0, cigarette smoke contains increasing amounts of unprotonated nicotine; with smoke pH at 6.9, about 10 percent of the nicotine is present in the smoke in free form; at pH 7.85 this rises to 50 percent (Brunnemann and Hoffmann, 1974). The free nicotine is present predominantly in the vapor phase of the smoke and is more quickly absorbed through the oral mucosa than nicotine in salt form (Armitage and Turner, 1970). Data are urgently needed for examining the change in pH of the smoke of cigarettes with additives.

Although most additives that are used as flavor-enhancing agents are sprayed onto tobacco in milligram amounts and may therefore generate at most microgram amounts of toxic or tumorigenic agents in the smoke, it is nevertheless important to document the fate of such compounds when they are added to cigarettes, cigars, or pipe tobacco.

Tobacco Blend   Most U.S. cigarettes manufactured worldwide are blended cigarettes. The composition of the tobacco blend has a major influence on the pH, toxicity, and tumorigenicity of the smoke. Many tobacco lines are available, including about 60 species and about 1,000 different tobacco varieties (Tso, 1972). The wealth of this source permits the manipulation of the tobacco plant and its components and leads to selective use of those portions of the plant that enhance or reduce specific agents in the smoke. This is then reflected in the toxicity and/or carcinogenicity of the smoke. For example, there are flue-cured tobacco lines that contain 0.2 to 4.75 percent nicotine and burley lines with 0.3 to 4.58 percent nicotine (Chaplin, 1975).

Furthermore, flue-cured tobacco leaves harvested from the lowest stalk position contain 0.08 to 0.65 percent nicotine, whereas those from the highest positions contain between 0.13 and 4.18 percent nicotine (Tso, 1977). The resulting smoke differs widely in its concentration of toxic and tumorigenn agents (Hoffmann and Hoffmann, 1994a). Another example is the BaP content of the smoke generated from leaves harvested from the lowest stalk position, which ranges between 14.9 and 18.2 ng per cigarette, contrasted with BaP in the smoke from the leaves of the highest stalk position, which ranges between 23.2 and 35.2 ng per cigarette (Rathkamp et al., 1973).

The first comparative study of the smoke of cigarettes made exclusively from bright, oriental, burley, and Maryland tobacco was published by Wynder and Hoffmann (1963). The BaP levels in the smoke per cigarette (without filter tip) were 53, 44, 24, and 18 ng, respectively. The tars from the smoke of cigarettes made with bright and oriental tobaccos were significantly more tumorigenic than the tars from burley and Maryland tobaccos (Wynder and Hoffmann, 1963). A large-scale study by NCI confirmed the observation that the smoke of burley tobacco is lower in BaP and other carcinogenic agents than the smoke of bright tobacco and that the tar has less tumorigenic activity than the tar from bright tobacco (National Cancer Institute, 1980).

During the past three decades, the nitrate content of the U.S. cigarette blend increased from 0.3 to 0.5 percent to 0.6 to 1.35 percent (U.S. Department of Health and Human Services, 1981; Fischer et al., 1990). During smoking, the nitrates in tobacco give rise to nitrogen oxides that scavenge C,H-radicals and thereby inhibit the pyrosynthesis of carcinogenic PAHs; at the same time, nitrogen oxides are involved in the formation of nitrosamines from secondary and tertiary amines in tobacco (Rathkamp and Hoffmann, 1970; Hoffmann et al., 1994). The result is that today the smoke of the U.S. blended cigarette has lower concentrations of PAHs but higher concentrations of N-nitrosamines than the smoke of the U.S. blended cigarette three decades ago. Figure 7 shows the decrease per cigarette of BaP from 50 ng in 1965 to 20 ng in 1992 and the concomitant increase of the levels of the organ-specific lung carcinogen 4-(methylnitrosamino)-1-(3-pyridyl)-1-butanone (NNK) from 110 ng in the late 1970's to 176 ng in 1992. These data pertain to the smoke of a leading United States nonfilter cigarette. NNK is formed from nicotine during tobacco processing and smoking (Hoffmann and Hoffmann, 1994a). In laboratory animals, carcinogenic PAHs induce primarily squamous cell carcinoma, whereas NNK elicits mainly adenocarcinoma in the peripheral lung. One major reason for the steep ascent of lung adenocarcinoma incidence in cigarette smokers in the United States compared with the more modest rise of squamous cell carcinoma may lie in the more intense smoking of the low-nicotine cigarette. The deeper inhalation of the smoke from these cigarettes has led to higher yields of NNK and lower yields of BaP in the smoke of the more recent cigarettes. This modification has created a different profile of smoke carcinogens that is likely reflected in the changed tumor morphology that has emerged since the 1960's (Wynder and Hoffmann, 1994).

Figure 7

BaP and NNK in mainstream smoke of a leading U.S. nonfilter cigarette, 1959-1992

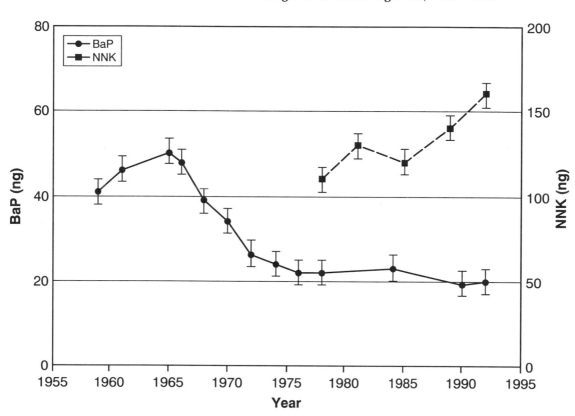

Source: Hoffmann and Hoffmann, 1994a.

SUMMARY   Table 5 indicates the potential roles that filter tips, perforated filter tips, cigarette paper, reconstituted tobacco, expanded tobacco, and an increase of the share of bright and burley tobacco in the cigarette blend have in affecting the smoke yields of selected toxic and tumorigenic agents. These observations have largely been taken into account with respect to the manufacture of blended U.S. filter cigarettes, which accounted for 97 percent of all cigarettes sold on the U.S. market in 1993. The result is a cigarette that delivers smoke with generally lower toxicity and tumorigenicity than products that were smoked 40 years ago. However, all the measurements on which this evaluation are based were obtained by standardized machine smoking with parameters that are not in line with the real practices of men and women who smoke the modern, low-yield, filter-tipped cigarettes (Russell, 1980; Herning et al., 1981; Kozlowski et al., 1982; Fagerström, 1982; Haley et al., 1985; Byrd et al., 1994). Is it thus safe to say that the modern cigarette is really less harmful?

Table 5

Changes in cigarette design and composition: Effects on smoke yields of selected toxic agents

Smoke Compound	Filter	Perforated Filter	Cigarette Paper	Reconstituted Tobacco	Expanded Tobacco	Bright Tobacco	Burley Tobacco
Tar	a	e	a	a	a	b	a
Nicotine	a	e	c	a	a	c	c
pH	NC	NC	NC	NC	NC	d	b
CO	c	a	NC	a	a	b	d
HCN	NC	a	NC	a	a	c	c
Volatile Aldehydes	NC	a	NC	a	a	b	a
Volatile Nitrosamines	e	e	NC	a	a	e	b
Phenol	e	e	NC	a	a	b	a
PAHs	a	e	NC	a	a	b	a
TSNAs	a	e	NC	f	f	e	b

a Significant decrease.
b Trend for increase.
c Can increase, can decrease.
d Trend for decrease.
e More than a 50-percent decrease.
f Unknown.

Key: CO = carbon monoxide; HCN = hydrocyanic acid; PAHs = polynuclear aromatic hydrocarbons; TSNAs = tobacco-specific N-nitrosamines; NC = no significant change.

How can the human risk from cigarette smoking truly be assessed? Should we not above all remember that the only way to prevent smoking-related diseases is abstinence from tobacco? Meanwhile, millions of smokers in the United States and worldwide continue to smoke cigarettes and to use other forms of tobacco because of their dependence on nicotine. Smoking cessation efforts have had success for many but are not likely to stem the tide of an enormous epidemic of smoking-related diseases that will be seen in the coming decades in those parts of the world that have hardly begun to tally the incidence and mortality from tobacco-related illness.

In the United States, we have today several sensitive techniques that can assist in determining uptake and even an individual's capacity for activating vs. detoxifying xenobiotics, such as the toxins and carcinogens from tobacco smoke (Bryant et al., 1988; Santella et al., 1992; Melikian et al., 1993; Hecht et al., 1994), but these sophisticated methods of risk assessment are research tools that for now do little to guide the consumer. One may agree with the content of an editorial published in the New York Times (1989) that read: "Obviously, no smoking is better than smoking, but the best should not be the enemy of the good. There is a strong social case for encouraging manufacturers to develop safer cigarettes that will sell." If we take this premise as a realistic approach to the tobacco and illness dilemma in our Nation, how can our regulatory agencies effectively protect the consumer and on what type of measurement should risk assessment from cigarette smoking be based? This is the question to be resolved. The authors hope that presentation of some historical background will assist with this aim.

QUESTION-AND-ANSWER SESSION

DR. HENNINGFIELD: Dr. Hoffmann, the influence of some parameters, such as increasing puff quantity, would be pretty obvious for their impact; you would take in more smoke. But what about the factor of changing the intensity of a puff? For example, the FTC method uses 35 mL over 2 seconds, or say about 18 mL per second. What would be the impact of tripling the intensity by going to, say, 60 mL per 1 second?

DR. HOFFMANN: This has been done by various groups, including Dr. Benowitz, Dr. Auston, and Dr. Ogg. All have shown that when you smoke more intensely (I think one report makes up to four or five puffs per minute, with puff volumes up to 55 mL), you obviously increase the smoke yields for cigarette smoke; based on epidemiological observations, but you inhale deeper.

Now, this is reflected in the yield of nicotine respectively as one of its major metabolites. And in fact, R.J. Reynolds Tobacco Company has recently shown a very low yielding cigarette. They determined 90 percent of all metabolites, and I think the results are in here. They have shown that with the very low yielding cigarettes, the smoker inhales more than one would expect from machine smoking data, based on the nicotine metabolites.

Machine smoking data may be all right for the cigarette without a filter tip, but based on all these studies (I think there are eight all total), the smoker of a low yielding cigarette inhales deeper and takes more puffs, smokes more intensely.

DR. RICKERT: Dr. Hoffmann, I think you were intimately involved in the NCI's less hazardous cigarette program a number of years ago. Why was that program abandoned?

DR. HOFFMANN: The timing was not right—I do not know the details. I work in the laboratory, and that is outside the field. It was purely politics.

DR. HARRIS: Dr. Hoffmann, you presented trends in some cigarette smoke components over time. What do you know, if anything, about gross characteristics of cigarette smoke, such as the trends in the pH of American cigarette smoke or in the oxidation reduction potential of smoke?

DR. HOFFMANN: The pH has increased slightly; it is slightly higher in filtered cigarettes, in perforated filter cigarettes, and in RT.

There has been a slight increase in unprotonated nicotine, but it is a minor difference, because it is still a blended cigarette. If you smoke a French cigarette, which are the black or burley type cigarettes, they have a pH of 7.5, or 40 percent of the nicotine is unprotonated; whereas, in our blended U.S. cigarettes, less than 5 percent is unprotonated. As an English study by Turner and others has shown, when you have unprotonated nicotine, most of it has a quicker result to the mucous membrane, especially of the oral cavity. In other words, when you have unprotonated nicotine, not in salt form but in free base, most of it is in the water phase, and therefore it is absorbed more quickly by the surface of the bronchial epithelium or the oral cavity.

Therefore, you would rarely see a Frenchman taking as deep inhalations as a smoker of a blended cigarette with an active filter tip. You watch a Paris cab driver and you will see that they never inhale; he just dangles the cigarette on the side of his mouth, because he would get a tremendous nicotine kick if he inhaled.

DR. HARRIS: Does the protonation state of nicotine, whether it is protonated or free base, affect the measurement method of nicotine as currently used by the FTC?

DR. HOFFMANN: No, the pH is not measured. I do not see the need because so far, in our U.S. blended cigarettes, there are no major differences. That may change, but at present, it is not.

DR. HUGHES: I noticed over time that the tar and nicotine yields have changed somewhat. What is your opinion about how feasible it is, using existing techniques, to change that ratio?

DR. HOFFMANN: The first study was performed in the United Kingdom by Russell. It demonstrated that the ratio of tar to nicotine, which was originally 100 to 6, has changed to 100 to 10. We see this in low yielding cigarettes. In other words, the nicotine is not reduced to the same extent that the tar is reduced.

DR. HUGHES: And how feasible would it be for the manufacturers to deliberately change that ratio at this point?

DR. HOFFMANN: They can do it easily by changing the tobacco variety, which is high in nicotine. We have heard about genetic engineering for a tobacco variety that is very high in nicotine. So that is possible. I mean, the manufacturer has everything in his hand to have high nicotine and low tar or vice versa.

In fact, for a brief time, there was a cigarette on the market that was free of nicotine. The nicotine was extracted from the tobacco with supercritical fluid transaction, and the tobacco was then used for cigarettes. So, the tobacco industry has a whole spectrum from high- to low-nicotine yield. That depends on what the consumer requests.

REFERENCES

Armitage, A.K., Turner, D.M. Absorption of nicotine in cigarette and cigar smoke through the oral mucosa. *Nature* 226: 1231-1232, 1970.

Benezet, H.J. Chemical control of pests in stored tobacco. *Recent Advances in Tobacco Science* 15: 1-25, 1989.

Bradford, J.A., Harlan, W.R., Hanmer, H.R. Nature of cigaret smoke. Technic of experimental smoking. *Industrial and Engineering Chemistry* 28(7): 836-839, 1936.

Brunnemann, K.D., Hoffmann, D. The pH of tobacco smoke. *Food and Cosmetics Toxicology* 12: 115-124, 1974.

Brunnemann, K.D., Hoffmann, D. Assessment of carcinogenic, volatile N-nitrosamines in tobacco and in mainstream and sidestream smoke of cigarettes. *Cancer Research* 37: 3218-3222, 1977.

Brunnemann, K.D., Hoffmann, D. Assessment of the carcinogenic N-nitrosodiethanolamine in tobacco products and tobacco smoke. *Carcinogenesis* 2: 1123-1127, 1981.

Brunnemann, K.D., Hoffmann, D. Decreased concentrations of N-nitrosodiethanolamine and N-nitrosomorpholine in commercial tobacco products. *Journal of Agricultural and Food Chemistry* 39: 207-208, 1991.

Brunnemann, K.D., Hoffmann, D., Gairola, C.G., Lee, B.C. Low ignition propensity cigarettes: Smoke analysis for carcinogens and testing for mutagenic activity of the smoke particulate matter. *Food and Chemical Toxicology* 32: 917-922, 1994.

Brunnemann, K.D., Kagan, M.R., Cox, J.E., Hoffmann, D. Analysis of 1,3-butadiene and other selected gas-phase components in cigarette mainstream and sidestream smoke by gas chromatography-mass selective detection. *Carcinogenesis* 11(10): 1863-1868, 1990.

Bryant, M.S., Vineis, P., Skipper, P.L., Tannenbaum, S.R. Hemoglobin adducts of aromatic amines: Associations with smoking status and type of tobacco. *Proceedings of the National Academy of Sciences of the United States of America* 85(24): 9788-9791, 1988.

Byrd, G.D., Robinson, J.H., Caldwell, W.S., deBethizy, J.D. Nicotine uptake and metabolism in smokers. *Recent Advances in Tobacco Science* 20: 5-31, 1994.

Chaplin, J.F. Genetic influence on chemical constituents of tobacco leaf and smoke. *Beitrage zur Tabakforschung* 8: 233-240, 1975.

CORESTA. Recommended Method No. 22. Routine analytical cigarette-smoking machine specifications, definitions and standard conditions. *CORESTA Information Bulletin* 124-140, 1991-1993.

DeBardeleben, M.Z., Claflin, W.E., Gannon, W.F. Role of cigarette physical characteristics on smoke composition. *Recent Advances in Tobacco Science* 4: 85-111, 1978.

Djordjevic, M.V., Fan, J., Ferguson, S., Hoffmann, D. Self-regulation of smoking intensity. Smoke yields of the low-nicotine, low-"tar" cigarettes. *Carcinogenesis* 16(9): 2015-2021, 1995.

Dobrowsky, A. The absorption of tobacco smoke: How far is the cigarette its own filter? *Tobacco Science* 4: 126-129, 1960.

Doll, R., Hill, A.B. Smoking and carcinoma of the lung. Preliminary report. *British Medical Journal* 2: 739-748, 1950.

Dontenwill, W.P. Tumorigenic effect of chronic cigarette smoke inhalation on Syrian golden hamsters. In: *Experimental Lung Cancer. Carcinogenesis and Bioassays*, E. Karbe and J.F. Park (Editors). New York: Springer-Verlag, 1974, pp. 331-359.

Fagerström, K.O. Effects of a nicotine-enriched cigarette on nicotine titration, daily cigarette consumption, and levels of carbon monoxide, cotinine, and nicotine. *Psychopharmacology* 77(2): 164-167, 1982.

Fischer, S., Spiegelhalder, R., Preussmann, R. Tobacco-specific nitrosamines in European and U.S. cigarettes. *Archiv fur Geschwulstforschung* 60: 169-177, 1990.

George, T.W., Keith, C.H. The selective filtration of tobacco smoke. In: *Tobacco and Tobacco Smoke. Studies in Experimental Tobacco Carcinogenesis*, E.L. Wynder and D. Hoffmann (Editors). New York: Academic Press, 1967, pp. 577-622.

Grise, V.N. Market growth of reduced tar cigarettes. *Recent Advances in Tobacco Science* 10: 4-14, 1984.

Haley, N.J., Sepkovic, D.W., Hoffmann, D., Wynder, E.L. Cigarette smoking as a risk factor for cardiovascular disease. VI. Compensation with nicotine availability as a single variable. *Clinical Pharmacology and Therapeutics* 38: 164-170, 1985.

Halter, H.M., Ito, T.I. Effect of tobacco reconstitution and expansion processes on smoke composition. *Recent Advances in Tobacco Science* 4: 113-132, 1979.

Hecht, S.S., Carmella, S.G., Foiles, P.G., Murphy, S.E. Biomarkers for human uptake and metabolic activation of tobacco-specific nitrosamines. *Cancer Research* 54(7 Suppl): 1912s-1917s, 1994.

Herning, R.I., Jones, R.T., Bachman, J., Mines, A.H. Puff volume increases when low-nicotine cigarettes are smoked. *British Medical Journal (Clinical Research Ed.)* 283(6285): 187-189, 1981.

Hoffmann, D., Brunnemann, K.D., Prokopczyk, B., Djordjevic, M.V. Tobacco-specific N-nitrosamines and Areca-derived N-nitrosamines: Chemistry, biochemistry, carcinogenicity and relevance to humans. *Journal of Toxicology and Environmental Health* 41: 1-52, 1994.

Hoffmann, D., Hoffmann, I. Tobacco consumption and lung cancer. In: *Lung Cancer*, H.H. Hansen (Editor). Boston: Kluwer Academic Publications, 1994a, pp. 1-42.

Hoffmann, D., Hoffmann, I. Recent developments in smoking-related cancer research. *Journal of Smoking Related Diseases* 5: 77-93, 1994b.

Jarvis, M.J., Russell, M.A. Tar and nicotine yields of U.K. cigarettes 1972-1983. Sales-weighted estimates from non-industry sources. *British Journal of Addiction* 80(4): 429-434, 1985.

Jenkins, R.W.J., Newman, R.H., Chavis, M.K. Cigarette smoke formation studies II. Smoke distribution and mainstream pyrolytic composition of added ^{14}C-menthol (U). *Beitrage zur Tabakforschung* 5: 299-301, 1970.

Kiefer, J.E., Touey, G.P. Filtration of tobacco smoke particles. In: *Tobacco and Tobacco Smoke. Studies in Experimental Tobacco Carcinogenesis*, E.L. Wynder and D. Hoffmann (Editors). New York: Academic Press, 1967, pp. 545-575.

Kozlowski, L.T., Rickert, W.S., Pope, M.A., Robinson, J.C., Frecker, R.C. Estimating the yields to smokers of tar, nicotine, and carbon monoxide from the "lowest yield" ventilated filter cigarette. *British Journal of Addiction* 77: 159-165, 1982.

Melikian, A.A., Prahalad, A.K., Hoffmann, D. Urinary *trans,trans*-muconic acid as an indicator of exposure to benzene in cigarette smokers. *Cancer Epidemiology, Biomarkers and Prevention* 3: 47-51, 1993.

Moore, G.E., Bock, F.G. Tar and nicotine levels of American cigarettes. *National Cancer Institute Monograph* 28: 89-94, 1968.

National Cancer Institute. *Bioassays of dl-Menthol for Possible Carcinogenicity*. Vol. 98. Carcinogenesis Technical Report Series. Bethesda, MD: National Intitutes of Health, 1979, pp. 1-123.

National Cancer Institute, Smoking and Health Program. *Toward Less Hazardous Cigarettes. The First Set of Experimental Cigarettes*. DHEW Publication No. (NIH) 76-905. Bethesda, MD: U.S. Department of Health, Education, and Welfare, Public Health Service, National Institutes of Health, 1976a.

National Cancer Institute, Smoking and Health Program. *Toward Less Hazardous Cigarettes. The Second Set of Experimental Cigarettes*. DHEW Publication No. (NIH) 76-1111. Bethesda, MD: U.S. Department of Health, Education, and Welfare, Public Health Service, National Institutes of Health, 1976b.

National Cancer Institute, Smoking and Health Program. *Toward Less Hazardous Cigarettes. The Third Set of Experimental Cigarettes*. DHEW Publication No. (NIH) 77-1280. Bethesda, MD: U.S. Department of Health, Education, and Welfare, Public Health Service, National Institutes of Health, 1977.

National Cancer Institute, Smoking and Health Program. *Toward Less Hazardous Cigarettes. The Fourth Set of Experimental Cigarettes*. Bethesda, MD: U.S. Department of Health, Education, and Welfare, Public Health Service, National Institutes of Health, 1980.

New York Times. Safer cigarettes (editorial). March 3, 1989. p. A38.

Norman, V. The effect of perforated tipping paper on the yields of various smoke components. *Beitrage zur Tabakforschung* 7: 282-287, 1974.

Owens, W.F., Jr. Effect of cigarette paper on smoke yield and composition. *Recent Advances in Tobacco Science* 4: 3-24, 1978.

Perfetti, T.A., Gordin, H.H. Just noticeable differences. Studies of mentholated cigarette products. *Tobacco Science* 29: 57-66, 1985.

Pfyl, B. Zur Bestimmung des Nikotins II. Mitteilung. *Zeitschrift für Lebensmittel-Untersuchung und-Forschung* 66: 501-510, 1933.

Pillsbury, H.C., Bright, C.C., O'Connor, K.J., Irish, F.W. Tar and nicotine in cigarette smoke. *Journal–Association of Official Analytical Chemists* 52: 458-462, 1969.

Pyriki, C. Verteilung von Nikotin im Rauch von Zigaretten. *Chemiker-Zeitung* 58: 279-280, 1934.

Rathkamp, G., Hoffmann, D. Inhibition of the pyrosynthesis of several selective smoke constituents. *Beitrage zur Tabakforschung* 5: 302-306, 1970.

Rathkamp, G., Tso, T.C., Hoffmann, D. Smoke analysis of cigarettes made from bright tobaccos differing in variety and stalk position. *Beitrage zur Tabakforschung* 7: 179-189, 1973.

Royal College of Physicians. *Smoking and Health*. London: Pitman, 1962.

Russell, M.A.H. The case for medium-nicotine, low-tar, low-carbon monoxide cigarettes. *Banbury Report* 3: 297-310, 1980.

Santella, R.M., Grinberg-Gunes, R.A., Young, T.L., Dickey, C., Singh, V.N., Wang, L.W., Perera, F.P. Cigarette smoking related polycyclic aromatic hydrocarbon-DNA adducts in peripheral mononuclear cells. *Carcinogenesis* 13: 2041-2045, 1992.

Spears, A.W. Effect of manufacturing variables on cigarette smoke composition. *CORESTA Bulletin d'Information* 65-78, 1974.

Tiggelbeck, D. Comments on selective cigarette-smoke filtration. *National Cancer Institute Monograph* 28: 249-258, 1968.

Tobacco Reporter Staff. Safe cigarette flavorings not a risk, says independent panel. *Tobacco Reporter* 121(7): 32-39, 1994.

Tso, T.C. The potential for producing safer cigarette tobacco. *Agriculture Science Review* 10: 1-10, 1972.

Tso, T.C. Simple correlation and multiple regression among leaf characteristics, smoke components, and biological responses of bright tobaccos. *Agricultural Research Service Technical Bulletin* 1551: 1-135, 1977.

U.S. Department of Agriculture. Percent of total cigarette production which are filter-tipped cigarettes. *Foreign Tobacco* 8: 40-41, 1993.

U.S. Department of Agriculture, Economic Research Service. *Tobacco Situation and Outlook Report*. TBS-229. Washington, DC: U.S. Department of Agriculture, 1994.

U.S. Department of Health, Education, and Welfare. *Smoking and Health. Report of the Advisory Committee to the Surgeon General of the Public Health Service.* Publication No. 1103. Rockville, MD: U.S. Department of Health, Education, and Welfare, Public Health Service, 1964.

U.S. Department of Health and Human Services. *The Health Consequences of Smoking: The Changing Cigarette. A Report of the Surgeon General.* DHHS Publication No. (PHS) 81-50156. Rockville, MD: U.S. Department of Health and Human Services, Public Health Service, Office on Smoking and Health, 1981.

U.S. Department of Health and Human Services. *The Health Consequences of Smoking: Nicotine Addiction. A Report of the Surgeon General, 1988.* DHHS Publication No. (CDC) 88-8406. Rockville, MD: U.S. Department of Health and Human Services, Public Health Service, Centers for Disease Control, Center for Health Promotion and Education, Office on Smoking and Health, 1988.

Williamson, J.T., Graham, J.F., Allman, D.R. The modification of cigarette smoke filters. *Beitrage zur Tabakforschung* 3: 233-242, 1965.

Wynder, E.L., Graham, E.A. Tobacco smoking as a possible etiologic factor in bronchiogenic carcinoma. A study of six hundred and eighty-four proved cases. *Journal of the American Medical Association* 143: 329-336, 1950.

Wynder, E.L., Hoffmann, D. Ein experimenteller Beitrag zur Tabakrauchkanzerogenese. *Deutsche Medizinische Wochenschrift* 88: 623-628, 1963.

Wynder, E.L., Hoffmann, D. Reduction of the tumorigenicity of cigarette smoke. *Journal of the American Medical Association* 192: 88-94, 1965.

Wynder, E.L., Hoffmann, D. (Editors). *Tobacco and Tobacco Smoke. Studies in Experimental Tobacco Carcinogenesis.* New York: Academic Press, 1967.

Wynder, E.L., Hoffmann, D. Smoking and lung cancer: Scientific challenges and opportunities. *Cancer Research* 54: 5284-5295, 1994.

Wynder, E.L., Taioli, E., Fujita, Y. Ecologic study of lung cancer risk factors in the U.S. and Japan with special reference to smoking and diet. *Japanese Journal of Cancer Clinics* 83: 418-423, 1992.

ACKNOWLEDGMENTS   The authors greatly appreciate the editorial assistance of Ilse Hoffmann and Jennifer Johnting. The authors' work cited in this article was supported by NCI grant CA-29580.

Attitudes, Knowledge, and Beliefs About Low-Yield Cigarettes Among Adolescents and Adults

Gary A. Giovino, Scott L. Tomar, Murli N. Reddy, John P. Peddicord, Bao-Ping Zhu, Luis G. Escobedo, and Michael P. Eriksen

INTRODUCTION   Per capita consumption of cigarettes in the United States increased rapidly from 1900 to 1963 (Miller, 1981; U.S. Department of Health and Human Services, 1989); however, since the January 1964 release of the first Surgeon General's report on smoking (U.S. Department of Health, Education, and Welfare, 1964), cigarette consumption has been declining (Miller, 1981; U.S. Department of Agriculture, 1987 and 1994). In 1994 per capita consumption was about the same as during World War II (Miller, 1981; U.S. Department of Agriculture, 1994). However, the prevalence of smoking was slightly higher in the 1940's (Centers for Disease Control and Prevention, 1994a; U.S. Department of Health and Human Services, 1988), indicating that smokers in the 1990's consumed more cigarettes per day than did smokers in the 1940's (Harris, 1994; U.S. Department of Health and Human Services, 1980).

Falls in per capita consumption of cigarettes seem linked to health concerns. For example, in the early 1950's, scientific and popular articles led to increasing concern about smoking-related cancers. American and British studies provided a scientific foundation for the mounting health concerns (Doll and Hill, 1950 and 1952; Levin et al., 1950; Wynder and Graham, 1950). Articles such as "Cancer by the Carton," published in the *Reader's Digest* (Norr, 1952), also carried the message to many people (U.S. Department of Health and Human Services, 1989).

One apparent result of these early health communications was the marked increase in the consumption of filter-tipped cigarettes. In the 1940's few people smoked those varieties (U.S. Department of Agriculture, 1962), but by 1992 about 97 percent of cigarettes sold had filters (Figure 1) (Federal Trade Commission, 1994). Switching to filtered cigarettes was promoted by slogans such as "Kent with the micronite filter is smoked by more scientists and educators than any other cigarette" (Anonymous, 1985).

The release of the first Surgeon General's report on smoking was a major turning point in public perception of the health threat of tobacco (U.S. Department of Health, Education, and Welfare, 1964; U.S. Department of Health and Human Services, 1989). In response, cigarette companies began introducing cigarettes in the 1960's and early 1970's that yielded,

Figure 1
Domestic market share of all filter-tipped cigarettes and those filter-tipped cigarettes yielding ≤15 mg tar: United States, 1946-1992

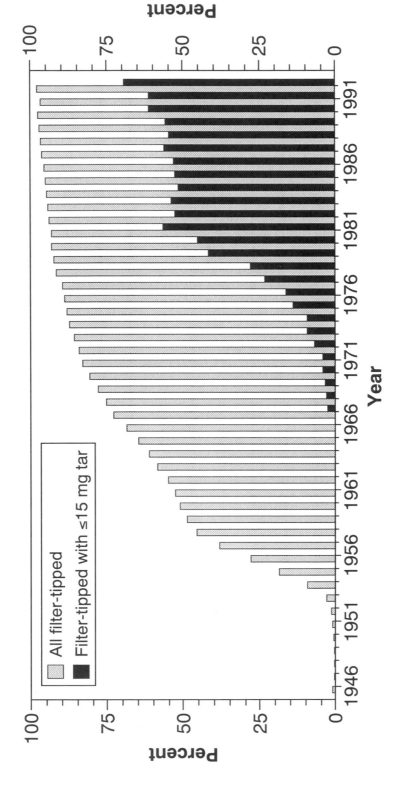

Sources: U.S. Department of Agriculture, 1962; Federal Trade Commission, 1994.

by the Federal Trade Commission (FTC) method (Pillsbury et al., 1969), 15 mg or less tar (Federal Trade Commission, 1994; Slade, 1989; Warner, 1985). By 1992 these so-called milder cigarettes had captured about 69 percent of the market (Federal Trade Commission, 1994).

The lower tar cigarettes were accompanied by advertisements such as the following:

> Vantage is changing a lot of my feelings about smoking. I like to smoke, and what I like is a cigarette that is not limited on taste. But I am not living in an ivory tower. I hear the things being said about high tar smoking as well as the next guy. So, I started looking for a low tar smoke that had some honest-to-goodness taste (Anonymous, 1977).

It is believed that the Vantage advertisements targeted "intelligent" smokers (Pollay, 1990).

Since 1974, FTC has collected data on advertising and promotion of cigarettes yielding 15 mg or less tar (Figure 2) (Federal Trade Commission, 1994). As pointed out by Davis (1987), for many years the proportion of advertising and promotional expenditures for lower tar cigarettes exceeded

Figure 2
Domestic market share and proportion of total advertising and promotional expenditures related to cigarettes yielding ≤15 mg tar, by year: United States, 1975-1992

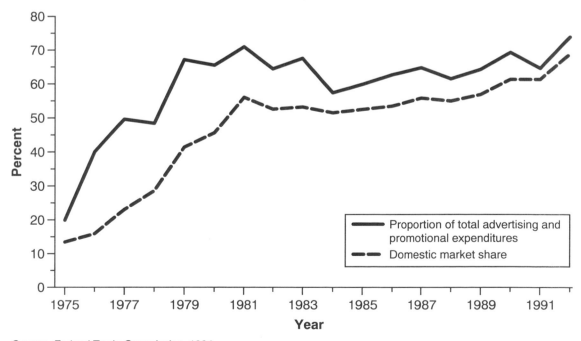

Source: Federal Trade Commission, 1994.

market share, suggesting an attempt to increase market share. As shown in Figure 2, the two proportions are converging. In 1992 lower tar cigarettes accounted for 69 percent of market share and 71 percent of advertising expenditures (Federal Trade Commission, 1994).

One major purpose of the marketing of these varieties of cigarettes appears to have been to alleviate smokers' health concerns (Pollay, 1990; Warner 1985). The advertisements seem to have achieved a large part of their goal. In 1993 a Gallup Organization poll posed the following question: "Besides selling the product, what message do you think cigarette advertising is trying to get across when it uses terms like low tar, low nicotine, or low yield?" (Gallup Organization, Inc., 1993, pp. 22). Fifty-eight percent of respondents (56 percent of smokers and 60 percent of nonsmokers) answered that the message indicates a positive health benefit, that is, that the brand is safer, healthier, less harmful, not as bad for you, or less cancerous (Gallup Organization, Inc., 1993).

MONITORING NATIONAL DATA Three national surveys helped shed light on the patterns in attitudes, knowledge, and beliefs about low-yield cigarettes: the 1986 Adult Use of Tobacco Survey (AUTS), the 1987 National Health Interview Survey (NHIS) Cancer Control Supplement, and the 1993 Teenage Attitudes and Practices Survey (TAPS). The 1986 AUTS was a national telephone survey of approximately 13,000 Americans ages 17 years and older (Pierce et al., 1990). The nationally representative sample of the 1987 NHIS included about 22,000 Americans ages 18 years and older who were interviewed primarily in their homes (Schoenborn and Boyd, 1989). The 1993 TAPS sample included about 13,000 people 10 to 22 years of age who were contacted via telephone or in their homes (Centers for Disease Control and Prevention, 1994b). The 1993 TAPS included a cross-sectional component of persons 10 to 15 years of age in 1993 and a followup component of a cohort of persons first interviewed in 1989 who were 15 to 22 years old in 1993 (Centers for Disease Control and Prevention, 1994b).

There are difficulties in using the 1993 TAPS data to make prevalence estimates. Some participants lost to followup were more likely to be smokers in 1989, a phenomenon that would be likely to decrease the overall prevalence estimate (Centers for Disease Control and Prevention, 1994b). The data used for this report are not used to generate smoking prevalence estimates; rather, they look at characteristics of persons who reported that they were currently smoking.

The 1986 AUTS and the 1987 NHIS questions used to determine tar levels assessed items such as brand name, filter vs. nonfilter, pack hardness, cigarette length, mentholation, and if the cigarette was regular, light, or ultralight. The tar level assigned is based on responses to the questions using FTC tables (Federal Trade Commission, 1985). The tar categories used for this report are (1) less than or equal to 6 mg, (2) 7 to 15 mg, and (3) 16 mg or more. (The actual cutpoints used here are 6.99 mg and 15.99 mg.)

SURVEY FINDINGS

**Use of Low-Tar
or Light Cigarettes**

The percentage distribution of tar yield of the usual brand of cigarettes smoked among current smokers by sex and age is shown in Figure 3. Female smokers were more likely to smoke lower tar yield brands than men. Smokers 18 to 24 years of age were less likely to use the lower tar brands than smokers ages 25 to 44 or 45 to 64. These patterns were similar to those found by the AUTS for both current and former smokers.

With regard to race and ethnicity (Figure 4), white Americans who smoked in 1987 were more likely to smoke lower tar and nicotine cigarettes (76.8 percent) than Hispanics (67.8 percent) or black Americans (52.4 percent). Education is a strong correlate of smoking cigarette brands with 15 mg or less tar (Figure 4). Beginning with persons who have completed 9 to 11 years of education, as education increased, smokers *were* more likely to smoke low-tar brands.

In the 1993 TAPS, adolescents and young adults who smoked and usually bought their own cigarettes were asked what brands they smoked. Furthermore, they were asked, "Is the brand you smoke regular, light, or

Figure 3
Prevalence (by percent) of current smokers' use of cigarette brands[a] with ≤15 mg tar, by sex and age: Ages 18 and older, United States, 1987

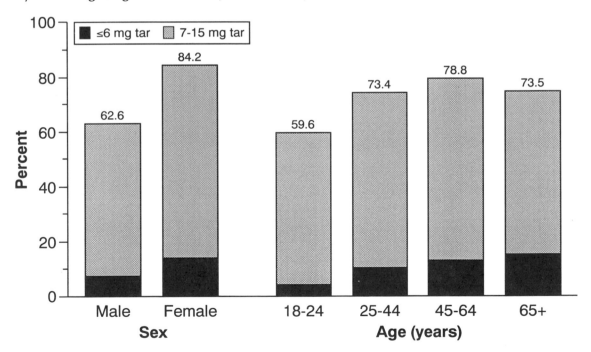

[a] *Self-reported usual brand.*

Source: National Center for Health Statistics, 1987.

Figure 4

Prevalence (by percent) of current smokers' use of cigarette brands[a] with ≤15 mg tar, by race and education: Ages 18 and older, United States, 1987

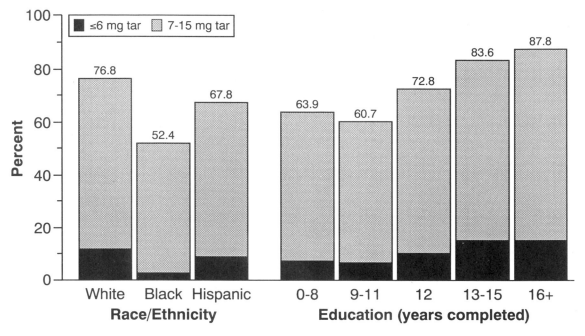

[a] *Self-reported usual brand.*

Source: National Center for Health Statistics, 1987.

ultralight?" Of note, "light" and "ultralight" are terms used in advertising and may not correlate precisely with tar and nicotine levels (Davis et al., 1990). However, these are terms that smokers frequently use in describing the brands they smoke.

There are two key findings from the TAPS data. First, among 10- to 18-year-olds and 19- to 22-year-olds, females were more likely than males to smoke light and ultralight cigarettes (Figure 5). Very few males smoked ultralight cigarettes. Second, the proportion of males and females using these brands increased with age. This pattern among young persons (increasing use of light and ultralight brands with increasing age) is reflected in both the 1987 NHIS and the 1993 TAPS.

The 1993 TAPS race and ethnicity findings are similar to those detected by the NHIS: White youth were most likely to smoke light cigarettes (52.6 percent), followed by Hispanic youth (44.5 percent), with much smaller proportions of black youth (15 percent) reporting use of these brands (Figure 6). Anecdotal evidence also indicates that African-American youth begin with higher tar cigarettes (Gallup International Institute, 1992).

Figure 5
**Prevalence (by percent) of use of light and ultralight cigarettes among current smokers,[a]
by sex and age: Ages 10 to 22, United States, 1993**

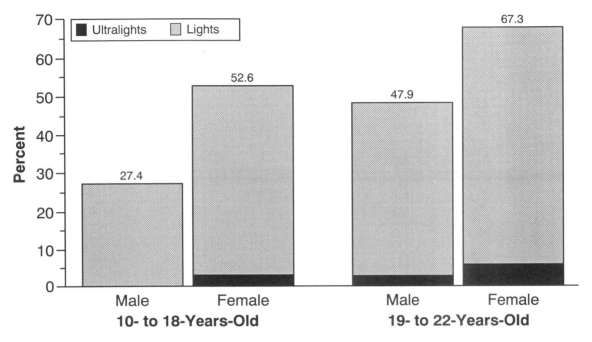

[a] *Who usually buy their own cigarettes.*
Source: Centers for Disease Control and Prevention, 1993.

In the 1993 TAPS, students were asked to rate how well they were doing in school; the categories used here were less than average, average, better than average, and much better than average. The percentage of young smokers who smoked light or ultralight cigarettes increased with level of performance in school: from 30 percent for those who performed less than average to 66 percent for those who performed much better than average (Figure 6).

Brand Switching   Brand switching is one measure of the perceived health risk associated with lower tar yield cigarettes. The 1986 AUTS asked the following question of current smokers: "Thinking of your entire smoking history, have you ever switched from one cigarette to another, just to reduce the amount of tar and nicotine?" Former smokers were asked, "Did you ever switch from one type of cigarette to another just to reduce the amount of tar and nicotine?" Approximately 38 percent of current smokers and 26 percent of former smokers answered "Yes."

The 1987 NHIS asked current smokers, "Have you ever switched to a low tar and nicotine cigarette just to reduce your health risk?" About 44 percent of current smokers answered that they had switched for that reason. As

Figure 6

Prevalence (by percent) of use of light and ultralight cigarettes among current smokers,[a] by race/ethnicity and school performance: Ages 10 to 22 years, United States, 1993

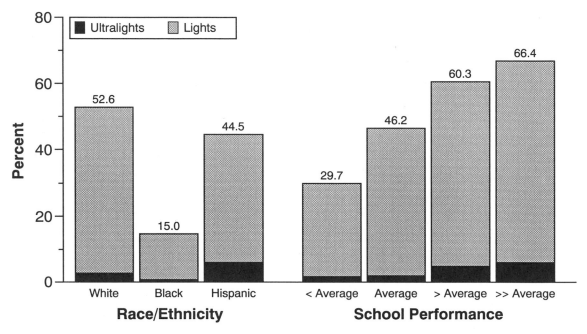

[a] *Who usually buy their own cigarettes.*

Source: Centers for Disease Control and Prevention, 1993.

shown in Figures 7 and 8, there are clear trends and differences by sex, age, race/ethnicity, and education. Figure 7 shows that females (48.4 percent) were more likely to switch than males (39.4 percent). Smokers in the 25-to-44 and 45-to-64 age groups were most likely to have switched to lower yield brands (45.2 and 45.9 percent, respectively), followed by smokers older than age 64 (41.3 percent) and those 18 to 24 years (36.4 percent). Figure 8 shows that whites (47 percent) were more likely to switch than Hispanics (30.9 percent) or African-Americans (30.8 percent), and the more educated were more likely to switch than the less educated.

Smokers of low-tar yield varieties were more likely to have switched. That is, among smokers consuming brands yielding 6 mg or less tar, 74 percent of current smokers in the 1986 AUTS had ever switched compared with 19 percent of smokers consuming cigarettes yielding 16 mg or more tar. These patterns were similar for both former smokers (as reported by the AUTS) and current smokers (as reported by the NHIS).

Persons who switched brands were more likely to smoke low-tar yield brands. For example, according to the 1986 AUTS, 22 percent of switchers smoked brands yielding 6 mg or less tar compared with 5 percent of people

Figure 7
**Percentage of current smokers who have ever switched brands,[a] by sex and age:
Ages 18 and older, United States, 1987**

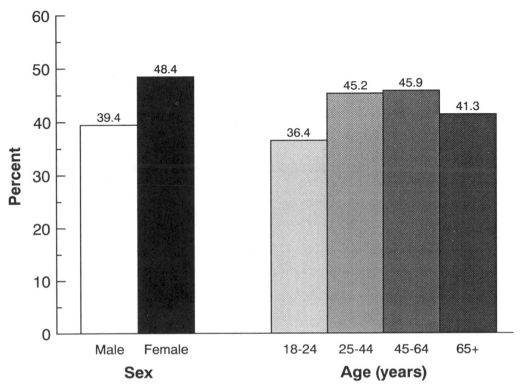

who had never switched. This suggests that many smokers switch to lower
tar brands rather than starting with those brands.

**HEALTH BELIEFS
AND SWITCHING** Survey data on health beliefs shed light on possible factors that
may drive or influence smokers' switching to lower tar cigarette
brands. The surveys indicate that current smokers of lower tar brands and
persons who had switched brands were more likely to acknowledge health
risks than those who smoked higher tar brands or who had not switched
brands. Figures 9 and 10 illustrate this relationship between tar yield of the
smoker's brand and beliefs that smoking is related to cancer and emphysema.

It is worth pointing out that the majority of smokers of high-tar
cigarettes, as well as smokers who have never switched, acknowledged the
health risks of smoking (Figure 10). However, there is an inverse gradient
for both variables.

Similarly, concerns about health risks decrease as tar yields rise (Table 1).
Among smokers who switched brands, 85 percent stated that they were

Figure 8

Percentage of current smokers who have ever switched brands,[a] by race/ethnicity and education: Ages 18 and older, United States, 1987

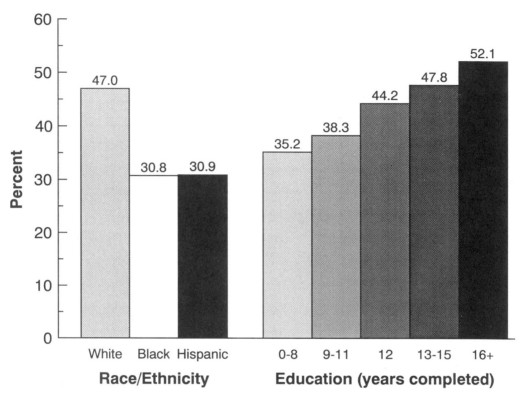

[a] To lower tar/nicotine brands to reduce their health risks.

Source: National Center for Health Statistics, 1987.

concerned about the health effects of smoking compared with 70 percent of those who had never switched. Furthermore, people in the lower tar yield categories and those who switched were more likely to respond that their health had been affected by their smoking, and they were more likely to report that a doctor had advised them to quit.

Moreover, people who smoke low-tar cigarettes and those who switched were more likely to acknowledge that some brands are more hazardous than others (Table 1). Smokers of low-tar brands were more likely to state that their brand is less hazardous compared with smokers of higher tar brands. Among switchers, 33 percent believed that their brand is less hazardous than other brands. For smokers who had never switched, only 16 percent held this belief.

In the 1993 TAPS, adolescents and young adults who smoked light and ultralight cigarettes were asked why they smoked those brands. Four reasons were most commonly cited: Thirty-three percent of respondents said that

Figure 9
Percentage of current smokers who believe that low-tar cigarettes pose reduced cancer risk, by tar yield and history of switching: Ages 18 and older, United States, 1987

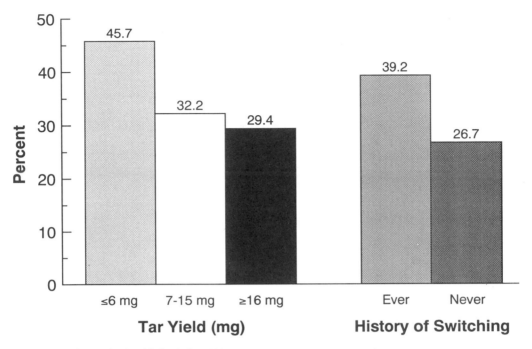

Source: *National Center for Health Statistics, 1987.*

they smoked light or ultralight cigarettes because they taste better, 29 percent said they are less irritating, 21 percent said they thought these cigarettes were healthier than other brands, and 19 percent said they "just liked them."

QUITTING SMOKING   The surveys revealed some interesting trends with regard to quitting. In the 1987 NHIS, participants were asked to identify techniques they had used in their efforts to quit smoking. Among participants who had switched brands, 38 percent said they had ever switched to lower tar and nicotine cigarette brands as a quitting strategy; 62 percent switched for other reasons (Table 2). Switchers were more likely to have tried these quitting strategies, with the exception of quitting cold turkey, than smokers who had never switched. This suggests that switchers were seeking help with quitting. In addition, those who smoked lower tar cigarettes were slightly more likely to have sought help during previous quit attempts than were persons who smoked higher tar cigarettes.

However, the data from the 1986 AUTS indicate that the prevalence of cessation increases with increasing tar yield (Figure 11). That is, ever-smokers who smoked higher tar yield brands were more likely to have quit than people who smoked lower tar brands. Respondents who had never switched were more likely to have quit smoking than switchers.

Figure 10
Percentage of current smokers who believe that cigarette smoking is related to emphysema, by tar yield[a] and history of switching[b]: Ages 18 and older, United States, 1987

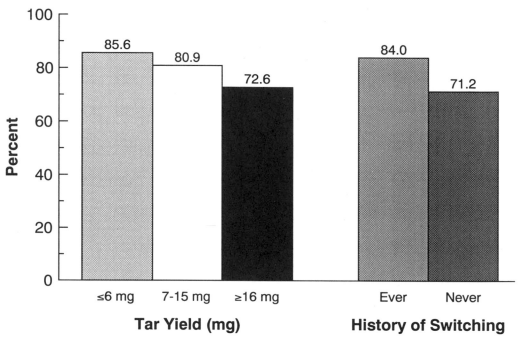

[a] *Of current brand.*
[b] *Ever switched to lower tar/nicotine brands to reduce health risks.*

Source: National Center for Health Statistics, 1987.

Table 1
Health concerns and beliefs of current smokers, by tar yield and history of switching[a], by percent: Ages 17 and older, United States, 1986

	Tar Yield (mg)			History of Switching	
	≤6	7-15	≥16	Ever	Never
Concerned About Health Effects	84	79	68	85	70
Some Brands More Hazardous Than Others	60	46	39	54	40
Their Brand Is Less Hazardous Than Others	48	26	12	33	16

[a] *Ever switched to reduce tar and nicotine.*

Source: Centers for Disease Control, 1986.

Table 2
Quit strategies ever used by current smokers, by tar yield and history of switching[a], by percent: Ages 18 and older, United States, 1987

	Tar Yield (mg)			History of Switching	
	≤6	7-15	≥16	Ever	Never
Switch to Low Tar	37	22	18	38	6
Special Filters	14	9	8	13	4
Gradual Reduction	39	34	36	42	27
Nicotine Gum	16	10	10	12	8
The Great American Smokeout	10	9	8	12	6
Cold Turkey	86	84	82	82	85
Book/Pamphlet	9	9	7	10	5
Relatives/Friends	18	18	18	20	13

[a] *Switching to lower tar and nicotine brand to reduce health risks.*

Source: National Center for Health Statistics, 1987.

Among persons who had ever been regular smokers, those who smoked low-tar cigarettes and those who switched to lower tar brands were more likely to have made a recent effort to quit smoking and relapsed and were less likely to be former smokers (data not shown). Among smokers who had never tried to quit, smokers of low-tar cigarettes and those who switched to low-tar cigarettes were more likely to have considered quitting (data not shown).

DISCUSSION   These data seem to reflect an interplay of the forces of motivation to quit and nicotine dependence (Russell, 1981). Smokers of lower tar cigarettes appear to be especially interested in quitting and are more actively seeking help than smokers of higher tar cigarettes. Perhaps when lower tar smokers were unsuccessful in their attempts to quit, they switched to a lower tar brand to allay their fears about the health consequences of continuing to smoke. The tacit health claims associated with advertisements of the lower tar brands may have allayed smokers' health concerns (Davis, 1987). Because of the cross-sectional nature of the data, however, further research on the topic is warranted.

Not all switching is a step toward quitting. Three of every five smokers who had ever switched to lower tar and nicotine brands did not do so as a quitting strategy. Both low-tar cigarette smokers and ever-switchers were more likely, compared respectively with high-tar smokers and persons who had never switched brands, to (1) acknowledge the dangers of smoking,

Figure 11
**Prevalence of cessation among ever-smokers, by tar yield and history of switching[a]:
Ages 17 and older, United States, 1986**

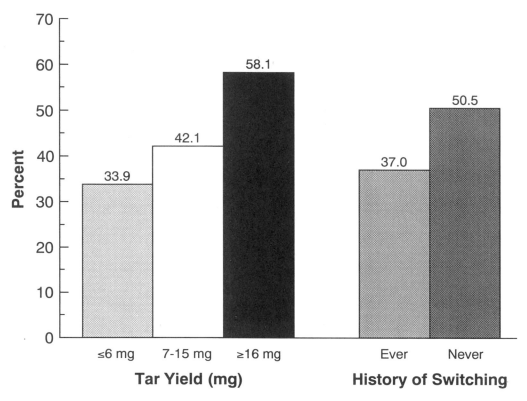

[a] *Ever switched to reduce tar/nicotine.*

Source: Centers for Disease Control, 1986.

(2) say that their health has been affected, (3) be concerned about health effects, and (4) believe that their cigarettes are safer.

The data on prevalence of cessation are especially intriguing, given that low-tar cigarette smokers and ever-switchers are better educated and it is known that persons with more years of education are less likely to be smokers and more likely to have quit (Centers for Disease Control and Prevention, 1994a; Giovino et al., 1994). These data and the Pollay (1990) observation that the tobacco industry seems to be targeting lower tar yield cigarettes toward more highly educated smokers deserve consideration. The innovation of quitting smoking, which started among persons with more education, may have been replaced by the innovation of switching to lower tar brands (Rogers, 1983; U.S. Department of Health and Human Services, 1989).

As stated by Samet (this volume), available evidence indicates that smoking lower tar cigarettes only minimally reduces smokers' health risks. The reduced prevalence of cessation among smokers who have switched brands and smokers of low-yield cigarettes, coupled with beliefs among some in the public that these cigarettes are safer, suggest that low-yield cigarettes have kept many smokers smoking who otherwise might have quit. The net effect of the introduction and mass marketing of these brands, then, may have been and may continue to be an increased number of smoking-attributable deaths.

QUESTION-AND-ANSWER SESSION

DR. SHIFFMAN: I don't know if you have these data, but I am wondering, when smokers in these surveys make a deliberate switch, do you have a sense of how big a jump they make in the FTC tar and nicotine values?

DR. GIOVINO: We have begun to look at the issue of the penultimate brand vs. the current or the last brand. The reason I can't give you a direct answer is because we looked at it as a function of whether or not they smoke more now or less now. And I will have to check this, but I think it was about .2 mg nicotine.

DR. HOFFMANN: We know now that nicotine is one major reason that people smoke or chew tobacco. Therefore, you could have classified your groupings according to nicotine, which I would have done, because that is why people smoke; it is not for the tar.

DR. GIOVINO: I think the analysis clearly could be done both ways, and I understand your reasoning. The reason that I felt comfortable with tar is because it is based on perceptions. A lot of this is based on perceptions of health risks.

My guess is that they are so highly correlated that the analysis would find very similar findings, and if the committee would like me to do that, we can certainly do that.

DR. PETITTI: This is a pretty technical question, but your last slide had a conclusion that low-tar smokers are less likely to be former smokers and switchers are less likely to be former smokers. I presume those are age adjusted?

DR. GIOVINO: We did age-specific analyses. We did not have time to do age-adjusted analyses. We used three age categories: 17 to 34 years, 35 to 64 years, and 65 plus years. For switching, the relationship held in every category; for low tar, it held in every category except the 17 to 34 category.

DR. BENOWITZ: I wonder if you have any information on smoking of the really ultralows, like 1 mg and below, because there is some evidence that the yields from those are really fundamentally different, and I will be talking about that later. But do you know anything about the characteristics of those smokers?

DR. GIOVINO: The numbers in those categories became very small. You know, at 6 mg or less, it was 10 or 12 percent. At 1 mg, the numbers would have been . . . .

DR. BENOWITZ: So, no one is smoking them.

DR. GIOVINO: Very small numbers, yes.

DR. FREEMAN: Do you have any guess or reason why young black males in particular are smoking so much less today, since it is obviously not a function of education. Do you have any sense of why that is happening?

DR. GIOVINO: What Dr. Freeman is referring to are the trends in the High School Senior data, in National Health Interview Survey data among people 18 to 24, in the National Household Survey on Drug Abuse data, the Youth Risk Behavior Survey data, the TAPS data, and others, that show that African-American youth are much less likely to smoke than white youth.

I will take 2 minutes, because it is an interesting study. It is not a school dropout effect, because when we look at dropouts, white kids who have dropped out are much more likely to smoke than African-American kids. Also, regardless of race and ethnicity, all kids who drop out are more likely to smoke.

We don't believe that it is because they have switched to other drugs. We have looked at Monitoring the Future data, and it does not look like cigarette smoking has been replaced by an increased use of alcohol and other drugs.

There are some data to suggest that differential misclassification may explain some of the difference. There was a paper by Karl Bauman in the *American Journal of Public Health* that showed that African-American youth may be a little more likely to differentially underreport in a household survey. Household surveys pose the most serious concerns about confidentiality, unless serious steps are taken to protect confidentiality.

We see lower smoking rates among blacks in school surveys, where there is greater privacy. And even in Bauman's household survey, mean validated tobacco use was three times higher in white youth than in African-American youth.

To answer your question in more detail, variables like discretionary income, parental education, importance of religion, and how well they do in school do not explain it. In other words, the trends seem to be down in African-Americans more than white youth in just about all the subcategories that we have carved out.

There are explanations, and some were presented in the 1994 Surgeon General's report: There have been changes in attitudes about smoking, and the attitudes held by African-American youth changed in a much more health-promoting direction than the attitudes among white youth. There appears to have been some sort of social climate change, such that cigarette smoking does not appear to be as socially acceptable among African-Americans; there are certainly some reports of grassroots involvement at the church and other levels.

There also appears to be a differential concern about the potential weight-controlling effects of cigarettes, with African-American youth being less obsessed with slimness than white youth.

It is a very intriguing phenomenon and one that we have examined in detail.

DR. FREEMAN: Is this reflected in the 18- to 24-year-old group?

DR. GIOVINO: The prevalence trends have definitely translated into the 18- to 24-year-old age group, and even in the 25 to 29 age group. African-Americans start smoking about a year later in life, but the differences we are seeing are not enough, and we are definitely seeing translation into the young adult population.

DR. STITZER: One more question on the youth. Your data seem to contradict the popular wisdom that youth begin with light cigarettes. I wondered if there were any data suggesting that they do play some role in initiation or original experimental use?

DR. GIOVINO: Some of that dogma, if I understand it right, is that it might have influenced young girls starting because they were less irritating, and that seems to be part of the scenario. Young girls are more likely to have used the lights or the ultralights, to the extent that the cross-sectional data can tell us exactly.

I find myself thinking this, and again, this is hypothesis generation: You see a lot more ads for regular cigarettes than you do for light cigarettes, especially if you think about Marlboros, Camels, Newports, etc. Regardless of the reason, it is possible that they start on the regulars, that the thought of quitting occurs to them, they have difficulty quitting and the thought is, "Well, I have got to do something here, so maybe I will switch." It is a hypothesis.

DR. KOZLOWSKI: A number of years ago, Fred Silverstein, Scott Feldon, and I published a paper in the *Journal of Health and Social Behavior* on the role of low-yield cigarettes and the recruitment to smoking, particularly in women, we found, in a school sample.

And you have to think that there were some young women who were particularly sensitive to the effects of smoking. Not all were. In other words, a small percentage of the market were under great social pressure to take up smoking, and the low-yield cigarette, smoked without vent blocking and so on, provided a nice trial-sized dose. So, it helped some people, but it was not across the board.

REFERENCES

Anonymous. Health claims made for filter cigarettes. *New York State Journal of Medicine* 85(7): 317, 1985.

Anonymous. Vantage is changing a lot of my feelings about smoking. *Time Magazine*, November 7, 1977. pp. 86-87.

Centers for Disease Control and Prevention. Adult Use of Tobacco Survey. Public use data tape, 1986.

Centers for Disease Control and Prevention. Teenage Attitudes and Practices Survey. Public use data tape, 1993.

Centers for Disease Control and Prevention. Cigarette smoking among adults—United States, 1993. *MMWR. Morbidity and Mortality Weekly Report* 43: 925-930, 1994a.

Centers for Disease Control and Prevention. Changes in cigarette brand preferences of adolescent smokers—United States, 1989-1993. *MMWR. Morbidity and Mortality Weekly Report* 43: 577-581, 1994b.

Davis, R.M. Current trends in cigarette advertising and marketing. *New England Journal of Medicine* 316: 725-732, 1987.

Davis, R.M., Healy, P., Hawk, S.A. Information on tar and nicotine yields on cigarette packages. *American Journal of Public Health* 80: 551-553, 1990.

Doll, R., Hill, A.B. Smoking and carcinoma of the lung. *British Medical Journal* 2: 740-748, 1950.

Doll, R., Hill, A.B. A study of the aetiology of carcinoma of the lung. *British Medical Journal* 2: 1271-1286, 1952.

Federal Trade Commission. *"Tar," Nicotine and Carbon Monoxide of the Smoke of 207 Varieties of Domestic Cigarettes*. Washington, DC: Federal Trade Commission, 1985.

Federal Trade Commission. *Federal Trade Commission Report to Congress for 1992*. Washington, DC: Federal Trade Commission, 1994.

Gallup International Institute. *Teen-age Attitudes and Behavior Concerning Tobacco. Report of the Focus Groups*. Princeton, NJ: The George H. Gallup International Institute, 1992.

Gallup Organization, Inc. *The Public's Attitudes Toward Cigarette Advertising and Cigarette Tax Increase*. Princeton, NJ: The Gallup Organization, Inc., 1993, pp. 22-24.

Giovino, G.A., Schooley, M.W., Zhu, B.P., Chrisman, J.H., Tomar, S.L., Peddicord, J.P., Merritt, R.K., Husten, C.G., Eriksen, M.P. Surveillance for selected tobacco-use behaviors—United States, 1900-1994. *MMWR. Morbidity and Mortality Weekly Report* 43(3): 1-43, 1994.

Harris, J.A. *Working Model for Predicting the Consumption and Revenue Impacts of Large Increases in the U.S. Federal Cigarette Excise Tax*. Working paper no. 4803. Cambridge, MA: National Bureau of Economic Research, 1994.

Levin, M.L., Goldstein, H., Gerhardt, P.R. Cancer and tobacco smoking: A preliminary report. *Journal of the American Medical Association* 143: 336-338, 1950.

Miller, R. U.S. cigarette consumption, 1900 to date. In: *Tobacco Yearbook*, W. Harr (Editor). Bowling Green, KY: Cockrel Corporation, 1981, p. 53.

National Center for Health Statistics. National Health Interview Survey Cancer Control Supplement. Public use data tape, 1987.

Norr, R. Cancer by the carton. *Reader's Digest* December: 7-8, 1952.

Pierce, J.P., Hatziandreu, E.H., Flyer, P., Hull, J., Maklan, D., Morganstein, D., Schreiber, G. *Report of the 1986 Adult Use of Tobacco Survey*. OM 90-2004. Rockville, MD: U.S. Department of Health and Human Services, Public Health Service, Centers for Disease Control, Office on Smoking and Health, 1990.

Pillsbury, H.C., Bright, C.C., O'Connor, K.J., Irish, F.W. Tar and nicotine in cigarette smoke. *Journal of Official Analytical Chemists* 52: 458-462, 1969.

Pollay, R.W. "The Functions and Management of Cigarette Advertising." Unpublished manuscript, University of British Columbia, 1990. 20 pp.

Rogers, E.M. (Editor). *Diffusion of Innovations*. New York: Free Press, 1983.

Russell, M.A. Dependence and motivation to stop smoking. In: *Smoking and Arterial Disease*, R.M. Greenhalgh (Editor). Bath, United Kingdom: Pitman Medical, 1981, pp. 285-288

Schoenborn, C.A., Boyd, G. *Smoking and Other Tobacco Use: United States, 1987*. Vital and Health Statistics. Series 10: Data From the National Health Interview Survey (No. 169). DHHS Publication No. (PHS) 89-1597. Rockville, MD: U.S. Department of Health and Human Services, Public Health Service, Centers for Disease Control, National Center for Health Statistics, 1989.

Slade, J. The tobacco epidemic: Lessons from history. *Journal of Psychoactive Drugs* 21: 281-291, 1989.

U.S. Department of Agriculture. *Tobacco Situation*. TS 99. Washington, DC: U.S. Department of Agriculture, Economic Research Service, 1962.

U.S. Department of Agriculture. *Tobacco Situation and Outlook Report*. TS 200. Washington, DC: U.S. Department of Agriculture, Commodity Economics Division, Economic Research Service, 1987.

U.S. Department of Agriculture. *Tobacco Situation and Outlook Report*. TS 226. Washington, DC: U.S. Department of Agriculture, Commodity Economics Division, Economic Research Service, 1994.

U.S. Department of Health and Human Services. *The Health Consequences of Smoking for Women. A Report of the Surgeon General*. Rockville, MD: U.S. Department of Health and Human Services, Public Health Service, Office of the Assistant Secretary for Health, Office on Smoking and Health, 1980.

U.S. Department of Health and Human Services. *The Health Consequences of Smoking: Nicotine Addiction. A Report of the Surgeon General, 1988*. DHHS Publication No. (CDC) 88-8406. Rockville, MD: U.S. Department of Health and Human Services, Public Health Service, Centers for Disease Control, Center for Health Promotion and Education, Office on Smoking and Health, 1988.

U.S. Department of Health and Human Services. *Reducing the Health Consequences of Smoking: 25 Years of Progress. A Report of the Surgeon General, 1989*. DHHS Publication No. (CDC) 89-8411. Rockville, MD: U.S. Department of Health and Human Services, Public Health Service, Centers for Disease Control, Center for Chronic Disease Prevention and Health Promotion, Office on Smoking and Health, 1989.

U.S. Department of Health, Education, and Welfare. *Smoking and Health: A Report of the Advisory Committee to the Surgeon General of the Public Health Service*. PHS Publication No. 1103. Rockville, MD: U.S. Department of Health, Education, and Welfare, Public Health Service, 1964.

Warner, K.E. Tobacco industry response to public health concern: A content analysis of cigarette ads. *Health Education Quarterly* 12: 115-127, 1985.

Wynder, E.L., Graham, E.A. Tobacco smoking as a possible etiological factor in bronchogenic carcinoma. A study of six hundred and eighty-four proved cases. *Journal of the American Medical Association* 143: 329-336, 1950.

Cigarette Smoke Components and Disease: Cigarette Smoke Is More Than a Triad of Tar, Nicotine, and Carbon Monoxide

Jeffrey E. Harris

INTRODUCTION   Cigarette smoke is a complex mixture of chemicals. Some smoke components, such as carbon monoxide (CO), hydrogen cyanide (HCN), and nitrogen oxides, are gases. Others, such as formaldehyde, acrolein, benzene, and certain N-nitrosamines, are volatile chemicals contained in the liquid-vapor portion of the smoke aerosol. Still others, such as nicotine, phenol, polyaromatic hydrocarbons (PAHs), and certain tobacco-specific nitrosamines (TSNAs), are contained in the submicron-sized solid particles that are suspended in cigarette smoke.

In view of this chemical complexity, cigarette smoke has multiple, highly diverse effects on human health. It is not unexpected that multiple chemicals in cigarette smoke can contribute to any single adverse health effect.

Thus, HCN may affect the human respiratory system by its toxic effects on the cilia that line the respiratory tract. At the same time, HCN may cross the placenta and have toxic effects on the growing fetus. In addition, HCN also may cause nerve damage in cigarette smokers with optic neuropathy (Costagliola et al., 1989). Although the PAHs and TSNAs in the particulate phase of cigarette smoke are known carcinogens, catechols and phenols in the particulate phase also are considered carcinogens or tumor promoters. Benzene and formaldehyde in the liquid-vapor portion of the smoke also may be carcinogenic.

Aside from specific chemical constituents, certain physical-chemical properties of smoke may participate in disease processes. Thus, the pH of the smoke may affect the site and degree of nicotine absorption as well as the smoker's depth of inhalation. The oxidation-reduction state of the smoke can be important because oxidants influence the maturing of cholesterol-laden plaques in the coronary arteries and other blood vessels. In short, cigarette smoke is far more than a triad of tar, nicotine, and carbon monoxide. This fact needs to be considered carefully in any discussion of the adequacy of current cigarette testing methods or current cigarette labeling practices.

MAINSTREAM VS. SIDESTREAM CIGARETTE SMOKE   Both smokers and nonsmokers can incur adverse health effects from the smoke of burning cigarettes. Smokers inhale mostly mainstream (MS) smoke, which is drawn through the burning tobacco column and filter tip and exits through the mouthpiece of the cigarette. Nonsmokers inhale mostly sidestream (SS) smoke, which is emitted into the surrounding air between puffs from the end of the smoldering cigarette. Sidestream smoke is the major source of environmental tobacco smoke (ETS).

Although SS and MS smoke have qualitatively similar chemical compositions, the respective quantities of individual smoke constituents can be quite different (U.S. Department of Health and Human Services, 1987 and 1989). For example, in studies of nonfilter cigarettes smoked by machines, the yield of CO in undiluted SS smoke was 2.5- to 4.7-fold that of MS smoke, whereas the corresponding SS/MS ratio for N-nitrosodimethylamine (NDMA), an animal carcinogen, was 0.2 (U.S. Department of Health and Human Services, 1989). In one compilation of toxic and tumorigenic agents in cigarette smoke, the SS/MS ratio ranged from 0.03 to 130 (Hoffmann and Hecht, 1990). In another study, the concentration of the carcinogen 4-aminobiphenyl in undiluted SS smoke was 32-fold that of MS smoke. The SS smoke from so-called reduced-yield cigarettes does not necessarily have reduced emissions of toxic and carcinogenic chemicals (Adams et al., 1987; Rando et al., 1992).

Whereas exposure to SS smoke depends on the distance from the burning cigarette and conditions of ventilation, the higher concentrations of certain toxic and carcinogenic chemicals in SS smoke result in measurable levels of these chemicals in nonsmokers exposed to ETS. For example, nonsmokers exposed to relatively high concentrations of SS smoke have detectable urinary levels of the metabolites of the tobacco-specific nitrosamine 4-(methylnitrosamine)-1-(3-pyridil)-1-butanone (NNK) (Hecht et al., 1993). Young children exposed to ETS via their smoking mothers have detectable levels of PAH-albumin adducts in their blood (Crawford et al., 1994).

Exposures to specific chemical agents in ETS can in turn produce pathological effects in humans and in animal models. The CO in SS smoke reduces the blood's ability to deliver oxygen to the heart, an effect that is especially important in patients with coronary heart disease (CHD) (Sheps et al., 1990). Secondhand cigarette smoke activates blood platelets, which in turn play a role in the development of atherosclerotic plaques in CHD (Glantz and Parmley, 1995).

The remainder of this chapter focuses on the chemical components of MS smoke and their health effects on cigarette smokers; however, the components of SS smoke and their health effects on nonsmokers cannot be ignored.

MAJOR HEALTH EFFECTS OF CIGARETTE SMOKE

The major health effects of cigarette smoke include:
- cancer;
- noncancerous lung diseases;
- atherosclerotic diseases of the heart and blood vessels; and
- toxicity to the human reproductive system.

Other health effects of cigarette smoke, such as retardation of healing of peptic ulcers and interaction with certain therapeutic drugs, are not considered in detail here.

The epidemiologic evidence on the degree (if any) to which filter-tipped and low-tar cigarettes have reduced the risks of smoking-related diseases are reviewed by Samet (this volume).

The psychoactive drug in cigarette smoke is nicotine. Cigarette smoking is a highly controlled form of self-administration of this drug. Nicotine use is self-reinforcing. Attempts to stop smoking lead to craving, withdrawal symptoms, and high rates of relapse (U.S. Department of Health and Human Services, 1988; Harris, 1993). The psychoactive effects of nicotine are discussed in detail in chapters by Benowitz (this volume) and Henningfield and Schuh (this volume).

CANCER   Cigarette smoking causes cancers of the lung, esophagus, larynx, oral cavity, bladder, and pancreas in male and female smokers. In fact, cigarette smoking is the major cause of lung cancer in the United States, accounting for 90 percent of cases in men and 79 percent in women (U.S. Department of Health and Human Services, 1989). Smoking is also reported to increase the risks of cancers of the kidney, liver, anus, penis, and uterine cervix as well as several forms of acute leukemia (Garfinkel and Bofetta, 1990; U.S. Department of Health and Human Services, 1982, 1989, and 1990).

Numerous epidemiological studies covering the experience of millions of men and women over many years show that smokers' risks of developing cancer increase with the number of cigarettes smoked daily, the lifetime duration of smoking, and early age of starting smoking. Smoking cessation gradually reduces cancer risk, although a persistent excess risk has been observed even two decades after cessation (U.S. Department of Health and Human Services, 1989 and 1990). Cigarette smoke interacts with other causative agents, including alcohol, asbestos, radon daughters, certain viruses, and certain workplace exposures, in the development of human cancers (U.S. Department of Health and Human Services, 1982, 1989, and 1990).

Condensates collected from cigarette smoke cause mutations and damage to DNA (deoxyribonucleic acid) in laboratory assays of mutagenesis (Gairola, 1982) as well as malignant transformation (in laboratory tests) of a chemical's ability to induce malignant changes in mammalian cells. The most widely used experimental system is the mouse skin bioassay, in which cancers are induced by the repeated application of condensates of cigarette smoke to the shaved skins of mice.

Humans naturally puff on cigarettes. The puffed smoke, in a volume of about 30 to 70 mL, is temporarily retained in the smoker's mouth, after which it may be inhaled deeply into the lungs. By contrast, some laboratory animals breath by panting, and others are obligate nose breathers. Even with installation of smoke through artificial airways, it can be quite difficult to get the animals to inhale deeply, as human smokers do. Accordingly, the distribution and retention of smoke components in the respiratory systems of laboratory animals may not mimic natural human smoking. Nevertheless, long-term smoke inhalation regularly induces tumors of the larynx in Syrian golden hamsters. Direct installation of cigarette tar into the airways of laboratory animals causes lung cancers (Hoffmann and Hecht, 1990; U.S. Department of Health and Human Services, 1982).

MS cigarette smoke contains more than three dozen distinct chemical species considered to be tumorigenic in humans or animals (Hoffmann and Hecht, 1990; U.S. Department of Health and Human Services, 1982 and 1989). Among the most prominent are PAHs such as benzo(a)pyrene (BaP); aza-arenes such as dibenzo-acridine; N-nitrosamines such as NDMA; aromatic amines such as 4-aminobiphenyl; aldehydes such as formaldehyde; other organics such as benzene; and certain inorganic compounds such as arsenic, nickel, and chromium. Some of these chemicals alone are capable of initiating tumors in laboratory animals; others can promote the development of previously initiated cancers. Still others indicate direct human epidemiological evidence of carcinogenicity.

Certain chemical components of smoke may contribute to specific cancers. For example, TSNAs may contribute to cancers of the lung, larynx, esophagus, and pancreas, whereas 4-aminobiphenyl and certain aryl amines may contribute to cancer of the bladder (Vineis, 1991). Benzene in cigarette smoke may play a role in smoking-induced leukemia (Melikian et al., 1993).

NONCANCEROUS LUNG DISEASES Cigarette smoking is the main cause of chronic obstructive lung disease (COLD), also called chronic obstructive pulmonary disease (U.S. Department of Health and Human Services, 1984a). Smoking accounts for 84 percent of COLD deaths in men and 79 percent in women (U.S. Department of Health and Human Services, 1989).

COLD is a slowly progressive illness that develops after repeated insults to the lung over many years. In the early years after starting to smoke, an individual may report no symptoms. However, even at this early stage breathing tests can often detect abnormalities in the small terminal airways of the lung (Beck et al., 1981; Seely et al., 1971; U.S. Department of Health and Human Services, 1984a), and these abnormalities have been directly observed in autopsy studies of young smokers who died suddenly (Niewoehner et al., 1974). For smokers in their twenties, there is already a dose-response relationship between the extent of abnormal lung tests and the number of cigarettes smoked daily. In random population surveys, from 17 to 60 percent of adult smokers younger than age 55 have detectable small airway dysfunction (U.S. Department of Health and Human Services, 1984a).

Over the course of an individual's two decades or more of smoking, a constellation of chronic respiratory changes develops. These chronic lung injuries include (1) mucus hypersecretion with chronic cough and phlegm; (2) airway thickening and narrowing, resulting in obstruction to airflow during expiration; and (3) emphysema, that is, abnormal dilation of the air spaces at the end of the respiratory tree, with destruction of the walls lining the air sacs, resulting in further airflow obstruction. These changes can cause significant respiratory impairment, disability, and death. Although individual patients vary in the relative contribution of these three changes, those with clinically severe COLD typically have all three.

Although a minority of cigarette smokers will develop clinically severe COLD, some chronic deterioration in lung structure or function is demonstrable in most long-term smokers (U.S. Department of Health and Human Services, 1984a). Some smokers show more chronic cough and phlegm, others more airway obstruction. In general, breathing function declines with the increase in a person's cumulative exposure to smoke, measured in pack-years (Dockery et al., 1988).

Cigarette smoke produces pathological changes in the lungs of smokers by a number of different mechanisms (U.S. Department of Health and Human Services, 1990). Cigarette smoke is toxic to the cilia that line the central breathing passages. These cilia, in combination with mucus secretions, defend against deep inhalation of foreign material (U.S. Department of Health and Human Services, 1984a). Smoking also induces many abnormalities in the inflammatory and immune systems within the lung (U.S. Department of Health and Human Services, 1985). In particular, cigarette smoke causes inflammatory cells to produce an enzyme called elastase, which in turn breaks down elastin, an important protein that lines the elastic walls of the air sacs (Fera et al. 1986; U.S. Department of Health and Human Services, 1984a). Moreover, oxidants present in cigarette smoke can inactivate a separate protective enzyme called alpha$_1$-antitrypsin, which inhibits the destructive action of elastase (Janoff, 1985; U.S. Department of Health and Human Services, 1984a).

Many organic and inorganic chemicals in the gaseous, volatile, and particulate phases of cigarette smoke appear to contribute to smoke's toxicity to the respiratory system, including hydrocarbons, aldehydes, ketones, organic acids, phenols, cyanides, acrolein, and nitrogen oxides. Some components contribute to the development of chronic mucus hypersecretion in the central airways, whereas others play a greater role in the production of small airway abnormalities and emphysematous injury to the peripheral air sacs. Oxidizing agents in smoke inhibit the enzymes that defend against the destruction of lung elastin (U.S. Department of Health and Human Services, 1984a).

ATHEROSCLEROTIC CARDIOVASCULAR DISEASES   Cigarette smoking is a major contributing cause to CHD, stroke, and other atherosclerotic diseases of the circulatory system (U.S. Department of Health and Human Services, 1984b and 1989).

Atherosclerosis is a chronic disease that can affect the arterial blood vessels in virtually every part of the human body. The most important form of atherosclerosis in the United States is coronary atherosclerosis. Its manifestations, which include angina, heart attack, heart failure, and sudden death, are described by the inclusive term coronary heart disease. Atherosclerosis involving the arteries supplying the brain is a form of cerebrovascular disease. Atherosclerosis involving the arteries to the limbs is called peripheral vascular disease (PVD).

In numerous epidemiologic studies of millions of people, cigarette smokers have been found to have higher rates of heart attack, sudden death, and other manifestations of CHD. They also have higher rates of stroke, PVD, and other atherosclerotic lesions (U.S. Department of Health and Human Services, 1984b and 1989; U.S. Department of Health, Education, and Welfare, 1979). In the Cancer Prevention Study II (CPS-II) of more than 1 million people followed from 1982 through 1986, men currently smoking had a 94-percent greater risk of CHD than lifelong nonsmokers, whereas women currently smoking had a 78-percent greater risk. In smokers younger than age 65, men had a 181-percent greater risk and women a 200-percent greater risk (U.S. Department of Health and Human Services, 1989).

Cigarette smoking is sometimes called an independent risk factor for CHD because smokers' CHD rates are found to be higher even when other risk factors such as gender, blood pressure, and cholesterol level are taken into account. It is sometimes called a modifiable risk factor because one can reduce or stop smoking. Although smoking obviously cannot be a cause of CHD in someone who never smoked, it can be an important contributor to CHD in a smoker. Among 548,000 deaths from CHD in the United States in 1985, an estimated 115,000 would not have occurred but for the presence of cigarette smoking (U.S. Department of Health and Human Services, 1989).

Cigarette smoke appears to enhance the atherosclerotic process by several different mechanisms (U.S. Department of Health and Human Services, 1990; Glantz and Parmley, 1995). Cigarette smoking affects cholesterol metabolism. Smokers repeatedly have been observed to have lower levels of the protective high-density lipoprotein (HDL) cholesterol (Willett et al., 1983), and smoking cessation raises HDL cholesterol (Rabkin, 1984). In animal models, cigarette smoke can damage the inner lining of blood vessels, thus enhancing the transfer of low-density lipoprotein (LDL) cholesterol particles across the arterial wall and into the developing cholesterol-laden plaque (Krupski et al., 1987; Zimmerman and McGeachie, 1987; Penn et al., 1994). Cigarette smoking also can affect the blood clotting system, including the adherence of blood platelets to the lining of arterial blood vessels (Pittilo et al., 1984; U.S. Department of Health and Human Services, 1984b; Burghuber et al., 1986) and the formation of blood clots that block a narrowed artery. Acrolein in cigarette smoke may be partly responsible for its platelet-adhering effects (Selley et al., 1990). Cigarette smoke also can cause spasm of the coronary arteries.

Many chemical components of cigarette smoke have been implicated in the development of atherosclerotic disease. Nicotine, the major psychoactive component of smoke, causes powerful changes in heart rate and blood circulation. Nicotine appears to cause injury to the arterial lining (Krupski et al., 1987). Carbon monoxide in cigarette smoke binds to the hemoglobin in red blood cells, thereby reducing the oxygen-carrying capacity of the blood (Sheps et al., 1990). PAHs, such as 7,12-dimethylbenz(*a,h*)anthracene and

BaP, have been found to accelerate the development of atherosclerosis in animal models; this suggests that cell injury and cell proliferation (or hyperplasia) may contribute to the development of the growing plaque (Glantz and Parmley, 1991). Hydrogen cyanide, nitrogen oxides, and chemical components of cigarette tar also have been implicated. Free radicals in cigarette smoke, which are highly reactive oxygen products, are damaging to the heart muscle cells (Church and Pryor, 1985).

CIGARETTE SMOKING AND HUMAN REPRODUCTION   Cigarette smoking adversely affects sexual and reproductive function in women in a number of different ways. Cigarette smoking appears to impair female fertility (Baird and Wilcox, 1985; Daling et al., 1987; Mattison, 1982; U.S. Department of Health and Human Services, 1980). Among the possible mechanisms are direct toxicity to eggs, interference with motility in the female reproductive tract, and alterations in immunity that predispose female smokers to infections that block the Fallopian tubes (Chow et al., 1988).

Maternal cigarette smoking has serious adverse effects on the outcome of pregnancy. These include retarded fetal growth; low birth weight; spontaneous abortion; certain complications of pregnancy, labor, and delivery, such as bleeding during pregnancy and prolonged premature rupture of membranes; and infant death (U.S. Department of Health and Human Services, 1980, 1989, and 1990; U.S. Department of Health, Education, and Welfare, 1979). Direct nicotine toxicity has been suggested as a mechanism for spontaneous abortion (U.S. Department of Health and Human Services, 1990). Although a smoking-induced reduction in maternal weight gain contributes to fetal growth retardation (U.S. Department of Health and Human Services, 1980; Werler et al., 1985), the evidence points to oxygen starvation of the fetus and placenta as important factors. Carbon monoxide in cigarette smoke can cross the placenta and bind to the hemoglobin in fetal blood. Smoking causes constriction of the umbilical arteries, impairing placental blood flow. Nicotine, which also crosses the placenta, can have a number of toxic effects on the fetus (U.S. Department of Health and Human Services, 1980). The carcinogen 4-aminobiphenyl crosses the placenta in a mother who smokes and adducts with the hemoglobin in the fetus' blood (Coghlin et al., 1991). Cyanide, another component of cigarette smoke, also has been implicated.

Women currently smoking enter nonsurgical menopause about 1 to 2 years earlier than nonsmokers (U.S. Department of Health and Human Services, 1990). Heavy smokers experience an even earlier menopause than light smokers. This effect has important consequences for women's health, because the rates of osteoporosis and atherosclerotic cardiovascular diseases increase after menopause. One proposed mechanism for early menopause is that PAHs in smoke are directly toxic to ovarian follicles (Mattison, 1980).

Cigarette smoking also may affect male reproductive performance. In several studies, men who report impotence (i.e., the inability to maintain an erection sufficient for intercourse) were more likely to be cigarette smokers. This association between smoking and impotence is particularly common among men who have high blood pressure or diabetes and appears to be a consequence of increased atherosclerotic disease in the blood vessels supplying the genitalia rather than an effect on sexual drive.

ABSOLUTE RISK VS. RELATIVE RISK   Human epidemiology can be used to estimate quantitatively the risk of specific diseases to human smokers. For example, in the CPS-II study of smoking practices and mortality rates among 1.2 million U.S. adults followed from 1982 through 1986, about 0.8 percent of current male smokers ages 65 or older died of lung cancer each year (U.S. Department of Health and Human Services, 1989), whereas the comparable annual lung cancer death rate was about 0.04 percent among men ages 65 or older who never smoked. These quantitative risk estimates are often termed "absolute risks." That the continuing smokers' risk of lung cancer was twentyfold that of nonsmokers is an expression of "relative risk."

Estimating relative risks from analyses of chemical composition of different cigarettes is far more complicated. For example, the smoke from cigarette A might contain 0.05 mg of BaP, a known carcinogen, whereas the smoke from cigarette B might contain 0.02 mg of BaP. To estimate human lung cancer risks from these data alone would require a number of assumptions relating the dose of BaP to the incidence lung cancer in humans. Whereas cigarette A had 2.5-fold as much BaP as cigarette B, it cannot be concluded automatically that the relative risk of getting lung cancer for those smoking cigarette A is 2.5-fold greater than those smoking cigarette B. The relative concentrations of benz(*a*)anthracene, another carcinogen in the PAH group, might be higher or lower.

Toxicity studies in nonhuman species also can give estimates of relative risk, but applying these estimates directly to humans requires caution. The fact that the smoke from cigarette C might produce twice as many revertants as cigarette D in a particular strain of the Ames salmonella assay is an indicator that C contains higher concentrations of certain mutagens. Likewise, if cigarette E produced three times as many tumors as cigarette F in a mouse skin carcinogenesis assay, we can conclude that cigarette E contains higher concentrations of certain carcinogens, including tumor initiators and tumor promotors (DuMouchel and Harris, 1983).

TAR, NICOTINE, CARBON MONOXIDE, AND OTHER SMOKE CONSTITUENTS   Some studies (e.g., Adams et al., 1987) suggest that the yields of most toxic agents in cigarette smoke are correlated with their tar, nicotine, and CO deliveries. Still other studies show the correlation to be weak at best. Kaiserman and Rickert (1992) found a 0.89 correlation between the declared tar level and the BaP delivery of 35 brands of Canadian cigarettes. However, for 16-mg tar brands, the measured BaP ranged from 15 to 28 ng per cigarette. Fischer and colleagues (1991) found no correlation between tar delivery and the concentration of certain TSNAs in 170 European cigarettes.

The lack of a perfect correlation between tar values and specific chemical yields is not simply an artifact of measurement error. As Hoffmann and colleagues (this volume) report, there are many alternative methods to reduce cigarette smoke constituents, including various filter designs, changes in paper porosity, mixing of tobacco species, and the use of reconstituted tobacco sheets and expanded tobacco. However, all these methods do not reduce every smoke constituent uniformly. For example, perforated filter tips selectively reduce the volatile and gaseous components of cigarette smoke, whereas reconstituted tobacco sheets reduce BaP and tar but not acrolein or acetaldehyde. Likewise, as reported by Hoffmann and coworkers (this volume), the increased burley tobacco content (and with it, the nitrate content) of at least one marketed cigarette resulted in an increase in the delivery of NNK, a tobacco-specific nitrosamine, over the course of three decades.

In a study of cigarette brands sold in the United Kingdom from 1983 through 1990, Phillips and Waller (1991, p. 469) concluded that, "with the exception of nitrogen monoxide, which is strongly dependent upon the type of tobacco, and the delivery of some phenols and PAHs, which may be affected to a minor extent by the design of cigarette," the three routinely monitored smoke components (tar, nicotine, and CO) provided "an adequate guide" to the yields of the other chemical entities examined. However, as the foregoing review of cigarette smoke constituents and disease suggests, the exceptions may prove the rule. It would be unscientific to claim that the absolute human risk or even the relative risk of a particular brand of cigarettes is lower merely because, on average, everything but TSNAs, phenols, and PAHs seems to be lower. With phenols and related flavorant compounds implicated in smoke-induced chromosomal damage (Jansson et al., 1988), it would seem that, at minimum, biological testing would be warranted.

As discussed elsewhere in this volume, the yields of nicotine and carbon monoxide are significantly influenced by the smoker's style or "topography" of smoking, including number of puffs, interval between puffs, velocity and volume of each puff, depth of draw, length of cigarette smoked, depth of inhalation into the lungs, and other factors. It is possible that these differences in smoking topography might selectively influence the yields of some smoke chemicals more than others. Fischer and colleagues (1989) found that TSNA yields depended on the total volume of smoke inhaled by the smoker and that total smoke volume was increased for smokers of low- and medium-tar cigarettes. Studies of smokers' exposure to specific carcinogenic compounds (e.g., by measurement of PAH adducts to DNA) do not always show a relationship between exposure and self-reported smoking intensity (Santella et al., 1992).

SMOKE CONSTITUENTS, CIGARETTE-RELATED DISEASE, AND MODIFIED LABELING OF CIGARETTES

Henningfield and colleagues (1994) recently proposed modified labeling of cigarettes. Their proposed new new cigarette label included a warning statement; categorization of nicotine yield; nicotine content; tar, nicotine, and CO deliveries (average and maximal); harmful additives; and information about factors affecting nicotine delivery. The use of a nicotine-yield category was intended to replace such marketing terms as "light" and "ultralight." These authors noted, "An additional strategy that could be used to assist consumers in making informed decisions would be to fully disclose the tobacco smoke constituents of potential health significance, analogous to harmful constituent disclosure of foods" (Henningfield et al., 1994, pp. 312-313).

The new nutritional labels mandated by the Food and Drug Administration (FDA) on all packaged foods contain information on a wide array of vitamins, minerals, cholesterol, total fat, and saturated fat. These labels reflect the product's characteristics. They make no pretense that any two individuals will eat breakfast cereal in the same way. Nor do they imply that each and every consumer will understand or want to understand each and every entry on the label.

In the same way, the author has designed a "mock" cigarette label (Figure 1) to indicate what such an FDA-style label for cigarettes might look like. This is a sample and is not intended to reflect any current brand on the market. The opening box gives an explanation as well as a warning about the ways in which a smoker can obtain higher yields by changing his or her style of smoking. Then some "basic cigarette facts" would be included, such as length, type of filter, and weight of tobacco. In addition to data on the range of yields of tar (total particulates less nicotine) and nicotine, the label would show the range of yields of important smoke chemicals.

The concept of full disclosure of cigarette characteristics is entirely consistent with the current Federal Trade Commission (FTC) method. In fact, the current FTC measurements of tar, nicotine, and CO are included in the proposed mock label. In addition, as we move to an era where both short- and long-term biological testing have become commonplace in industry, one might imagine a rating system based on the Ames test, skin painting, and other studies. Illustrative results for such biological testing are included in the mock label.

One might object that such detailed disclosure of cigarette characteristics will confuse the smoker. Such an assertion is unscientific and unfair. To publish a label that discloses, for example, the tobacco-specific nitrosamine contents of a particular brand of cigarettes is no more confusing or complicated than printing a label that discloses the riboflavin and potassium yields of a particular brand of breakfast cereal. It would be remarkable to discover cereal manufacturers or consumer advocates arguing that the vitamin contents or trace metal levels of cereals should be withheld from consumers because vitamin E and zinc levels might correlate—at least roughly—with dietary fiber contents.

To a limited degree, researchers have studied consumers' responses to advertised tar and nicotine ratings of cigarettes. But there are no data—at least in the public domain—on the possible effects of providing consumers with additional cigarette-specific information of the type considered in the mock label.

Figure 1
"Mock" cigarette label

Our tar/nicotine label has changed! The Food and Drug Administration now requires each pack of HARRIS *Ultras* to display the deliveries of the most important chemicals in your cigarette smoke. Your own smoke intake of these chemicals may vary from low to high depending on the size of your puffs, the number of puffs per minute, the depth of your draw, and how far you smoke your cigarette down to the filter overwrap. For a factsheet about the new cigarette label, write to: New Cigarette Label Factsheet, P.O. Box 7551, Brookline, MA 02146.

Basic Cigarette Facts

Cigarette Length	100 mm
Cigarette Diameter	8 mm
Length of Filter Plus Plugwrap	20 mm
Total Cigarette Weight	1.20 gm
Tobacco Weight	0.90 gm
Type of Filter	Cellulose Acetate
Design of Filter	Perforated
U.S.-Grown Tobacco	55%
Cigarettes Per Pack	20

Delivery Per Cigarette	**Low**	**High**
Nicotine	1.0 mg	1.5 mg
Carbon Monoxide	14 mg	20 mg
Carcinogenic PAHs	0.1 µg	0.2 µg
Tobacco-Specific Nitrosamines	0.3 µg	2.0 µg
Hydrogen Cyanide	0.4 mg	0.6 mg
Acrolein	60 µg	140 µg
Formaldehyde	20 µg	100 µg
Nitrogen Oxides	0.1 mg	0.4 mg
Catechols	200 µg	400 µg
Phenols	45 µg	60 µg
Nickel	0.1 µg	0.2 µg
Total Particulates Less Nicotine	6 mg	16 mg
Redox Potential of Smoke	160 mV	240 mV
pH of Whole Smoke	5.8	6.0

Biological Test Results

Ames Salmonella	+
Tracheal Installation	++
Mammalian Cell Transformation	+
Syrian Golden Hamster Inhalation	+
Mouse Skin Carcinogenesis	++
Antielastase Test	++++

INGREDIENTS: Domestic flue-cured, Burley, and oriental leaf tobaccos; flavorants (including menthol in HARRIS ULTRAGREENS), and humectants, including diethylene glycol. Citric acid added to cigarette paper. Residues of maleic hydrazide (a suckercide used in tobacco growing) less than 1 part per million.

WARNING: Keep out of reach of children!

Key: PAHs = polyaromatic hydrocarbons.

In any case, smokers constitute only the demand side of the cigarette market. On the supply side are a handful of cigarette manufacturers who, so far as is known, go to considerable lengths to determine the detailed characteristics of competitors' products. From time to time, a cigarette manufacturer will disclose the level of a particular chemical in a particular brand. One classic example is the claim by one manufacturer, in the early 1960's, that a particular brand delivered smoke with reduced phenol, an announcement that coincided with scientific reports that the phenol in cigarette smoke inhibited the cilia lining in the respiratory tract. However, without systematic and complete disclosure requirements, such "competition" will remain haphazard at best. In 1989 the tar content was listed on only 14 percent and the nicotine content on only 11 percent of U.S. cigarette packages (Davis et al., 1990).

Enhanced and complete disclosure of cigarette characteristics by a standardized label would create a basis for more effective competition among manufacturers. If Hoffmann and colleagues' (this volume) data are generalizable, then the growing trend toward use of burley tobaccos in American cigarettes might have resulted in increased deliveries of TSNAs, even as other smoke constituents have declined. Without specific disclosure of tobacco-specific nitrosamines, it is unclear how this deleterious trend would be reversed or even detected. As economists know, competition among manufacturers over a specific brand characteristic, such as a cigarette's TSNA delivery, does not require that the average smoker—or even most smokers— know what a "nitrosamine" is.

QUESTION-AND-ANSWER SESSION

DR. HOFFMANN: We go through stages in all research; so we go through stages in tobacco research. The first stage was to identify those agents that, in the laboratory animal, cause disease. The second stage we are in now is a biomarker stage. This gives us 4-aminobiphenol, bihemoglobin, and tobacco-specific nitrosamines.

I do think we are now in a better position to judge the relationship between smoke components and disease. One should not forget that we have now moved past the stage of biomarkers where it is solely the identification of agents, and I do think one should not have such a negative outlook.

DR. HARRIS: Yes. I did not include as possible endpoints by which to compare individual cigarettes the possibility that these components may be found bound to the hemoglobin and red cells, or circulating proteins, or albumen in the blood. It is a fact that certain biomarkers, certain hydrocarbons, 4-aminobicarbons, and other compounds, have been now found bound to blood proteins or other compounds, not only among those who smoke cigarettes, but recently, in the *Journal of the National Cancer Institute*, among those who are exposed passively to cigarette smoke.

Whether those can be used for a comparative analysis of different cigarettes, I do not know. But I would, in order at least to be provocative or speculative, state that we will soon be entering an era when we can make comparisons among cigarettes by more than merely standards of chemical constituents.

DR. KOZLOWSKI: I imagine that the HARRIS ULTRA is an ultralow-tar cigarette, and it is perforated. And so, like other current 1-mg tar cigarettes, it might be 80 or 90 percent perforated, so you get air dilution of between 80 and 90 percent. I am disappointed that the label, in talking about compensatory smoking factors, does not mention the issues of vent blocking and staying away from the vents, because in fact, increased puff numbers would have a relatively small effect, if this 90-percent dilution factor was not eliminated.

DR. HARRIS: In designing that mock label, I did not attempt to be scientifically precise as to absolutely everything one would put in about proper directions for use or factors that might affect yield. Actually, your yields could vary, and then afterward put in a perforated tip. If you will look carefully, it was a 6-mg tar cigarette but with very high nicotine— 1 mg of nicotine.

One could argue, however, that if one is to continue to publish what basically are the FTC data, expanded possibly to include a high or low range, or to include other constituents, that there ought to be something about directions for appropriate use.

DR. HEADEN: Dr. Harris, in proposing a possible design for a cigarette label, I would like to know your opinion of who you think the audience is for that label. Is it the tobacco industry and other regulators who might possibly be able to interpret the information that you have? Is it the consumer, who might smoke that cigarette, many of whom have lower educational levels, or would it be both?

DR. HARRIS: I think it would have to be considerate of everyone and, although it may sound as if I would add the results of additional constituents just to satisfy some intellectually rarified audience, I raise the question, why do we put such a large array of constituents on our ordinary food supply? Some people might argue that we should not insult consumers by assuming that they cannot pick and choose, to understand or use meaningfully some forms of information rather than others. At this point, unless there is a solid confirmation that all those constituents of smoke, or characteristics of cigarettes, are simply summarized by the amount of tar, one wonders whether the lack of that information is at least deceiving some people. That is the best I can do to answer that.

DR. SONDIK: Dr. Harris, the label is intriguing, and I would not want to spend too much time on it, but a couple of points might differentiate it from the FDA label, which I happen to believe is one of the major advances in nutrition. The FDA label is designed to aid people in developing their diets. Their diet consists of all types of food, and the idea is to integrate all of these things together, which is the idea behind putting all of these different measurements on it, not just a single measurement, such as calories, for example, or total fat.

The second thing is, that label must have education along with it. And that is part of the program in NCI, the Department of Agriculture, the FDA, and others who are involved in a very intense education program—to try to be sure that the public knows how to interpret a label like this. So, in a sense, that label is more complex and aimed at a variety of types of decisions.

I would think that a label such as you proposed would be aimed at perhaps a single decision, which is whether or not this is a useful thing for me to do, trading off whatever my immediate gain might be, and pleasure, vs. long-term health effects. Is there a way of getting that onto the label?

DR. HARRIS: I do not know. It also has occurred to me that once more dimensions to cigarettes are specifically disclosed, that would be the basis of further competition among cigarette manufacturers. So, the manufacturers would then be seeing not only whether a cigarette is low or high in tar, nicotine, and carbon monoxide, but in other specific components, too. That means that while the consumer does not specifically choose among high- or low-benzo(*a*)pyrene cigarettes, the disclosure of such contents provides an incentive for manufacturers to try to reduce that component. This is the same way that the disclosure of saturated fat contents in certain breakfast cereals or other foods, even without consumer knowledge, provides an incentive for some manufacturers to try to reduce that content. Nevertheless, it provides some incentive on the supply side, not just the demand side.

DR. BENOWITZ: I know that you are not intending to be totally comprehensive about your mock insert, or label, and I think it is worthwhile keeping in mind the parallel with foods. If you are talking about limiting intake, there really are only two contents that we know about that might limit intake. One is the amount of the tobacco in the cigarette, which you did put down, and the other is the amount of nicotine contained in there, which is something that people do not often think about. But the amount of nicotine in tobacco limits what a person can get. And the intake of nicotine is not necessarily correlated at all with the yield.

So, I think that when we think about any sort of labeling for content, the nicotine content, which is the maximum available dose one could get, should really be a part of it.

DR. HARRIS: I noticed that that was in your original proposal, and I am not an expert on the degree to which nicotine content is very limiting for how many smokers. I would rather defer that to a later discussion, as to how important that is.

REFERENCES

Adams, J.D., O'Mara-Adams, K.J., Hoffmann, D. Toxic and carcinogenic agents in undiluted mainstream smoke and sidestream smoke of different types of cigarettes. *Carcinogenesis* 8(5): 729-731, 1987.

Baird, D.D., Wilcox, A.J. Cigarette smoking associated with delayed conception. *Journal of the American Medical Association* 253: 2979-2983, 1985.

Beck, G.J., Doyle, C.A., Schachter, E.N. Smoking and lung function. *American Review of Respiratory Disease* 123: 149-155, 1981.

Burghuber, O.C., Punzengruber, C., Sinzinger, H., Haber, P., Silberbauer, K. Platelet sensitivity to prostacyclin in smokers and non-smokers. *Chest* 90(1): 34-38, 1986.

Chow, W.-H., Daling, J.R., Weiss, N.S., Voigt, L.F. Maternal cigarette smoking and tubal pregnancy. *Obstetrics and Gynecology* 7: 167-170, 1988.

Church, D.F., Pryor, W.A. Free-radical chemistry of cigarette smoke and its toxicological implications. *Environmental Health Perspectives* 64: 111-126, 1985.

Coghlin, J., Gann, P.H., Hammond, S.K., Skipper, P.L., Taghizadeh, K., Paul, M., Tannenbaum, S.R. 4-Aminobiphenyl hemoglobin adducts in fetuses exposed to the tobacco smoke carcinogen in utero. *Journal of the National Cancer Institute* 83(4): 274-280, 1991.

Costagliola, C., Rinaldi, M., Giacoia, A., Rosolia, S., Cotticelli, C., Rinaldi, E. Red cell glutathione as a marker of tobacco smoke-induced optic neuropathy. *Experimental Eye Research* 48(4): 583-586, 1989.

Crawford, F.G., Mayer, J., Santella, R.M., Cooper, T.B., Ottman, R., Tsai, W.Y., Simon-Cereijido, G., Wang, M., Tang, D., Perera, F.P. Biomarkers of environmental tobacco smoke in preschool children and their mothers. *Journal of the National Cancer Institute* 86(18): 1398-1402, 1994.

Daling, J., Weiss, N., Spadoni, L., Moore, D.E., Voigt, L. Cigarette smoking and primary tubal infertility. In: *Smoking and Reproductive Health*, M.J. Rosenberg (Editor). Littleton, MA: PSG Publishing, 1987, pp. 40-46.

Davis, R.M., Healy, P., Hawk, S.A. Information on tar and nicotine yields on cigarette packages. *American Journal of Public Health* 80(5): 551-553, 1990.

Dockery, D.W., Speizer, F.E., Ferris, B.G., Jr., Ware, J.H., Louis, T.A., Spiro, A. III. Cumulative and reversible effects of lifetime smoking on simple tests of lung function in adults. *American Review of Respiratory Disease* 137(2): 286-292, 1988.

DuMouchel, W.H., Harris, J.E. Bayes methods of combining the results of cancer studies in humans and other species. *Journal of the American Statistical Association* 78: 293-308, 1983.

Fera, T., Abboud, R.T., Richter, A., Johal, S.S. Acute effect of smoking on elastaselike activity and immunologic neutrophil elastase levels in broncheolar lavage fluid. *American Review of Respiratory Disease* 133: 568-573, 1986.

Fischer, S., Spiegelhalder, B., Preussmann, R. Influence of smoking parameters on the delivery of tobacco-specific nitrosamines in cigarette smoke—a contribution to relative risk evaluation. *Carcinogenesis* 10: 1059-1066, 1989.

Fischer, S., Spiegelhalder, B., Preussmann, R. Tobacco-specific nitrosamines in commercial cigarettes: Possibilities for reducing exposure. *IARC Scientific Publications* 105: 489-492, 1991.

Gairola, C.G. Genetic effects of fresh cigarette smoke in Saccharomyces cerevisiae. *Mutation Research* 102: 123-136, 1982.

Garfinkel, L., Bofetta, P. Association between smoking and leukemia in two American Cancer Society prospective studies. *Cancer* 65: 2356-2360, 1990.

Glantz, S.A., Parmley, W.W. Passive smoking and heart disease: Epidemiology, physiology, and biochemistry. *Circulation* 83: 1-12, 1991.

Glantz, S.A., Parmley, W.W. Passive smoking and heart disease: Mechanisms and risk. *Journal of the American Medical Association* 273: 1047-1053, 1995.

Harris, J.E. Smoking and nothingness. In: *Deadly Choices: Coping with Health Risks in Everyday Life*. New York: Basic Books, 1993, pp. 151-177.

Hecht, S.S., Carmella, S.G., Murphy, S.E., Akerkar, S., Brunnemann, K.D., Hoffmann, D. A tobacco-specific lung carcinogen in the urine of men exposed to cigarette smoke. *New England Journal of Medicine* 329(21): 1543-1546, 1993.

Henningfield, J.E., Kozlowski, L.T., Benowitz, N.L. A proposal to develop meaningful labeling for cigarettes. *Journal of the American Medical Association* 272(4): 312-314, 1994.

Hoffmann, D., Hecht, S.S. Advances in tobacco carcinogenesis. *Handbook of Experimental Pharmacology*, Vol. 94, No. I, C.S. Cooper and P.L. Grover (Editors). Berlin: Springer-Verlag, 1990.

Janoff, A. Elastases and emphysema: Current assessment of the protease-antiprotease hypothesis. *American Review of Respiratory Disease* 132: 417-433, 1985.

Jansson, T., Curvall, M., Hedin, A., Enzell, C.R. In vitro studies of the biological effects of cigarette smoke condensate. III. Induction of SCE by some phenolic and related constituents derived from cigarette smoke. A study of structure-activity relationships. *Mutation Research* 206(1): 17-24, 1988.

Kaiserman, M.J., Rickert, W.S. Carcinogens in tobacco smoke: Benzo(a)pyrene from Canadian cigarettes and cigarette tobaccos. *American Journal of Public Health* 82: 1023-1026, 1992.

Krupski, W.C., Olive, G.C., Weber, C.A., Rapp, J.H. Comparative effects of hypertension and nicotine on injury-induced myointimal thickening. *Surgery* 102: 409-415, 1987.

Mattison, D.R. Morphology of oocyte and follicle destruction by polycyclic aromatic hydrocarbons in mice. *Toxicology and Applied Pharmacology* 53: 249-259, 1980.

Mattison, D.R. The effects of smoking on fertility from gametogenesis to implantation. *Environmental Research* 28: 410-433, 1982.

Melikian, A.A., Prahalad, A.K., Hoffmann, D. Urinary *trans, trans*-muconic acid as an indicator of exposure to benzene in cigarette smokers. *Cancer Epidemiology, Biomarkers and Prevention* 2(1): 47-51, 1993.

Niewoehner, D.E., Kleinerman, J., Rice, D.B. Pathologic changes in the peripheral airways of young cigarette smokers. *New England Journal of Medicine* 291: 755-758, 1974.

Penn, A., Chen, L.C., Snyder, C.A. Inhalation of steady-state sidestream smoke from one cigarette promotes atherosclerotic plaque development. *Circulation* 90: 1363-1367, 1994.

Phillips, G.F., Waller, R.E. Yields of tar and other smoke components from UK cigarettes. *Food and Chemical Toxicology* 29(7): 469-474, 1991.

Pittilo, R.M., Clarke, J.M., Harris, D., Mackie, I.J., Rowles, P.M., Machin, S.J., Woolf, N. Cigarette smoking and platelet adhesion. *British Journal of Haematology* 58(4): 627-632, 1984.

Rabkin, S.W. Effect of cigarette smoking cessation on risk factors for coronary atherosclerosis: a control clinical trial. *Atherosclerosis* 53(2): 173-184, 1984.

Rando, R.J., Menon, P.K., Poovey, H.G., Lehrer, S.B. Assessment of multiple markers of environmental tobacco smoke (ETS) in controlled, steady-state atmospheres in a dynamic test chamber. *American Industrial Hygiene Association Journal* 53(11): 699-704, 1992.

Santella, R.M., Grinberg-Funes, R.A., Young, T.L., Dickey, C., Singh, V.N., Wang, L.W. Perera, F.P. Cigarette smoking related polycyclic aromatic hydrocarbon-DNA adducts in peripheral mononuclear cells. *Carcinogenesis* 13(11): 2041-2045, 1992.

Seely, J.E., Zuskin, E., Bouhys, A. Cigarette smoking: Objective evidence for lung damage in teenagers. *Science* 172: 741-743, 1971.

Selley, M.L., Bartlett, M.R., McGuiness, J.A., Ardlie, N.G. Effects of acrolein on human platelet aggregation. *Chemico-Biological Interactions* 76(1): 101-109, 1990.

Sheps, D.S., Herbst, M.C., Hinderliter, A.L., Adams, K.F., Ekelund, L.G., O'Neil, J.J., Goldstein, G.M., Bromberg, P.A., Dalton, J.L., Pallenger, M.N., Davis, S.M., Koch, G.G. Production of arrythmias by elevated carboxyhemoglobin in patients with coronary artery disease. *Annals of Internal Medicine* 113(5): 343-351, 1990.

U.S. Department of Health and Human Services. *The Health Consequences of Smoking for Women. A Report of the Surgeon General.* Rockville, MD: U.S. Department of Health and Human Services, Public Health Service, Office of the Assistant Secretary for Health, Office on Smoking and Health, 1980.

U.S. Department of Health and Human Services. *The Health Consequences of Smoking: Cancer. A Report of the Surgeon General.* DHHS Publication No. (PHS) 82-50179. Rockville, MD: U.S. Department of Health and Human Services, Public Health Service, Office on Smoking and Health, 1982.

U.S. Department of Health and Human Services. *The Health Consequences of Smoking: Chronic Obstructive Lung Disease. A Report of the Surgeon General.* DHHS Publication No. (PHS) 84-50205. Rockville, MD: U.S. Department of Health and Human Services, Public Health Service, Office on Smoking and Health, 1984a.

U.S. Department of Health and Human Services. *The Health Consequences of Smoking: Cardiovascular Disease. A Report of the Surgeon General.* DHHS Publication No. (PHS) 84-50204. Rockville, MD: U.S. Department of Health and Human Services, Public Health Service, Office on Smoking and Health, 1984b.

U.S. Department of Health and Human Services. *The Health Consequences of Smoking: Cancer and Chronic Lung Disease in the Workplace. A Report of the Surgeon General.* DHHS Publication No. (PHS) 85-50207. Rockville, MD: U.S. Department of Health and Human Services, Public Health Service, Office on Smoking and Health, 1985.

U.S. Department of Health and Human Services. *The Health Consequences of Involuntary Smoking. A Report of the Surgeon General.* DHHS Publication No. (CDC) 87-8398. Rockville, MD: U.S. Department of Health and Human Services, Public Health Service, Centers for Disease Control, Center for Health Promotion and Education, Office on Smoking and Health, 1987.

U.S. Department of Health and Human Services. *The Health Consequences of Smoking: Nicotine Addiction. A Report of the Surgeon General, 1988.* DHHS Publication No. (CDC) 88-8406. Rockville, MD: U.S. Department of Health and Human Services, Public Health Service, Centers for Disease Control, Center for Health Promotion and Education, Office on Smoking and Health, 1988.

U.S. Department of Health and Human Services. *Reducing the Health Consequences of Smoking: 25 Years of Progress. A Report of the Surgeon General, 1989.* DHHS Publication No. (CDC) 89-8411. Rockville, MD: U.S. Department of Health and Human Services, Public Health Service, Centers for Disease Control, Center for Chronic Disease Prevention and Health Promotion, Office on Smoking and Health, 1989.

U.S. Department of Health and Human Services. *The Health Benefits of Smoking Cessation. A Report of the Surgeon General, 1990.* DHHS Publication No. (CDC) 90-8416. Rockville, MD: U.S. Department of Health and Human Services, Public Health Service, Centers for Disease Control, Center for Chronic Disease Prevention and Health Promotion, Office on Smoking and Health, 1990.

U.S. Department of Health, Education, and Welfare. *Smoking and Health. A Report of the Surgeon General.* DHEW Publication No. (PHS) 79-50066. Rockville, MD: U.S. Department of Health, Education, and Welfare, Public Health Service, Office of the Assistant Secretary for Health, Office on Smoking and Health, 1979.

Vineis, P. Black (air-cured) and blond (flue-cured) tobacco and cancer risk. I: Bladder cancer. *European Journal of Cancer* 27(11): 1491-1493, 1991.

Werler, M.M., Pober, B.R., Holmes, L.B. Smoking and pregnancy. *Teratology* 32: 473-481, 1985.

Willett, W., Hennekens, C.H., Castelli, W., Rosner, B., Evans, D., Taylor, J., Kass, E.H. Effects of cigarette smoking on fasting triglyceride, total cholesterol, and HDL-cholesterol in women. *American Heart Journal* 105(3): 417-421, 1983.

Zimmerman, M., McGeachie, J. The effect of nicotine on aortic endothelium: A comparative study. *Atherosclerosis* 63: 33-41, 1987.

ACKNOWLEDGMENT   Financial support from the National Cancer Institute is acknowledged, but the contents of this manuscript are the author's sole responsibility.

The Changing Cigarette and Disease Risk: Current Status of the Evidence

Jonathan M. Samet

INTRODUCTION   Since the early 1950's when filter tip cigarettes were first widely introduced, the cigarette has evolved continually through modifications intended to reduce yields of tar and nicotine (U.S. Department of Health and Human Services, 1991). Following the introduction of the filter tip cigarette, sales-weighted averages of tar and nicotine deliveries show a temporal trend of declining yield, which continues to the present (Figure 1). In the face of continued modifications of the cigarette and the seemingly associated changes in exposure of smokers to cigarette smoke components, questions have been raised concerning the implications of the changing cigarette for disease risks in smokers.

Only epidemiologic studies can provide information on modification of the risks of smoking as the cigarette has evolved, and only epidemiologic data

Figure 1
Tar and nicotine content of U.S. cigarettes, sales-weighted average basis, 1957-1987

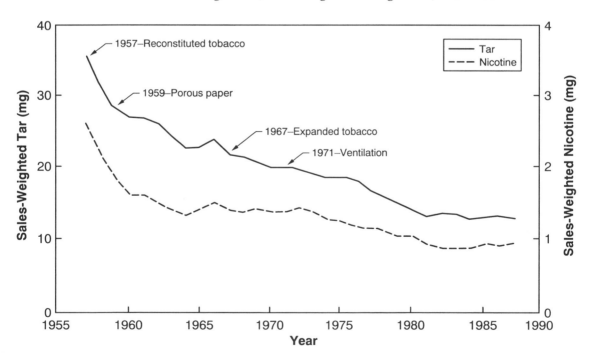

Source: U.S. Department of Health and Human Services, 1989.

77

can measure the risks of cigarettes under the "natural" circumstances of use. However, the dynamic nature of the exposure (Figure 1) challenges the epidemiologic researcher to classify accurately the pattern of cigarette use when changes are made that may not be indexed by tar and nicotine yields measured with a smoking machine.

In considering the health implications of the changing cigarette, the concepts of exposure and dose are fundamental. Exposure has been defined by the National Research Council (1991) as the amount of material potentially available for interaction with a human, that is, material in contact with a person at a boundary, whether that boundary be the skin, lung, or the alimentary tract. On the other hand, dose is the amount of material that enters the organism. Dose may be further classified as the internal dose (i.e., the amount of material deposited) or as the biologically effective dose (i.e., the amount of material delivered to some biologically relevant site). Changes in the cigarette can be interpreted as potentially leading to changes in exposure; the health consequences of changing exposure vary with any resultant changes in dose of components of cigarette smoke that cause disease.

The physiological functioning of the lung is also relevant to understanding the linkages in changes in the cigarette to changes in exposure and dose. The lung is a complex organ with several different "compartments," including the upper airway that extends from the nose and mouth to the larynx; the airways of the lung itself, which include the trachea, bronchi, and bronchioles; and the parenchyma of the lung, which includes the interstitium and the airspaces, or alveoli. The lung behaves as a filter that absorbs and deposits gaseous and particulate components of smoke throughout its surfaces during the act of smoking. The sites and extent of deposition of inhaled mainstream components vary, depending on solubility and other characteristics of gas phase components and the sizes of the particles. Cigarette smoke is a dynamic mixture in the respiratory tract, changing with humidification of the mixture, growth of particles, and changing composition as components are selectively removed by the filtration process (U.S. Department of Health and Human Services, 1984). These physiological considerations imply that there is no simple relationship, linear or nonlinear, between reported tar and nicotine yields—a measure of exposure—and biologically effective doses of toxic smoke components delivered to the sites of injury in the respiratory tract.

The measures of cigarette smoking used in epidemiologic research on smoking and health can be classified as estimating either exposure or dose. The most widely used measures, for example, information on cigarette smoking (duration of smoking, number of cigarettes smoked per day, and type or brand of cigarettes smoked), are exposure measures. Biomarkers that can be interpreted as indicators of dose include levels of carboxyhemoglobin, nicotine, and cotinine (U.S. Department of Health and Human Services, 1990). Thus, for epidemiological purposes, researchers use exposure measures, typically obtained by questionnaire, and dose measures, based on biomarkers. For example, cigarettes smoked per day is an exposure measure, whereas pack-years (packs smoked per day multiplied by the number of years smoked) is a cumulative exposure measure. An estimate of kilograms of tar deposited in the lung is an absorbed dose measure; nanograms of benzo(*a*)pyrene, for example, reaching basal cells might be considered a biologically effective dose for carcinogenesis. New markers take dose measures to the molecular level (Vineis and Caporaso, 1995).

To assess the consequences of changes in the cigarette, it is necessary to have information on how changes in tar and nicotine yield, as assessed by the Federal Trade Commission (FTC) method, affect dose measures, extending to the molecular level. Any new approach to testing cigarette yields should be designed to be informative both as an exposure measure and as an indicator of biologically relevant doses of cigarette smoke components.

EPIDEMIOLOGIC EVIDENCE ON THE CHANGING CIGARETTE AND DISEASE RISKS

Overview

Epidemiologic evidence is available on the effect of the changing cigarette on all-cause mortality and on three major categories of disease caused by cigarette smoking: lung and other cancers, nonmalignant respiratory diseases, and cardiovascular disease (CVD). *The Health Consequences of Smoking: The Changing Cigarette. A Report of the Surgeon General* (U.S. Department of Health and Human Services, 1981) addressed the changing cigarette, covering the relevant toxicologic and epidemiologic evidence. This chapter considers key epidemiologic publications since that report but does not provide a systematic overview of the many studies on the changing cigarette.

The principal study designs that have been used to address the health consequences of the changing cigarette are the ecological study, a descriptive approach conducted at the group level, and cohort and case-control studies, analytic approaches conducted at the individual level. Cross-sectional studies have proven informative in investigating nonmalignant respiratory diseases. The ecological approach is exemplified by a comparison of temporal changes in rates of smoking-related diseases with patterns of consumption of various types of cigarettes. The American Cancer Society (ACS) studies of large groups of volunteer participants are cohort studies; the participants were enrolled, information about smoking was obtained on enrollment and periodically thereafter, the population was followed over time, and mortality was ascertained. Some of the earliest evidence on smoking and lung cancer was obtained in the classic case-control studies conducted by Doll and Hill (1950) and Wynder and Graham (1950). In these studies, the smoking habits of patients hospitalized with lung cancer were compared with the smoking habits of control patients having another disease.

Evidence from epidemiologic studies has well-known strengths and limitations (Rothman, 1986). Epidemiologic research has had a central role in characterizing the consequences of the changing cigarette because it supplies direct information on the consequences of varying tar and nicotine yield products. Thus, the findings inherently consider compensatory changes in inhalation patterns or in numbers of cigarettes smoked and provide the evidence needed to answer the question of immediate public health relevance: whether disease risk varies with cigarette tar and nicotine yield as determined by the FTC method.

Exposure misclassification is a potential threat to the validity of studies of the changing cigarette. Typically, the exposure of smokers to cigarettes of varying tar and nicotine yields is estimated based on information on brands and types of cigarettes smoked. However, smokers may not be able to provide a fully accurate history of brands used throughout their lifetimes; therefore, estimates of tar and nicotine yield are potentially subject to error (U.S. Department of Health and Human Services, 1990). The consequences of misclassification include biased estimates of the effect of tar and nicotine yields and reduction of statistical power. Additional methodological concerns include the possibility of selection bias if smokers affected by symptoms or disease tend to switch to lower yield products; another concern is confounding by other aspects of lifestyle if smokers of lower yield cigarettes differ substantially in lifestyle characteristics from those smoking higher yield products. However, the research challenge of studying the consequences of the changing cigarette is no different from the challenge posed by other complex mixtures of inhaled agents, and epidemiologic research has the advantage of integrating the effects of the mixture, even though individual components may be interacting in ways that are difficult to characterize.

Lung Cancer   The ACS's Cancer Prevention Study I (CPS-I) provided early evidence on the risks of lower tar and nicotine cigarettes (Hammond et al., 1976). CPS-I included about 1 million volunteers who were followed from 1960 to 1972. Mortality was examined by three categories of tar intake—high, medium, and low. For all causes of mortality and for lung cancer mortality, the standardized mortality ratios declined as estimated tar or nicotine intake declined (Table 1). The findings were similar for males (Table 1) and for females (data not shown). However, comparison with mortality in never-smokers shows that smokers of even the lowest tar and nicotine products nonetheless had substantially higher mortality rates.

Other studies have had similar findings for lung cancer. Wynder and colleagues at the American Health Foundation have conducted an ongoing case-control study of smoking and lung cancer that provides information on cigarette type and lung cancer risk over decades since the 1950's. Reports from this study have consistently shown that smokers of lower tar products, indexed in a variety of ways, have reduced lung cancer risk (Wynder et al., 1970; Wynder and Kabat, 1988). For example, in a recent report based on cases from the late 1970's and early 1980's, risks were examined separately for persons with squamous cell and small cell carcinomas of the lung (Kreyberg I) and adenocarcinoma of the lung (Kreyberg II) (Wynder and Kabat, 1988). Smoking was classified as 100 percent filter, 100 percent nonfilter, or intermediate, by number of switchers from nonfilter to filter. For smokers of filter cigarettes only, risks were approximately 10 to 30 percent less than those of smokers of nonfilters only (Table 2).

Table 1

Standardized mortality ratios for men in Cancer Prevention Study I for total mortality, lung cancer, and coronary heart disease (CHD) by tar and nicotine intake

	Tar and Nicotine Intake		
Deaths	High[a]	Medium[b]	Low[c]
Total Deaths			
1960-1966	1.00	0.90	0.88
1967-1972	1.00	0.98	0.81
Lung Cancer			
1960-1966	1.00	0.96	0.83
1967-1972	1.00	0.94	0.79
CHD			
1960-1966	1.00	0.91	0.93
1967-1972	1.00	1.03	0.82

[a] *High = 2.0 to 2.7 mg nicotine and 25.8 to 35.7 mg tar.*
[b] *Medium = intermediate.*
[c] *Low = <1.2 mg nicotine and tar generally <17.6 mg.*

Source: Hammond et al., 1976.

Table 2

Adjusted odds ratios and 95-percent confidence intervals for males in the American Health Foundation case-control study, by level of filter smoking

	Tumor Type			
	Kreyberg I		Kreyberg II	
Pattern of Smoking	Odds Ratio	95% Confidence Interval	Odds Ratio	95% Confidence Interval
Nonfilter Only	1.00	—	1.00	—
Switchers (1-9 years)	0.83	0.59 - 1.17	0.96	0.61 - 1.51
Switchers (10+ years)	0.66	0.49 - 0.90	0.79	0.53 - 1.18
Filter Only	0.69	0.37 - 1.27	0.87	0.43 - 1.54

Source: Wynder and Kabat, 1988.

A multicenter case-control study conducted in Europe during the late 1970's also provided information on cigarette type and lung cancer risk (Lubin et al., 1984). In this study, risk for lung cancer increased progressively in both males and females as the proportion of filter use declined from 100 percent. Findings were similar in a case-control study that was conducted in New Mexico from 1980 through 1983, although a linear dose-response relationship between lung cancer risk and the extent of filter cigarette smoking was not observed (Pathak et al., 1986). Other recent case-control studies have provided comparable results (Wilcox et al., 1988; Kaufman et al., 1989).

Temporal patterns of lung cancer rates also have been interpreted as indicating lower lung cancer risks among smokers of lower tar and nicotine cigarettes. It has been suggested that the recent decline in lung cancer mortality rates among younger males may reflect changes in the cigarette (World Health Organization, 1986). This downturn has been observed in the United States and other countries (Gilliland and Samet, 1994).

Nonmalignant Respiratory Diseases
Cigarette smoking has diverse effects on the structure and function of the lung and is a cause of chronic bronchitis and chronic obstructive pulmonary disease (COPD) (U.S. Department of Health and Human Services, 1984). The persistent obstruction to airflow in the lung that is the hallmark of COPD reflects underlying changes in the small airways of the lung and emphysema, which is the permanent destruction of the air spaces of the lung. Chronic bronchitis, a condition of chronic sputum production, reflects hyperplasia of the lining of the airways of the lung and mucous gland proliferation. Compared with nonsmokers, smokers have a greater frequency of cough and production of phlegm, manifestations of the inflammation of the lung and increased mucus production secondary to smoking, and wheezing; smokers also have lower lung function.

A significant number of adults in the United States have COPD, which now causes more than 60,000 deaths annually (U.S. Department of Health and Human Services, 1984). The natural history of this disorder has been described through longitudinal investigations that have monitored lung function over time in smokers and nonsmokers (U.S. Department of Health and Human Services, 1984; Sherman et al., 1993). In nonsmokers, lung function increases through late adolescence and early adulthood, maintains a plateau across the third and fourth decades, and then begins to decline. In smokers, the decline begins at a younger age and tends to be steeper. The rate of decline increases with the number of cigarettes smoked per day but varies widely among smokers. With continued smoking, those with more rapid rates of decline eventually deteriorate to a level of lung function associated with impairment, and COPD is diagnosed. Although cessation earlier in the evolution of the disease is followed by return of the rate of decline to that of nonsmokers (U.S. Department of Health and Human Services, 1990), smoking cessation at this point in the natural history of the disease is not followed by improvement in lung function.

Findings have been reported that provide insights concerning tar and nicotine yields and respiratory symptoms and lung function level. Auerbach and colleagues (1979) quantitated smoking-related changes in the lungs of men having autopsies at a Veterans Administration hospital in New Jersey. In a rigorously investigated series of autopsied lungs, these investigators showed that smokers from a period during which cigarettes had comparatively high yields of tar and nicotine (1955 to 1960) had more changes in the airways at various smoking levels compared with smokers from a later period (1970 to 1977). They interpreted this temporal pattern as indicating that cigarettes with lower tar and nicotine yields had less effect on lungs than did higher yield cigarettes.

A number of studies have shown that smokers of lower yield cigarettes have comparatively lower rates of respiratory symptoms. Respiratory questionnaire data collected in the late 1970's from approximately 6,000 Pennsylvania women are illustrative (Schenker et al., 1982). The brand of cigarettes currently smoked was determined and used with FTC tar yield information to classify the smokers by tar exposure. Tar yield was positively associated with cough and phlegm but not with wheezing or shortness of breath. For cough and phlegm, there were consistent exposure-response relationships with an approximate doubling of symptom frequency from the lowest to the highest exposure category (Table 3). The findings of other studies are similar. For example, a large study of civil servants in the United Kingdom, the Whitehall study, showed that the percentage of smokers reporting phlegm increased with tar yield within each stratum of cigarettes smoked per day, even the lowest (Higenbottam et al., 1980).

Table 3

Absolute and relative risks of chronic cough and chronic phlegm in Pennsylvania women by smoking status, cigarettes smoked per day (CPD), and tar yield of current brand

Smoker Classification	Chronic Cough		Chronic Phlegm	
	Risk	Relative Risk	Risk	Relative Risk
Never-Smokers	0.038	1.00	0.033	1.00
Ex-Smokers	0.056	1.46	0.052	1.58
Current Smokers				
1-14 CPD				
7 mg tar	0.073	1.92	0.067	2.04
15 mg tar	0.103	2.71	0.085	2.56
22 mg tar	0.137	3.61	0.103	3.12
15-24 CPD				
7 mg tar	0.136	3.58	0.155	4.67
15 mg tar	0.185	4.87	0.190	5.74
22 mg tar	0.240	6.32	0.226	6.82
25+ CPD				
7 mg tar	0.273	7.18	0.234	7.05
15 mg tar	0.353	9.29	0.281	8.48
22 mg tar	0.430	11.32	0.327	9.87

Source: Schenker et al., 1982.

Respiratory morbidity also has been investigated. Followup of outpatient visits by enrollees in a Kaiser-Permanente group over 1 year showed that there was a reduced risk for pneumonia and influenza but not other respiratory conditions, associated with use of low-tar and -nicotine products (Petitti and Friedman, 1985a). However, in comparison with nonsmokers, smokers using low-tar and -nicotine cigarettes had an increased risk for pneumonia, influenza, and COPD.

Not all studies show less disease associated with lower yield cigarettes. One recent study from Finland found that symptom levels in young smokers who were just initiating smoking did not depend greatly on tar yield (Rimpela and Teperi, 1989). In this 6-year followup study, the youths were surveyed on several occasions, and the relationship between tar yield and symptom onset was determined. There was little evidence of less symptom occurrence in the new smokers using low-tar cigarettes in comparison with those smoking higher tar cigarettes. Moreover, symptoms were far more frequent in the smokers of low-tar cigarettes in comparison with nonsmokers. In a randomized trial in the United Kingdom, lower tar cigarettes were not associated with either lower symptom frequency or higher level of ventilatory function, as assessed by measuring the peak expiratory flow rate (Withey et al., 1992a and 1992b). The investigators monitored urinary nicotine metabolites and concluded that compensation led to comparable levels across the trial period.

The evidence does not suggest a relationship between tar yield and lung function level. For example, in the Whitehall study (Higenbottam et al., 1980), there was no cross-sectional relationship between tar yield and level of the forced expiratory volume in 1 second. In the Normative Aging Study (Sparrow et al., 1983), a longitudinal study of U.S. veterans, tar yield of the usual brand of cigarettes smoked was not associated with decline of forced expiratory volume in 1 second.

Cardiovascular Disease   Harris (this volume) discusses mechanisms by which cigarette smoking causes CVD. Through some of these mechanisms, cigarette smoking is anticipated to increase the incidence of new cases (i.e., to cause more disease), whereas other mechanisms are anticipated to exacerbate the status of those who already had disease (U.S. Department of Health and Human Services, 1990). Thus, factors promoting atherogenesis would increase incidence, whereas factors such as sympathomimetic stimulation by nicotine or impairment of oxygen delivery by carbon monoxide might be expected to have more immediate effects and contribute to morbidity and mortality among those with coronary artery disease.

Strong evidence does not exist for either lower incidence or less morbidity from coronary heart disease (CHD) among smokers of lower yield cigarettes. In the American Cancer Society's CPS-I study (Hammond et al., 1976), smokers of lower tar products did have lower mortality from heart disease (Table 1). On the other hand, two case-control studies carried out during the 1980's, one involving men (Kaufman et al., 1989) and the other involving women (Palmer et al., 1989), did not show evidence of reduced risk for smokers smoking lower nicotine products. Both studies included persons with a first and nonfatal myocardial infarction. In the 1980-1981 study of men younger than 54, neither nicotine nor carbon monoxide yields of current brand were associated with risk of myocardial infarction (Table 4). From 1985 to 1988, a similar case-control study of women as old as 65 with nonfatal myocardial infarction also showed no relationship between nicotine or carbon monoxide yields of current brand of cigarettes and risk of myocardial infarction (Table 5).

The study of Kaiser-Permanente enrollees also supplied relevant information (Petitti and Friedman, 1985b). Hospitalization for a variety of cardiovascular outcomes was assessed in relation to type of cigarettes smoked, after adjusting for other predictors. Using a multivariate regression model, the investigators found relatively small increases in risk for hospitalization as tar yield increased.

Table 4
Relative adjusted risk of myocardial infarction in men by nicotine and carbon monoxide yield of cigarettes smoked

Smoker Status	Relative Risk	95% Confidence Interval
Never-Smoker	1.0	2.5 - 6.7
Current Smoker		
Nicotine yield (mg)		
< 0.8	3.8	2.3 - 6.5
0.8-0.9	4.1	2.5 - 6.7
1.0-1.1	3.4	2.2 - 5.3
1.2-1.4	2.4	1.5 - 3.8
≥ 1.5	3.2	1.9 - 5.6
Carbon monoxide yield (mg)		
< 10	3.5	1.9 - 6.6
10-14	4.4	2.6 - 7.5
15-17	3.2	2.1 - 5.0
18	2.9	1.8 - 4.5
≥ 19	3.3	1.8 - 6.0

Source: Kaufman et al., 1983.

Table 5

Relative adjusted risk of myocardial infarction in women by nicotine and carbon monoxide yield of cigarettes smoked

Smoker Status	Relative Risk	95% Confidence Interval
Never-Smoker	1.0	–
Current Smoker		
Nicotine yield (mg)		
< 0.40	4.7	2.8 - 8.0
0.40-0.63	3.3	2.3 - 4.8
0.64-0.75	3.2	2.2 - 4.5
0.75-1.00	4.7	3.4 - 6.5
1.01-1.06	3.6	2.6 - 5.0
1.07-1.29	5.1	3.4 - 7.5
≥1.30	4.2	2.4 - 7.2
Carbon monoxide yield (mg)		
< 4.8	4.9	2.9 - 8.2
4.8-9.1	4.4	2.4 - 4.9
9.2-11.1	3.8	2.7 - 5.4
11.2-14.4	3.8	2.7 - 5.2
14.5-15.0	4.1	2.9 - 5.7
15.1-18.0	4.2	2.9 - 6.2
> 18.0	4.8	2.8 - 8.1

Source: Palmer et al., 1989.

CONCLUSIONS   *The Health Consequences of Smoking: The Changing Cigarette: A Report of the Surgeon General* (U.S. Department of Health and Human Services, 1981) offered conclusions on these three major classes of disease. Do these conclusions remain tenable in light of more recent evidence?

With regard to cancer, the report concluded that:

> Today's filter-tipped, lower 'tar' and nicotine cigarettes produce lower rates of lung cancer than do their higher 'tar' and nicotine predecessors. Nonetheless, smokers of lower 'tar' and nicotine cigarettes have much higher lung cancer incidence and mortality than do nonsmokers (U.S. Department of Health and Human Services, 1981, p. 18).

The more recent case-control evidence remains consistent with the first component of this conclusion.

With regard to COPD, the report concluded that it was unknown whether risk was lower for smokers of low-tar and -nicotine cigarettes compared with risk for smokers of higher tar and nicotine cigarettes. There is no consistent evidence that risk for this disease is associated with the tar and nicotine yield of the cigarettes smoked.

> For CVD, the 1981 conclusion remains appropriate: . . . the overall changes in the composition of cigarettes that have occurred during the last 10 to 15 years have not produced a clearly demonstrated effect on cardiovascular disease, and some studies suggest that a decreased risk of CHD may not have occurred (U.S. Department of Health and Human Services, 1981, p. 125).

Our research needs have changed little from the agenda set out in that report 15 years ago. The report called for further surveillance of the characteristics of smoke in relation to the type of cigarettes, further characterization of compensatory changes in smoking, better understanding of doses of tobacco smoke components delivered to the lung, and additional epidemiologic research. Ongoing characterization of the health consequences of the changing cigarette should be implemented and maintained through cohort studies such as CPS-I or case-control methods. New biomarkers of exposure and dose should be applied to better understand the relationships of FTC tar and nicotine yields with biologically effective doses of smoke components.

QUESTION-AND-ANSWER SESSION

DR. PETITTI: It actually does amaze me that the conclusions of this report are the same as they were in 1981. It also amazes me how little information has developed in this field over the past 14 years.

I wanted you to comment on an issue that was, I think, not particularly well addressed in the 1981 report and has troubled me about the epidemiological data. It has to do with the tendency to examine the risk of lung cancer in strata defined by number of cigarettes smoked per day. When you define smoking by number of cigarettes smoked per day, you do take into account compensation by inhalation and amount smoked, but you don't take into account any kind of compensation that might occur because of a tendency to smoke an increased number of cigarettes per day and smoking a lower yield brand. That would suggest that in order to take that into account in the epidemiology, you would have to move people to a different category of number of cigarettes smoked per day.

Do you think that epidemiology can address this issue, and how do you think that places limitations on the first conclusion related to lung cancer, particularly?

DR. SAMET: It is a good question and I think much of the discussion about smokers' behavior that will follow will get at just how complex the physiology is and how difficult it is to make these determinations in the laboratory.

Then, if you think about trying to develop approaches that might be used in epidemiological studies, based around questionnaires to try to develop tools that would provide a better measure of dose, which I think is what you are calling for, it becomes very difficult.

You know, using some of our nested approaches, one might begin to use biomarkers within studies, within cohort studies, probably particularly, to sort this out. But I think you are pointing to a significant limitation of approaching this question in large population studies.

DR. BENOWITZ: The biggest effect was clearly in the lung cancer data, and the lung cancers occurred as a result of cigarettes smoked a long time ago. Is there any evidence that there is any difference in risk if you looked at modern or filtered cigarettes?

DR. SAMET: Let me see if I can rephrase the question. Are you asking, has there been an attempt to assess whether some estimate of tar dose, or tar received, is a better predictor of lung cancer risk than simply proportion of filter use?

DR. BENOWITZ: Yes. What I am wondering is, is there any relevance to the data when people were mostly smoking nonfiltered cigarettes to today's cigarette market, where they are filtered? Can the whole thing be done just by adding a filter?

DR. SAMET: Probably the right answer to the question is: I do not know. But if we think we could begin to use the information from studies of smokers of old nonfiltered products, through smokers of newer products, to try and define some kind of an exposure-response relationship, then I suppose it could be done. But I think that, if we were to do that, it would be subject to a great deal of uncertainty.

DR. HARRIS: I noticed that one of the studies omitted from your review was the second American Cancer Study, CPS-II, which followed people from 1982 to 1986. I am wondering if anyone knows whether that study will be analyzed in terms of the yield or type of cigarette and health outcomes.

DR. SAMET: There has already been a paper describing the demographics of tobacco use in that study and predictors of tar yield by various demographic predictors. I would anticipate seeing such an analysis eventually.

DR. WOOSLEY: We have already heard this morning how the marketing and the promotion of the low-tar and -nicotine cigarettes have been toward the more highly educated portion of the population. We have already seen how they responded to that by switching. We have already heard how they have expressed greater concern for their overall health.

I have a serious concern. Do you feel the data have adequately addressed the possibility that you are looking at a subset of the population who have done something else to modify their health risks and, therefore, have looked at a selected population with decreased negative outcomes because of these other factors, and that we really have not seen any influence of the cigarettes themselves?

DR. SAMET: I referred to that set of concerns under the rubric of selection bias. That is, people may select themselves to products based on either their response to what they were smoking or other characteristics that are relevant—an argument in epidemiology called confounding.

I think you are right; these are concerns. I think, on the other hand, in many of the studies there have been attempts to "adjust," to the extent one can, for such differences in the characteristics of those using different types of products. As you look across the consistency of the evidence in different populations with different approaches to controlling for such factors, and different study designs, a consistency emerges, I think at least for lung cancer, that would suggest some modest reduction of risk for those using the lower delivery products.

Could there be some element of residual bias in there? I certainly could not exclude it. But when we weigh the evidence in an attempt to understand those other factors, the socioeconomic indices and other measures in different studies would support that conclusion.

DR. BENOWITZ: I think that is the most important issue that we have to address here today. If labeling something low-tar and -nicotine implies improved health compared with higher tar and nicotine, I think those confounders have the most impact on that decision.

DR. HOFFMANN: With regard to Dr. Benowitz' question to me, it is rather interesting to see that multiple studies have shown that the increase in adenocarcinoma today is much higher than previously, because the nature has changed. So, to me, this has something to do with the cigarette. You get more adenocarcinoma in the peripheral lung than in former times; it is a ratio of 20 to 1 squamous cells, and today you have 1 to 1. So, I think at least the type of lung cancer that appears today has something to do with the change in cigarettes.

DR. SAMET: But certainly the histologic distribution of lung cancers has changed and I agree; we would like to know why.

DR. DEBETHIZY: Your data about the relationship between nicotine and cardiovascular disease are curious to me, because most of the data in the literature show that people who smoke low-yielding cigarettes actually absorb less nicotine. Could you comment on the fact that you do not see any dose-response relationship there?

DR. SAMET: I am not sure how you would like me to comment. I am describing the findings of a case-control study that describes how risks of nonfatal myocardial infarction varied with the level of nicotine or carbon monoxide intake, as estimated by what brand was being smoked at the time of the infarct.

These are not biomarker data, so there is no inference in these particular subjects as to what the level of nicotine or carbon monoxide may have been. The question is, again, looking at the yield or brand as an estimate of exposure, there was simply no relationship observed in these observational studies.

DR. HUGHES: In most of these studies, the control group is labeled nonsmokers. Is that usually never-smokers?

DR. SAMET: In most of the studies that are labeled nonsmokers, that is a never-smoker group. You basically will see two contrasts: vs. never-smokers or, in some of the studies, the contrast has been made between sort of the lower exposure group vs. the higher exposure group.

DR. HUGHES: The reason I asked that is, it seems to me that using controls of ex-smokers would be important for two reasons. One, it would be a control for the confounds that Dr. Woosley mentioned earlier. Second, all your studies have to do with switching cigarettes. None of them has to do with the alternative of either quitting or switching to a low-nicotine cigarette. Are there data to inform the consumer of the question, how much do I want to improve my health by quitting, vs. how much do I improve my health by switching to a low-tar cigarette?

DR. SAMET: Certainly, there are abundant data on how risks of diseases vary following cessation. I do not want to complicate this, and it was the subject of the 1990 Surgeon General's report. These risks vary in complex ways for different diseases, depending on the age at which the smoker stopped smoking and the duration of successful abstinence from smoking.

So, it is somewhat difficult to capture a single number that describes the risk in ex-smokers. It has to be done in a far more complex way. But, on the other hand, there are data sets, like the American Cancer Society data sets, that would allow one to describe how risks change following smoking cessation, for example. And it would be possible to derive some quantitative contrast between what might happen to smokers of different ages, different prior smoking histories, with switching products vs. cessation.

DR. RICKERT: On your emphysema slide, the one that dealt with the changes in lung function, there was a label that said, "never smoked and not susceptible to the effects of tobacco smoke." Do you have any idea what proportion of the population of smokers fell into the category "not susceptible"?

DR. SAMET: Such numbers are not readily available. I think most people who work in this field would guess that with regard to COPD, perhaps 20 to 25 percent of continued smokers seemed to fall into this group of rapid lung function decline.

DR. RICKERT: Are there any postulated mechanisms why smokers should be in that group?

DR. SAMET: There are many postulated mechanisms, some of which Dr. Harris already surveyed. They are essentially mechanisms having to do with the balance between factors in the lung that injure it and those that protect it, and how that balance may be shifted in individual smokers, either by virtue of genetics or aspects of smoking, toward destruction rather than susceptibility. It is the subject of a great deal of research.

DR. HEADEN: The next Surgeon General's report will be on smoking and tobacco use among ethnic minorities. I want to remind the group that some smoking patterns among ethnic minorities, particularly African-Americans, differ substantially from smoking patterns of whites. For example, African-Americans have extremely low daily rates of smoking, but they smoke very high tar and nicotine cigarettes. Thus, it suggests that perhaps we need some new data, oversampling for African-Americans and perhaps other ethnic groups, particularly males, to find out what the relationships would be for these subgroups.

DR. SAMET: I would certainly agree.

REFERENCES

Auerbach, O., Hammond, C., Garfinkel, L. Changes in bronchial in relation to cigarette smoking, 1955-1960 vs. 1970-1977. *New England Journal of Medicine* 300: 381-386, 1979.

Doll, R., Hill, A.B. Smoking and carcinoma of the lung. *British Medical Journal* 2: 739-748, 1950.

Gilliland, F.D., Samet, J.M. Incidence and mortality for lung cancer: Geographic, histologic, and diagnostic trends. *Cancer Surveys* 19: 175-195, 1994.

Hammond, E.C., Garfinkel, L., Seidman, H., Lew, E.A. Tar and nicotine content of cigarette smoke in relation to death rates. *Environmental Research* 12(3): 263-274, 1976.

Higenbottam, T., Clark, T.J., Shipley, M.J., Rose, G. Lung function and symptoms of cigarette smokers related to tar yield and number of cigarettes smoked. *The Lancet* 1(8165): 409-411, 1980.

Kaufman, D.W., Helmrich, S.P., Rosenberg, L., Miettinen, O.S., Shapiro, S. Nicotine and carbon monoxide content of cigarette smoke and the risk of myocardial infarction in young men. *New England Journal of Medicine* 308(8): 409-413, 1983.

Kaufman, D.W., Palmer, J.R., Rosenberg, L., Stolley, P., Warshaver, E., Shapiro, S. Tar content of cigarettes in relation to lung cancer. *American Journal of Epidemiology* 129(4): 703-711, 1989.

Lubin, J.H., Blot, W.J., Berrino, F., Flamant, R., Gillis, C.R., Kunze, M., Schmahl, D., Visco, G. Patterns of lung cancer risk according to type of cigarette smoked. *International Journal of Cancer* 33(5): 569-576, 1984.

National Research Council, Committee on Advances in Assessing Human Exposure to Airborne Pollutants. *Human Exposure Assessment for Airborne Pollutants.* Washington, DC: National Academy Press, 1991.

Palmer, J.R., Rosenberg, L., Shapiro, S. "Low yield" cigarettes and the risk of nonfatal myocardial infarction in women. *New England Journal of Medicine* 320: 1569-1573, 1989.

Pathak, D.R., Samet, J.M., Humble, C.G., Skipper, B.J. Determinants of lung cancer risk in cigarette smokers in New Mexico. *Journal of the National Cancer Institute* 76(4): 597-604, 1986.

Petitti, D.B., Friedman, G.D. Respiratory morbidity in smokers of low- and high-yield cigarettes. *Preventive Medicine* 14: 217-225, 1985a.

Petitti, D.B., Friedman, G.D. Cardiovascular and other diseases in smokers of low yield cigarettes. *Journal of Chronic Disease* 38: 581-588, 1985b.

Rimpela, A., Teperi, J. Respiratory symptoms and low tar cigarette smoking—a longitudinal study on young people. *Scandinavian Journal of Social Medicine* 17: 151-156, 1989.

Rothman, K.J. *Modern Epidemiology.* Boston, MA: Little, Brown and Company, 1986.

Schenker, M.B., Samet, J.M., Speizer, F.E. Effect of cigarette tar content and smoking habits on respiratory symptoms in women. *American Review of Respiratory Disease* 125: 684-690, 1982.

Sherman, C.B., Tollerud, D.J., Heffner, L.J., Speizer, F.E., Weiss, S.T. Airway responsiveness in young black and white women. *American Review of Respiratory Disease* 148(1): 98-102, 1993.

Sparrow, D., Stefos, T., Bosse, R., Weiss, S.T. The relationship of tar content to decline in pulmonary function in cigarette smokers. *American Review of Respiratory Disease* 127(1): 56-58, 1983.

U.S. Department of Health and Human Services. *The Health Consequences of Smoking: The Changing Cigarette. A Report of the Surgeon General.* DHHS Publication No. (PHS) 81-50156. Rockville, MD: U.S. Department of Health and Human Services, Public Health Service, Centers for Disease Control, Office on Smoking and Health, 1981.

U.S. Department of Health and Human Services. *The Health Consequences of Smoking: Chronic Obstructive Lung Disease. A Report of the Surgeon General.* DHHS Publication No. (PHS) 84-50205. Rockville, MD: U.S. Department of Health and Human Services, Public Health Service, Centers for Disease Control, Office on Smoking and Health, 1984.

U.S. Department of Health and Human Services. *Reducing the Health Consequences of Smoking: 25 Years of Progress. A Report of the Surgeon General.* DHHS Publication No. (CDC) 89-8411. Rockville, MD: U.S. Department of Health and Human Services, Public Health Service, Centers for Disease Control, Centers for Chronic Disease Prevention and Health Promotion, Office on Smoking and Health, 1989.

U.S. Department of Health and Human Services. *The Health Benefits of Smoking Cessation. A Report of the Surgeon General.* DHHS Publication No. (CDC) 90-8416. Rockville, MD: U.S. Department of Health and Human Services, Public Health Service, Centers for Disease Control, Centers for Chronic Disease Prevention and Health Promotion, Office on Smoking and Health, 1990.

U.S. Department of Health and Human Services. *Strategies To Control Tobacco Use In the United States: a blueprint for public health action in the 1990's*, D.M. Burns, J.M. Samet, and E.R. Gritz (Editors). NIH Publication No. 92-3316. Rockville, MD: U.S. Department of Health and Human Services, Public Health Service, National Institutes of Health, National Cancer Institute, 1991.

Vineis, P., Caporaso, N. Tobacco and cancer: Epidemiology and the laboratory. *Environmental Health Perspectives* 103(2): 156-160, 1995.

Wilcox, H.B., Schoenberg, J.B., Mason, T.J., Bill, J.S., Stemhagen, A. Smoking and lung cancer: Risk as a function of cigarette tar content. *Preventive Medicine* 17(3): 263-272, 1988.

Withey, C.H., Papacosta, A.O., Swan, A.V., Fitzsimons, B.A., Burney, P.G., Colley, J.R., Holland, W.W. Respiratory effects of lowering tar and nicotine levels of cigarettes smoked by young male middle tar smokers. I. Design of a randomised controlled trial. *Journal of Epidemiology and Community Health* 46(3): 274-280, 1992a.

Withey, C.H., Papacosta, A.O., Swan, A.V., Fitzsimons, B.A., Ellard, G.A., Burney, D.G., Colley, J.R., Holland, W.W. Respiratory effects of lowering tar and nicotine levels of cigarettes smoked by young male middle tar smokers. II. Results of a randomised controlled trial. *Journal of Epidemiology and Community Health* 46(3): 281-285, 1992b.

World Health Organization. *Tobacco Smoking. IARC Monographs on the Evaluation of the Carcinogenic Risk of Chemicals to Humans.* Lyon, France: International Agency for Research on Cancer, 1986.

Wynder, E.L., Graham, E.A. Tobacco smoking as a possible etiologic factor in bronchiogenic carcinoma. A study of six hundred and eighty-four proved cases. *Journal of the American Medical Association* 143: 329-346, 1950.

Wynder, E.L., Kabat, G.C. The effect of low-yield cigarette smoking on lung cancer risk. *Cancer* 62: 1223-1230, 1988.

Wynder, E.L., Mabuchi, K., Beattie, E.J. The epidemiology of lung cancer. Recent trends. *Journal of the American Medical Association* 213: 2221-2228, 1970.

Biomarkers of Cigarette Smoking

Neal L. Benowitz

INTRODUCTION   This chapter addresses the following question: To what extent do smoking-machine-derived tar, nicotine, and carbon monoxide ratings of cigarettes predict how much of those substances smokers actually absorb into their bodies?

Two issues need to be clarified. First is the difference between delivery and content: What a cigarette delivers to the smoker is not the same as what is present in the cigarette tobacco. Second is the issue of compensation vs. regulation or titration: Kozlowski and Pillitterri (this volume) focus on compensation—the individual's smoking behavioral response to a change in a cigarette brand; this chapter focuses on cigarettes that people have self-selected to smoke. Whether behavioral adjustment to nicotine yields indicates regulation or titration or compensation is not important. What is important is the relationship between what people choose to smoke and their intake of various tobacco-derived toxins.

USE OF VARIOUS BIOMARKERS   The biomarkers most widely used to quantitate exposure to tobacco smoke include nicotine, its metabolite cotinine, carbon monoxide, and with less success, thiocyanate. Recent investigation has focused on various hemoglobin and DNA (deoxyribonucleic acid) adducts and excretion of nitrosamines in the urine. These latter measures represent important future directions, but there are inadequate data in large enough populations to make conclusions about the relationship between these measures and U.S. Federal Trade Commission (FTC) yields. The use of mutagenic activity of the urine is discussed to address the utility of the tar-to-nicotine ratio that is computed from the "FTC method" in predicting relative human exposure to tar and nicotine. This is an important consideration in estimating human risks from different types of cigarettes.

NICOTINE ABSORPTION FROM CIGARETTES   Nicotine is rapidly absorbed from cigarettes. It enters arterial circulation first, then venous circulation; nicotine levels then fall relatively quickly as it is redistributed from the bloodstream to various body tissues. Subsequently, nicotine levels fall off with an elimination half-life of about 2 hours (Benowitz, 1988).

The intake of nicotine from a single cigarette can be approximated by measuring the nicotine blood concentration profile after a person smokes a single cigarette. The area under the plasma concentration-time curve is a reflection of systemic dose. The 24-hour nicotine consumption also can be estimated. Volunteer smokers have been studied smoking cigarettes on a research ward, where blood levels could be sampled frequently. Blood levels rise with smoking in the morning, more or less plateau through the latter part of the day, and then fall overnight (Benowitz and Jacob, 1984a). Carbon monoxide levels also build up during the day, plateau, and then fall overnight. By sampling blood periodically throughout the day for measurement of nicotine levels, it is possible to estimate daily exposure to nicotine in human smokers.

The metabolic disposition of nicotine in humans has been determined based on urine-recovery studies plus infusion studies of nicotine and cotinine (Figure 1) (Benowitz et al., 1994). On average, about 70 to 80 percent of nicotine is converted to cotinine, which is the main proximate metabolite. Most studies of nicotine intake from cigarettes producing different yields have used cotinine as the marker of nicotine intake. Cotinine is extensively metabolized, primarily to *trans*-3'-hydroxycotinine. Nicotine, cotinine, and hydroxycotinine also are conjugated as glucuronides. In the urine, a relatively small amount of cotinine is excreted unchanged compared with the total amount generated. However, in general, urine cotinine is well correlated with plasma cotinine so that urine cotinine can be used as a surrogate for plasma cotinine concentration (Jarvis et al., 1984). Saliva cotinine also is highly correlated with plasma cotinine and has been used in the same way.

Plasma cotinine levels fluctuate somewhat throughout the day. There is about a 15-percent change in cotinine levels from morning to night,

Figure 1

Quantitative scheme of nicotine metabolism, based on average excretion of metabolites as percentage of systemic dose during transdermal nicotine application

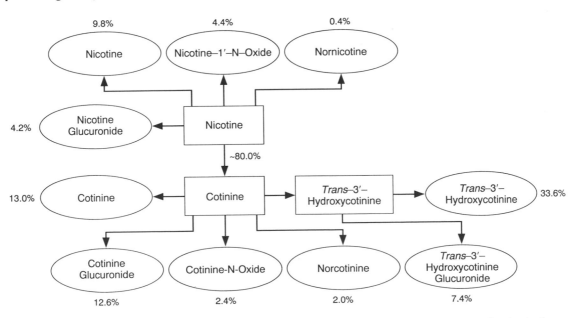

Note: *Compounds in ovals indicate excretion in urine, and associated numbers indicate percentage of systemic dose of nicotine.*

Source: *Benowitz et al., 1994.*

reflecting the approximately 16-hour half-life of cotinine (Benowitz et al., 1983a). Because of the relatively small circadian variation, cotinine levels can be measured at various times of the day, and this value can be used as representative of the average daily cotinine level.

It is possible, by measuring all the metabolites in the urine, to account for an average of 90 percent of the nicotine dose (Benowitz et al., 1994). An approach to estimating nicotine consumption is to measure all the metabolites in the urine and sum them up. At steady state (where the rates of intake of drug and generation of metabolism are the same as rates of elimination of drug and metabolites), this sum of all metabolites in a 24-hour urine excretion reflects the amount of nicotine that a person takes in each day.

NICOTINE CONTENT OF TOBACCO VS. FTC YIELD As noted earlier, cigarette content is not the same as cigarette yield or delivery. Figure 2 shows data from a 1983 study (Benowitz et al., 1983b) that investigated the nicotine content of tobacco. The nicotine concentration of tobacco averaged 1.6 percent. There was no relationship between nicotine content in the whole tobacco rod and the FTC-predicted nicotine yield. There was a significant inverse relationship between the concentration of nicotine and the FTC nicotine yield. Thus, the yield as measured by smoking machine gives no information whatsoever about the content of nicotine or other potential toxins in the tobacco. The content of nicotine in the tobacco simply represents the ultimate limit of the nicotine dose. The FTC method provides no information about the amount of nicotine that could be obtained from the tobacco if a person smoked it in a way to optimize intake.

QUANTITATING NICOTINE INTAKE IN SMOKERS There are four general methods for quantitating the intake of nicotine from tobacco: (1) In circadian fashion, measure blood nicotine levels during cigarette smoking (Benowitz and Jacob, 1984a and 1984b). If the clearance of nicotine also is measured by intravenous infusion of nicotine, blood levels during smoking can be converted to an absolute daily dose of nicotine. (2) The same can be done with blood level data after a person has smoked one or two cigarettes (Benowitz et al., 1991). (3) Blood cotinine levels during ad libitum cigarette smoking have been used widely to estimate nicotine intake, which is discussed below. (4) Finally, as mentioned by Byrd and colleagues (1995), measuring urine nicotine and metabolites during ad libitum smoking can be used to estimate nicotine intake. These four ways can be used to address the question of how much nicotine is being taken into the body from smoking.

Table 1 presents a summary of data on the dose per cigarette from the first three methods. The first method was used to study 44 smokers, measuring blood levels during 24 hours of smoking, at steady state (Benowitz and Jacob, 1984a, 1984b, and 1985). The dose was estimated to be about 1 mg per cigarette, with a range of 0.37 to 1.60 mg per cigarette.

Figure 2
Nicotine content of cigarettes as compared with FTC-determined values (regression analysis)

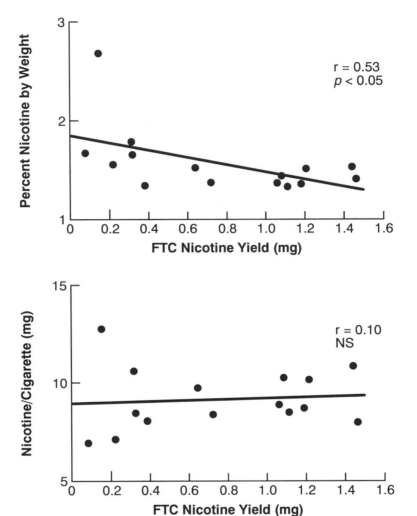

Note: "Nicotine intake per cigarette (mg)" indicates total amount of nicotine in the length of cigarette tobacco rod smoked in the standard FTC smoking machine assay.

Key: NS = not significant.

Source: Benowitz et al., 1983b.

The second method is based on studies of persons smoking one or two cigarettes (Benowitz et al., 1994). This method produced an average dose of 2.3 mg per cigarette, with a range of 0.37 to 3.47 mg. The study paradigm was one in which smokers were deprived overnight and given only one or two cigarettes to smoke in the morning. These were the only cigarettes allowed all day. The unusually high dose per cigarette most likely reflected

Table 1
Summary of absolute bioavailability of nicotine from cigarette smoking studies

| Method | N | Systemic Dose (mg/cigarette) | | | Reference |
		Average	Standard Deviation	Range	
1	22	1.04	0.36	0.37-1.60	Benowitz and Jacob, 1984a
	11	1.00	0.15	0.87-1.48	Benowitz and Jacob, 1984b
	11	0.90	0.15	—	Benowitz and Jacob, 1985
2	10	2.29	1.00	0.37-3.47	Benowitz et al., 1991
3	20	0.87	0.41	0.22-1.92	Benowitz and Jacob, 1994

the smokers' anticipation of no more cigarettes becoming available that day. This finding illustrates the tremendous range of nicotine intake a smoker has when there is a need, or an anticipated need, for nicotine. The intake of nicotine per cigarette in this study was double that typically consumed from ad libitum daily smoking. Consistent with this observation was another study in which subjects tripled their intake of nicotine per cigarette by smoking more intensely when the number of cigarettes allowed to be smoked per day was limited (Benowitz et al., 1986a).

The third method, that is, measuring blood cotinine concentrations, resulted in an estimated dose of about 0.9 mg of nicotine per cigarette, with a range of 0.22 to 1.92 mg per cigarette (Benowitz and Jacob, 1994). What is the quantitative relationship between nicotine intake and yield? Figure 3 shows nicotine intake data from volunteer smokers studied whose plasma nicotine levels were measured while they smoked their usual brand of cigarettes ad libitum while in a research ward (Benowitz and Jacob, 1984a). There was no correlation between the FTC-measured nicotine yield and study-measured intake of nicotine. The only yield that turned out to be accurate was 1 mg, which is fortuitous because it represents the average consumption. Also, most smokers of nonfiltered cigarettes took in less nicotine than predicted from the FTC yield. People who smoked low-yield cigarettes took in, on average, more nicotine than predicted by FTC yield. It is possible that in the 1940's and 1950's, when people smoked cigarettes with a nominal yield of 2.5 mg or higher of nicotine, they may in fact have been undersmoking those cigarettes and taking in considerably less smoke per cigarette than they do now. That behavior might explain the change in lung cancer pathology over the years. That is, a change in depth of inhaling and intensity of smoking may affect the location of the lung tumor.

Figure 3

Regression analysis of relationship between nicotine intake per cigarette and machine-determined nicotine yield

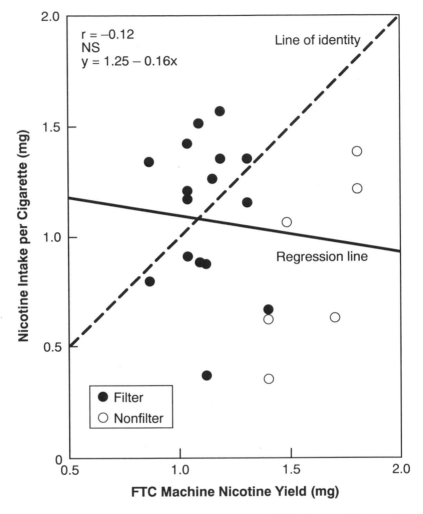

Key: *solid line = regression line; broken line = line of identity, which indicates points at which measured nicotine intake per cigarette equals machine-determined nicotine yield; NS = not significant.*

Source: *Benowitz and Jacob, 1984a.*

COTININE LEVELS AND NICOTINE INTAKE   What is the quantitative relationship between cotinine levels and the intake of nicotine from smoking? To address this question, dual infusions of deuterium-labeled nicotine and cotinine were given to smokers (Benowitz and Jacob, 1994). From resultant blood level data, it was possible to calculate the percentage of nicotine that is converted to cotinine and the clearance of cotinine per se. From these parameters can be derived a factor (K) that relates a given blood level of cotinine at steady state to a given daily intake of nicotine, a factor that averages 0.08. Thus, for a typical smoker with a level of 300 ng/mL, nicotine intake is estimated to be 24 mg per day. Based on average cigarette consumption, that represents an intake of about 1 mg of nicotine per cigarette. This K factor did not vary as a function of whether a person was a smoker or nonsmoker, brands of cigarette smoked, or gender. Thus, the author is aware of no bias in using this K factor to estimate the dose of nicotine based on a plasma cotinine concentration.

Data from a study of 136 smokers entering a smoking cessation program are shown in Figure 4 (Benowitz et al., 1983b). There was a weak relationship between FTC yield and cotinine level. The slope of this relationship was shallow and, in this study, not significant. From the lowest to the highest yield of cigarettes, there was only a 5- to 10-percent change in cotinine level, reflecting a 5- to 10-percent change in nicotine intake. There was a much stronger correlation between cigarettes per day and cotinine level (or nicotine intake). Thus, the greater the number of cigarettes a person smokes, the more nicotine is taken in. This is important because some studies, such as that of Rosa and colleagues (1992), purport to show a strong relationship between

Figure 4

Afternoon blood cotinine concentrations (Group 1) as compared by regression analysis with the number of cigarettes smoked per day (Panel A) and with the FTC-determined nicotine values (Panel B)

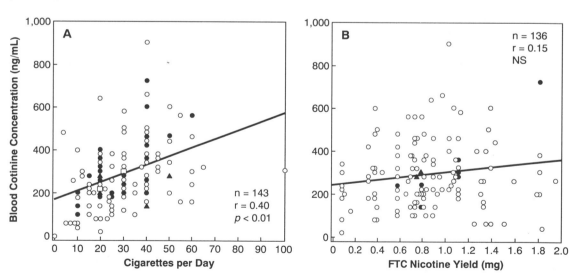

Note: *These smokers' values were so similar that plots of individual values overlapped. The total number of subjects shown in Panel B is lower because data for a few subjects were incomplete. Morning blood cotinine concentrations (Group 2, not shown) were on average slightly lower but had similar correlations with the number of cigarettes (r = 0.45) and the FTC yield (r = 0.06).*

Key: *NS = not significant; ○ = 1 observation; ● = 2 observations; ▲ = 3 observations; □ = 4 observations.*

Source: *Benowitz et al., 1983b.*

predicted nicotine intake and cotinine levels. But nicotine intake was calculated by Rosa and colleagues as the multiple of cigarettes per day times FTC yield. The strength of the relationship between this hybrid parameter and FTC yield derives primarily from the cigarettes-per-day term rather than from the FTC-yield term.

Figure 5 presents data by Gori and Lynch (1985) based on a population of more than 800 smokers recruited at shopping malls. These were not smokers who were trying to stop smoking. Plasma cotinine and nicotine concentrations were measured. The average cotinine concentration was about 300 ng/mL. Again, there was only a shallow slope in the relationship between FTC nicotine and cotinine level, with little difference in cotinine level comparing the lowest and the highest FTC nicotine yields.

Figure 5

Mean plasma nicotine and cotinine concentrations as a fraction of FTC nicotine yield of cigarettes smoked: n = 865

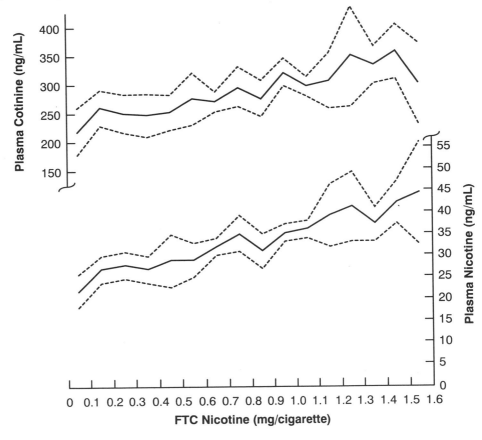

Key: *solid line = mean; broken line = 95-percent confidence intervals.*

Source: *Gori and Lynch, 1985.*

ULTRALOW-YIELD CIGARETTES   Yields from the ultralow cigarette may differ from yields from other cigarettes. Figure 6 shows data from another study of smokers of cigarettes of different yields compared by category of FTC nicotine (Benowitz et al., 1986b). The high-yield category was 1.0 mg of nicotine or higher; the low was 0.60 to 0.99 mg; the very low was 0.20 to 0.59 mg; and the ultralow was less than 0.20 mg nicotine per cigarette by FTC method.

Figure 6

Expired carbon monoxide, plasma thiocyanate, blood nicotine, and cotinine concentrations in 248 habitual smokers of cigarettes according to FTC yield

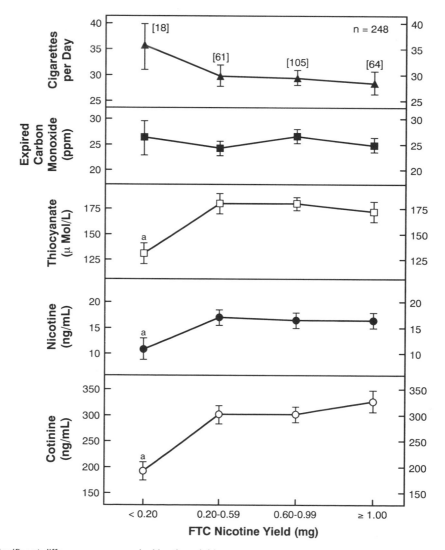

[a] *Significant difference compared with other yields.*

Key: ppm = parts per million.

Source: Benowitz et al., 1986b.

101

The ultralow cigarettes are typically rated 1 mg of tar or less. Smokers of ultralow-yield cigarettes smoked on average a few more cigarettes per day than other smokers. This appears to be one way in which these smokers are compensating for lower nicotine yields. Of note, carbon monoxide levels were similar for all yields. Thiocyanate, nicotine, and cotinine levels were the same for smokers of cigarettes with nicotine yields of 0.20 mg and higher. Only in the ultralow group was there any reduction in nicotine exposure, about 30 percent. Thus, cotinine levels produced by smoking ultralow-yield cigarettes, instead of averaging 300 ng/mL, averaged about 200 ng/mL. Gori and Lynch (1983) presented similar findings in a larger group of smokers. Smokers of the low-yield cigarette brand had the same mean cotinine levels as smokers of all other cigarette brands. In contrast, smokers of ultralow-yield cigarettes had lower cotinine levels, averaging about 200 ng/mL. Note that 200 ng/mL still corresponds to a daily intake of 16 mg of nicotine per day. If the FTC yield of 0.1 mg nicotine per cigarette were correct, one would need to smoke 160 cigarettes per day to achieve an intake of 16 mg. These smokers were not smoking 160 cigarettes per day. Thus, the FTC information on the ultralow-yield cigarette does not provide meaningful quantitative information, although there may be a difference between the ultralow- and higher yield cigarettes.

NICOTINE INTAKE AND MACHINE-DETERMINED YIELD Table 2 provides a summary of several studies of nicotine intake vs. machine-derived yields. These are studies that have examined the relationship between FTC machine yield and nicotine intake measured either by cotinine concentrations or by nicotine concentration. Rickert and Robinson (1981) reported plasma cotinine concentrations vs. machine nicotine yield and found no relationship. Russell and coworkers (1980) studied 330 subjects and found a weak relationship between plasma nicotine concentration and yield. Benowitz and colleagues (1983b) studied 272 smokers interested in smoking cessation and found no significant relationship between plasma cotinine and yield. Ebert and coworkers (1983) found a shallow relationship between plasma nicotine and yield. Gori and Lynch (1985) found a very shallow slope with 865 subjects but also found significant relationships because of the large number of subjects. In a study by Benowitz and colleagues (1986b), cotinine concentrations were virtually the same for any cigarette with a yield of 0.2 mg and more and were a third less for the ultralow cigarettes. In a study by Russell and coworkers (1986), the 392 smokers studied showed a shallow relationship between cotinine level and nicotine yield. Rosa and colleagues (1992) found a shallow slope relating cotinine level vs. FTC yield, similar to that of other studies. However, when Rosa and coworkers (1992) combined cigarettes per day times FTC yield, they found a strong relationship, which they interpreted as supporting the utility of the machine test method. In 298 Hispanics, Coultas and coworkers (1993) showed findings similar to those of the other studies.

The Byrd and colleagues study (1995) was the only study with different results: thirty-three volunteers were asked to provide 24-hour urine samples in which nicotine and metabolites were measured. The nicotine intake was

Table 2
Studies of nicotine intake compared with machine nicotine yield

Study	Population	Nicotine Yields (mg)	Results
Rickert and Robinson, 1981	84 during routine medical exams	0.25-1.3	PCOT vs. Mach-N r = 0.08
Russell et al., 1980	330 from smokers' clinics or research volunteers	0.5-3.5	PNIC vs. Mach-N r = 0.21[a]
Benowitz et al., 1983b	272 seeking smoking cessation therapy	<0.1-1.9	BCOT vs. FTC-N r = 0.15 (n = 137) r = 0.06 (n = 123)
Ebert et al., 1983	76—mix of smoking cessation, hospital employees, ambulatory patients	0.1-1.5	PNIC vs. FTC-N r = 0.25[a]
Gori and Lynch, 1985	865 recruited from shopping malls; 10 or more cigarettes per day	0.1-1.6	PNIC vs. FTC-N r = 0.37[a] PCOT vs. FTC-N r = 0.23[a]
Benowitz et al., 1986b	248 seeking smoking cessation (137 from previous study)	0.1-1.9	BCOT values similar for FTC-N 0.21 to > 1.0 BCOT 2/3 of others for FTC-N < 0.20
Russell et al., 1986	392 from smokers' clinics	—	BCOT vs. Mach-N r = 0.13[a] BNIC vs. Mach-N r = 0.26[a]
Rosa et al., 1992	125 attending military medical center	0.38-1.38	BCOT vs. Mach-N r = 0.30
Coultas et al., 1993	298 from Hispanic household survey	—	SCOT vs. FTC-N r = 0.12
Byrd et al., 1995	33 volunteers	0.13-1.3	Urine N + metabolites vs. FTC-N N/24 hr: r = 0.68[a] N/cig: r = 0.79[a]

[a] $p < 0.05$.

Key: PCOT = plasma cotinine concentration; Mach-N = smoking-machine-determined nicotine yield; PNIC = plasma nicotine concentration; BCOT = blood cotinine concentration; FTC-N = machine yield by FTC method; BNIC = blood nicotine concentration; SCOT = saliva cotinine concentration; N = nicotine.

taken on the basis of total recovery. This study found a strong relationship between yield and nicotine intake per cigarette per day that was totally different from any other study's findings. There are serious methodological concerns that might affect these conclusions. First, there were only 33 subjects, and recruitment procedures were unclear. In contrast, data already presented involving 2,000 individuals have shown a weak or no relationship between cotinine and FTC nicotine yields, so there is a problem of generalizability of the Byrd data. Second, an examination of particular data in the 1-mg tar group results in an average intake of 9 mg nicotine. However, the studies of Gori and Lynch (1985) and Benowitz and colleagues (1986b) showed an average cotinine concentration of 200 ng/mL for large groups of smokers of the same ultralow-yield cigarettes. A cotinine level of 200 ng/mL would correspond to an average daily intake of 15 or 16 mg, not the 9 mg reported by Byrd and colleagues (1995). Thus, even if only one group is studied, the subjects are not representative of the much larger numbers of subjects that have been studied by other investigators.

CARBON MONOXIDE AND FTC YIELD   Gori and Lynch (1985) have provided data on carbon monoxide levels in a large group of smokers of cigarettes of different yields (Figure 7). Their study and other studies have found virtually no relationship between carbon monoxide levels and FTC yields, even for the ultralow group. Thus, FTC carbon monoxide yield appears to be of no value in predicting human carbon monoxide exposure.

TAR-TO-NICOTINE RATIO   The tar-to-nicotine ratio also must be considered. Some authors have argued that even if there is only a small reduction of nicotine, because the machine tar-to-nicotine ratios are lower for low-yield cigarettes, there is a disproportionately greater overall health benefit due to reduced tar exposure (Russell et al., 1986). The question is whether machine-determined tar-to-nicotine ratios predict ratios of exposure in human smokers.

The author attempted to examine this question by studying mutagenic activity of urine by Ames test. This test involves culturing salmonella bacteria that are unable to generate histidine and therefore cannot grow. However, if the bacteria are mutated so that they can make histidine, they can grow. Growth can be quantitated by the number of colonies on a culture plate, and the number of colonies can be used as a measure of mutagenic activity of chemicals that were added to the salmonella culture before incubation. It is well known that the urine of cigarette smokers is mutagenic, presumably reflecting exposure to chemicals found primarily in cigarette smoke tar (Yamasaki and Ames, 1977).

Figure 8 shows urine mutagenicity data from one individual smoking his or her own brand of cigarettes who switched to a Camel (1 mg nicotine) cigarette, then switched to a True (0.4 mg nicotine) cigarette, and followed with a period of no smoking (abstinence). Urine mutagenicity was fairly stable for the individual, and there was no difference between smoking the Camel and True cigarettes.

Figure 7
Mean expired air carbon monoxide values as a function of FTC carbon monoxide yield of cigarettes smoked

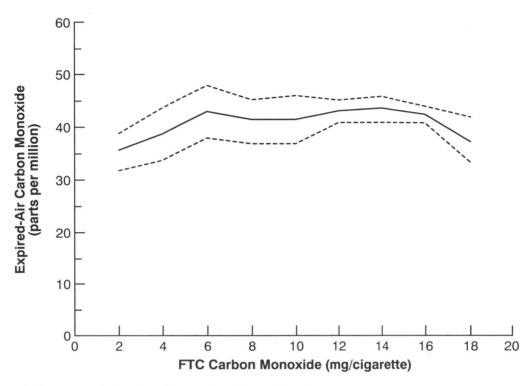

Key: solid line = mean; broken line = 95-percent confidence intervals.

Source: Gori and Lynch, 1985.

Figure 9 shows data from a crossover study of urine mutagenicity and nicotine intake from smokers smoking their own brand, high-yield (Camel), and low-yield cigarettes (True) (Benowitz et al., 1986b). The mutagenic activity of the urine was lower for both Camel and True compared with the usual brand, most likely because smokers did not like these other brands of cigarettes as much as they liked their own. However, the mutagenicity values for Camel and True were similar. The ratio of mutagenic activity over the 24-hour period under the nicotine plasma concentration-time curve (the latter being an estimate of daily nicotine intake) was used as a surrogate for tar-to-nicotine ratio and was the same in all conditions, although the machine-predicted ratios were 14.8 for smoker's own, 15.1 for Camel, and 11.5 for True. Thus, the in vivo tar-to-nicotine ratio did not correspond to differences in the machine-determined tar-to-nicotine ratios for different brands.

Figure 9 also shows similar data when switching to Carlton, which is an ultralow-yield cigarette. There was a small difference in the ratio of mutagenic

Figure 8

Urinary mutagenicity based on 24-hour urine collections in a habitual smoker smoking his or her own brand, Camel (high-yield), and True (low-yield) cigarettes

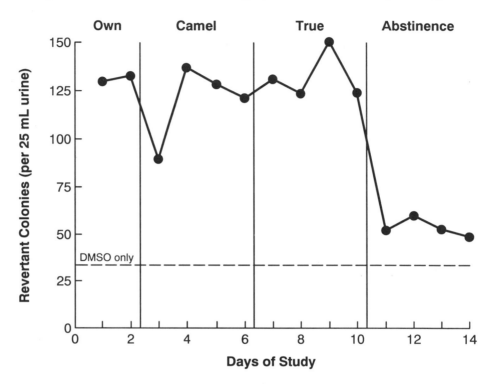

Note: *Mutagenic activity tends to be constant from day to day and falls to the DMSO control value (similar to that of nonsmokers) rapidly after stopping smoking.*

Key: *DMSO = dimethyl sulphoxide.*

Source: *Benowitz, 1989.*

activity to tar for Carlton compared with other cigarettes, but the difference was not near the values of 13.5, 15.4, and 7.3, which were predicted by FTC values.

The data of Rickert and Robinson (1981) shown in Table 3 explain the discrepancy between measured and predicted tar-to-nicotine ratios. These data, based on smoking machine tests, show that when cigarettes are smoked more intensely, the tar-to-nicotine ratio of low-yield cigarettes increases substantially. Thus, when smokers compensate for low-yield cigarettes by smoking them more intensely, the tar-to-nicotine ratio increases. Therefore, tar-to-nicotine ratios published by the FTC method cannot be used to make estimates of what the overall tar exposure will be for actual smokers.

CONCLUSIONS   The suggestion that there is a meaningful quantitative relationship between FTC-measured yields and actual intake is misleading. There do appear to be differences in nicotine exposure comparing high- vs. low-yield

Figure 9
Average urine mutagenicity and ratio of mutagenic activity to nicotine exposure for subjects in high-low yield (Group 1) and high-ultralow yield (Group 2) studies

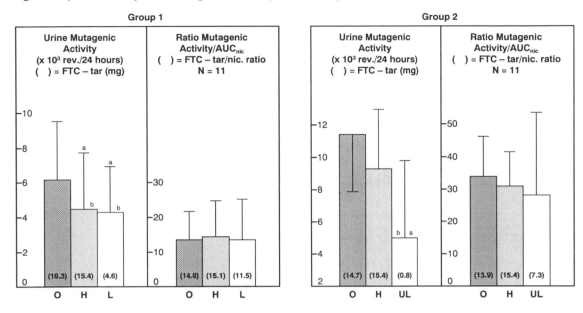

[a] *Indicates significant difference (p < .05, repeated measures analysis of variance) compared with own brand.*
[b] *Indicates significant difference compared with high-yield cigarettes.*

Note: Despite lower ratios of tar and nicotine based on FTC testing for low- and ultralow-yield cigarettes, ratios of mutagenic activity to nicotine exposure were not different while subjects smoked high-, low-, or ultralow-yield cigarettes. Also, bars indicate standard error of the mean.

Key: AUC_{nic} = ratio of mutagenic activity to nicotine exposure; rev = revertant colonies; nic = nicotine; O = smoker's own brand; H = high-yield cigarettes (Camel); L = low-yield cigarettes (True); UL = ultralow-yield cigarettes (Cambridge or Carlton).

Source: Benowitz et al., 1986b.

Table 3
Influence of intensity of smoking on tar-to-nicotine ratio, based on smoking machine studies

Group	N	Standard Yield (mg)		Tar-to-Nicotine Ratio Under Different Smoking Conditions		
		Tar	Nicotine	Standard	Moderate	Intensive
I	4	< 2	< 2	9.2	9.9	11.1[a]
II	10	2 - 5	0.2 - 0.5	10.3	11.7[a]	12.2[a]
III	8	5 - 10	0.5 - 0.9	11.3	11.9	12.6[a]
IV	9	10 - 14	0.8 - 1.0	12.7	13.3[a]	12.4
V	5	14 - 17	0.9 - 1.0	15.7	16.5[a]	14.7

[a] *p < 0.05 compared with standard smoking machine conditions.*

Key: N = number of brands tested.

Source: Rickert et al., 1983.

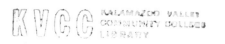

cigarettes, but the differences are small and not quantitatively proportional to nominal yield. Tar and nicotine ratings are poor predictors of human intake, except for those cigarettes that happen to be rated by smoking machines as 1 mg nicotine per cigarette, in which case that rating fortuitously fits the population average. Tobacco manufacturers have stated that the FTC method was never intended to measure intake in any individual. The author agrees. However, data for 2,000 people summarized here indicate that the FTC method does not work for the general population of smokers either.

In general, the FTC method underestimates human exposure. Smoking-machine-derived tar-to-nicotine ratios, which have been used to argue the benefit of switching to low-yield cigarettes, are not of value because these ratios change with changes in smoking behavior. On the other hand, because there is some relationship between yields and nicotine, and although the slope of that relationship is shallow, it is not recommended that smokers regress to smoking higher yield cigarettes.

QUESTION-AND-ANSWER SESSION

DR. RICKERT: When we first looked at this back in 1981, there was absolutely no relationship between yields and uptake as measured by cotinine. And then, as you follow the studies from 1981 through to 1994, there seems to be a growing tendency toward an association of some sort, and at the end you pointed out there was a shallow slope. Is this just a spurious change with time, or do you feel this may be related to changes in product characteristic because, obviously, the product that was smoked in 1981 is not the product that is smoked in 1994.

DR. BENOWITZ: Yes, when you look at the earlier studies, they show basically the same slope that studies that were done in 1989 and 1990 are showing. So, I think when we have a large enough population, we are probably seeing it even back in the 1980's. Prior to that, I have no idea.

DR. BOCK: Dr. Benowitz, you were quoted as saying something to the effect that compensation over the long term does not appear to be persistent. Is that your opinion?

DR. BENOWITZ: That statement was made in dealing with the question of when people are shifting from one cigarette to a lower yield cigarette, will there be permanent overcompensation? And the only studies that I found (I think Dr. Kozlowski is going to talk about these) looked at carbon monoxide levels and the amount of compensation. At least in one study, carbon monoxide levels went up and then went down again.

But if you look at the issue of compensation broadly, how do you interpret the fact that people smoke a cigarette with an FTC yield of .2 the same as the one that has the FTC nicotine yield of 1.5, and they have the same nicotine cotinine levels? If you do not call it compensation, you have to think of something to call it.

At some point in time, I do think people will be limited by how much smoke they take into their lungs. I do not think it is relevant to modern cigarettes as currently marketed, but it could be relevant to a low-nicotine cigarette.

DR. BOCK: You made a distinction just now and said "overcompensation." Is that what you intend to imply?

DR. BENOWITZ: Yes.

DR. BOCK: Because there is a little bit of a difference between overcompensation and compensation.

DR. BENOWITZ: Yes, I know. It is a good point.

DR. HATSUKAMI: In the studies where you looked at the FTC yield and the actual intake, have any of the studies differentiated people who actually initiated with low-tar and low-nicotine cigarettes and those who switched? Are there any differences in terms of slopes between those two groups of people?

DR. BENOWITZ: I have never seen that, but obviously that is a very interesting question in terms of initiation. The earlier data that we heard from Dr. Giovino suggest that most low-yield cigarette smokers are people who switched from higher yield, which I think is quite interesting. But I do not know the percentage of people who start with low-yield cigarettes. It would be a good question.

DR. DEBETHIZY: Would you say that, on average, the people who smoke lower yielding cigarettes absorb less nicotine?

DR. BENOWITZ: Yes, but the slope is very shallow.

DR. DEBETHIZY: So, if people are smoking very low-yielding cigarettes, they are absorbing less nicotine and the data do speak to that. So, compensation is incomplete; there is not a flat line.

One of the studies that you pointed out up there said that people absorbed, on average, 1 mg of nicotine from cigarettes. And I think that it is important to point out that people who smoke lower yielding cigarettes do absorb less nicotine.

DR. BENOWITZ: Yes, although it is unclear where the break is. Some of our data have suggested that the break is actually with the very, very low-yield cigarettes, rather than the cigarettes most people smoke. But I would accept the fact that there is a shallow relationship. Understand, however, that you are talking about a 10-percent variation in nicotine intake, going across yields from 0.1 to 1.6. So, there is some reduction in nicotine intake per cigarette on average, but it is very small.

DR. DEBETHIZY: The other point I want to make is, you do rightfully point out that I will discuss a little later why our study, which is the Byrd study, may be unique from the plasma cotinine studies, in the fact that it is done with a completely different method and what we think is a more precise method.

DR. WOOSLEY: I think the point you make is that the predictive accuracy of any yield numbers, except at the low end of the scale, is useless, and I think that is the most important message that I got out of your presentation.

The other message I have gotten out of the presentation was that this indicates that the differences in mortality that we saw earlier, which had the potential to be confounded, are very likely to be confounded because of the lack of a difference in exposure that your data indicate.

DR. BENOWITZ: I would certainly agree with that. On the coronary heart disease data, for example, with the low-yield cigarettes, I think you can virtually assume that their exposure to everything was substantially the same. It is no surprise that there is no protective effect of smoking low-yield cigarettes for heart disease.

DR. RICKERT: How relevant do you feel the absorption of nicotine is to the levels of other harmful constituents, such as benzo(*a*)pyrene and biphenyl, which are probably more related to disease processes than nicotine per se?

DR. BENOWITZ: I think there is considerable variability, and one has to look at that issue. I don't think there are enough data to know for the range of products.

REFERENCES

Benowitz, N.L. Pharmacologic aspects of cigarette smoking and nicotine addiction. *New England Journal of Medicine* 319: 1318-1330, 1988.

Benowitz, N.L. Dosimetric studies of compensatory cigarette smoking. In: *Independent Scientific Committee on Smoking and Health: Nicotine, Smoking, and the Low Tar Programme, London, November 18-20, 1986*, N. Wald and P. Froggatt (Editors). Oxford: Oxford University Press, 1989, pp. 133-150.

Benowitz, N.L., Hall, S.H., Herning, R.I., Jacob, P. III, Jones, R.T., Osman, A.-L. Smokers of low-yield cigarettes do not consume less nicotine. *New England Journal of Medicine* 309: 139-142, 1983b.

Benowitz, N.L., Jacob, P. III. Daily intake of nicotine during cigarette smoking. *Clinical Pharmacology and Therapeutics* 35: 499-504, 1984a.

Benowitz, N.L., Jacob, P. III. Nicotine and carbon monoxide intake from high- and low-yield cigarettes. *Clinical Pharmacology and Therapeutics* 36: 265-270, 1984b.

Benowitz, N.L., Jacob, P. III. Nicotine renal excretion rate influences nicotine intake during cigarette smoking. *Journal of Pharmacology and Experimental Therapeutics* 234: 153-155, 1985.

Benowitz, N.L., Jacob, P. III. Metabolism of nicotine to cotinine studied by a dual stable isotope method. *Clinical Pharmacology and Therapeutics* 56(5): 483-493, 1994.

Benowitz, N.L., Jacob, P. III, Denaro, C., Jenkins, R. Stable isotope studies of nicotine kinetics and bioavailability. *Clinical Pharmacology and Therapeutics* 49: 270-277, 1991.

Benowitz, N.L., Jacob, P. III, Fong, I., Gupta, S. Nicotine metabolic profile in man: Comparison of cigarette smoking and transdermal nicotine. *Journal of Pharmacology and Experimental Therapeutics* 268: 296-303, 1994.

Benowitz, N.L., Jacob, P. III, Kozlowski, L.T., Yu, L. Influence of smoking fewer cigarettes on exposure to tar, nicotine, and carbon monoxide. *New England Journal of Medicine* 315: 1310-1313, 1986a.

Benowitz, N.L., Jacob, P. III, Yu, L., Talcott, R., Hall, S., Jones, R.T. Reduced tar, nicotine, and carbon monoxide exposure while smoking ultralow- but not low-yield cigarettes. *Journal of the American Medical Association* 256: 241-246, 1986b.

Benowitz, N.L., Kuyt, F., Jacob, P. III, Jones, R.T., Osman, A.-L. Cotinine disposition and effects. *Clinical Pharmacology and Therapeutics* 34: 604-611, 1983a.

Byrd, G.D., Robinson, J.H., Caldwell, W.S., DeBethizy, J.D. Comparison of measured and FTC-predicted nicotine uptake in smokers. *Psychopharmacology* 122: 95-103, 1995.

Coultas, D.B., Stidley, C.A., Samet, J.M. Cigarette yields of tar and nicotine and markers of exposure to tobacco smoke. *American Review of Respiratory Disease* 148: 435-440, 1993.

Ebert, R.V., McNabb, M.E., McCusker, K.T., Snow, S.L. Amount of nicotine and carbon monoxide inhaled by smokers of low-tar, low-nicotine cigarettes. *Journal of the American Medical Association* 250: 2840-2842, 1983.

Gori, G.B., Lynch, C.J. Smoker intake from cigarettes in the 1 mg Federal Trade Commission tar class. *Regulatory Toxicology and Pharmacology* 3: 110-120, 1983.

Gori, G.B., Lynch, C.J. Analytical cigarette yields as predictors of smoke bioavailability. *Regulatory Toxicology and Pharmacology* 5: 314-326, 1985.

Jarvis, M., Tunstall-Pedoe, H., Feyerabend, C., Vesey, C., Salloojee, Y. Biochemical markers of smoke absorption and self reported exposure to passive smoking. *Journal of Epidemiology and Community Health* 38(4): 335-339, 1984.

Rickert, W.S., Robinson, J.C. Estimating the hazards of less hazardous cigarettes. II. Study of cigarette yields of nicotine, carbon monoxide, and hydrogen cyanide in relation to levels of cotinine, carboxyhemoglobin, and thiocyanate in smokers. *Journal of Toxicology and Environmental Health* 7: 391-403, 1981.

Rickert, W.S., Robinson, J.C., Young, J.C., Collishaw, N.E., Bray, D.F. A comparison of the yields of tar, nicotine, and carbon monoxide of 36 brands of Canadian cigarettes tested under three conditions. *Preventive Medicine* 12: 682-694, 1983.

Rosa, M., Pacifici, R., Altieri, I., Pichini, S., Ottaviani, G., Zuccaro, P. How the steady-state cotinine concentration in cigarette smokers is directly related to nicotine intake. *Clinical Pharmacology and Therapeutics* 52: 324-329, 1992.

Russell, M.A., Jarvis, M.J., Feyerabend, C., Saloojee, Y. Reduction of tar, nicotine and carbon monoxide intake in low tar smokers. *Journal of Epidemiology and Community Health* 40(1): 80-85, 1986.

Russell, M.A.H., Jarvis, M., Iyer, R., Feyerabend, C. Relation of nicotine yield of cigarettes to blood nicotine concentrations in smokers. *British Medical Journal* 5: 972-976, 1980.

Yamasaki, E., Ames, B.N. Concentration of mutagens from urine by absorption with the nonpolar resin XAD-2: Cigarette smokers have mutagenic urine. *Proceedings of the National Academy of Sciences of the United States* 74: 3555-3559, 1977.

ACKNOWLEDGMENTS   This research was supported by grants DA-02277, CA-32389, DA-01696, and RR-00083 from the National Institutes of Health. The author thanks David Greene for editorial assistance.

Pharmacology and Markers: Nicotine Pharmacology and Addictive Effects

Jack E. Henningfield and Leslie M. Schuh

INTRODUCTION   Dosing characteristics of cigarette brands are estimated using machines that smoke representative cigarettes from each brand according to a protocol termed the Federal Trade Commission (FTC) method (Peeler, this volume; Pillsbury, this volume). This technology and methodology provide tar- and nicotine-dosing estimates of cigarettes that are misleading to consumers and do not accurately predict what level of tar and nicotine intake consumers will obtain by smoking a given brand of cigarettes (Henningfield et al., 1994). An understanding of the dependence-producing and other behavior-modifying effects of cigarette smoke is necessary to understand why the FTC method is a poor predictor of the nicotine, tar, and carbon monoxide levels people obtain from cigarettes. Cigarette smoking behavior is influenced by nicotine dose, and smokers tend to maintain nicotine intake within upper and lower boundaries (Kozlowski, 1989). In brief, nicotine produces dose-related tolerance, physical dependence, and discriminative effects (i.e., effects that people can feel, which modify mood and physiology), and smokers change their behavior in response to these effects. Unlike human smokers, machines are not nicotine dependent, nor do they modify their behavior based on the flavor of the smoke.

The FTC method was developed in the 1960's to provide a relative ranking of nicotine, tar, and carbon monoxide yields from various cigarettes (Peeler, this volume; Pillsbury, this volume). This ranking has provided consumers with the false sense that they can tell precisely the amount of these substances they will obtain from a given cigarette. Since the 1960's there have been many advances in the understanding of nicotine and smoking behavior that can be useful in reforming this methodology. This chapter provides an overview of relevant research, including (1) physiological and behavioral pressures to sustain nicotine intake; (2) the relationship between smoking and nicotine dose; (3) determinants of compensatory behavior, including the role of nicotine and other factors, such as flavor; and (4) measurement of smoking and nicotine intake.

CIGARETTE SMOKING AS DRUG DEPENDENCE   Several findings bear on the issue of the strength of dependence on cigarettes. Although 70 to 90 percent of smokers are interested in quitting, only one in three succeeds before age 65 (Fiore, 1992). There is good and bad news about coronary bypass surgery and even a lung removal. The good news is

Addiction Severity   that these traumatic events are among the most powerful incentives to quit smoking. If one intervenes with patients who undergo these procedures, about one-half of them quit. However, the bad news is that the other half or more soon return to smoking (U.S. Department of Health and Human Services, 1988). There are two lessons here. First, incentives and motivation are important factors in the treatment of nicotine and other drug dependencies. Second, incentives and motivation have limitations; even the threat of death is not sufficient for half these smokers to stop smoking.

This is a tenacious addiction in which, despite so many people wanting and trying to quit, fewer than 1 in 10 has a 1-year success, and this means that only 2 to 3 percent of smokers stop smoking each year (Fiore, 1992). Indeed, as Kozlowski and colleagues (1989) show, more than half of heroin and cocaine users and alcoholics rate smoking cigarettes as harder to give up than these other drugs. Thus, there are strong biological pressures in nicotine-dependent humans that do not exist in machines to sustain addictive levels of nicotine intake.

Clinical Characteristics　As with dependence on other drugs, cigarette smoking tends to be a progressive, chronic, relapsing disorder (U.S. Department of Health and Human Services, 1988). The most notable distinction between cigarette smoking and other drug dependencies is that a much higher percentage of people who start smoking escalate and graduate to dependent levels than with other addictive drugs. About 1 in 10 smokers in this country is a low-level smoker, termed a "chipper," who smokes 5 or fewer cigarettes per day (U.S. Department of Health and Human Services, 1988); most of the rest show evidence of dependence. This is in contrast to alcohol use, where 10 to 15 percent of alcohol drinkers are problem drinkers; the rest generally drink in moderation and at times of their own choosing (U.S. Department of Health and Human Services, 1988).

People do not start smoking a pack of cigarettes per day. They likely would become ill at that level of nicotine intake. Rather, they start out with low levels. Over months and years, most people progress to higher and higher nicotine intake. They become tolerant; that is, nicotine loses effectiveness with its continued presence in the body, and it is necessary to increase the dose to maintain its effectiveness after repeated administrations. Eventually, smokers do more than simply tolerate high nicotine doses; they need continued nicotine to feel normal and function satisfactorily. At this point, smokers may go to great lengths to continue smoking and sustain their nicotine intake within upper and lower boundaries so that their intake does not fall low enough that they experience withdrawal symptoms or high enough to produce adverse effects (Kozlowski, 1989).

An important aspect of the chronic nature of tobacco dependence is related to daily patterns of nicotine blood levels. When smokers wake up in the morning, some residual nicotine remains in their blood from smoking on the previous day. Blood concentrations rise as they smoke until, by midafternoon, most smokers' intake equals metabolism and excretion, and nicotine level stabilizes. Levels fall rapidly overnight, and the cycle resumes the next day. Thus, blood concentrations never reach zero unless the person quits smoking for more than a few days. Moreover, cotinine, an active nicotine metabolite, has a half-life of about 20 hours (Cummings and Richard, 1988; Jarvis, 1989; Jarvis et al., 1987) and therefore persists in the body even longer.

It is difficult to disrupt these patterns when people have access to cigarettes. In a study by Benowitz and colleagues (1986a), people switched from 30 to 5 cigarettes per day. Because they tended to smoke these 5 cigarettes much more intensely, they reduced carbon monoxide levels by only one-half and nicotine levels by only about one-third. Thus, nicotine intake remained high enough to sustain dependence.

After quitting smoking, most people relapse quickly, and about one-third of the people who have quit smoking and remained abstinent for 1 year relapse (Fiore, 1992). As with alcohol and heroin, most nicotine relapses occur during the first 3 months of abstinence (Hunt et al., 1971). In fact, the determinants of relapse (e.g., degree of dependence and negative emotional states) and remission (e.g., substance-associated health problems and learning to manage cravings) are also similar across these three classes of drug dependence (U.S. Department of Health and Human Services, 1988).

Relapse to nicotine dependence has been studied in greater detail than relapse to heroin, cocaine, and alcohol dependence. Data from a Mayo Clinic study showed that, with minimal treatment intervention, one-quarter of the people relapsed in 2 days and about one-half in the first week (Kottke et al., 1989). More recent data on people who quit on their own showed that about two-thirds relapse within 3 days (Hughes et al., 1992). The withdrawal syndrome can be debilitating in its own right, but in the long run, its worst health consequences may be that most efforts to quit smoking never survive the withdrawal phase (Hughes et al., 1992), thereby dooming one-half of persistent smokers to die prematurely because of their tobacco use (Peto et al., 1994). Much of the benefit of current nicotine medications is providing adequate nicotine replacement for that formerly provided by cigarettes to help more people remain nonsmokers during the important first few weeks of tobacco abstinence.

NICOTINE DELIVERY SYSTEMS Tobacco products come in many different forms. All have toxicities and dependence potential, and there is variation related to the type of tobacco product and route of administration. Although the focus here is on cigarettes, at some point similar issues must be addressed with other tobacco products that currently have no dosage labeling. For example, moist snuff products vary widely in their nicotine-dosing capabilities, and there is evidence that the variation is accomplished primarily by manipulation of the pH level of the products by tobacco manufacturers (Henningfield et al., 1995; Djordjevic et al., 1995), but neither tobacco companies nor governmental agencies provide any form of nicotine dosage information to consumers except in cigarette advertising.

The cigarette, which may be conceived of as a nicotine dispenser with smoke as the vehicle, is the most toxic and dependence-producing form of nicotine delivery. Nicotine is volatilized at the tip of a burning cigarette from which it is carried by particulate matter (tar droplets) deep into the lungs with inspired air. The nearly 2,000 °F microblast at the cigarette's tip is also the source of carbon monoxide and many other toxicologically significant pyrolysis products. Nicotine is rapidly absorbed in the alveoli of the lungs, concentrated in the pulmonary veins as a bolus, and pumped by the left ventricle of the heart throughout the body. Absorption characteristics are similar to those of gases, such as oxygen, that are exchanged in the lung from inspired air to venous blood (Henningfield et al., 1993). Thus, smoke inhalation produces arterial boli that may be 10 times more concentrated than the levels measured in venous blood (Henningfield et al., 1990 and 1993).

Psychoactive effects have rapid onset and short duration, dissipating within a few minutes. This short duration requires the user to self-administer the drug repeatedly, perhaps taking hundreds of puffs per day. The cigarette allows the smoker very fine, "fingertip," dose control. The powerful engulfing sensory effects are also important in dependence. It is not just the drug but the conditions and the cues that become associated with the drug that make nicotine dependence so tenacious. Finally, the cigarette is a convenient, portable system that permits easily repeated dosing.

Benowitz (this volume) reviewed the pharmacokinetics of various nicotine delivery systems. Briefly, a cigarette produces a rapid spike of nicotine in the arterial blood. Smokeless tobacco products are also rapid, especially the higher pH tobacco products, and they require little practice for the user to achieve high nicotine levels. Whereas the nicotine dose obtained from a cigarette is largely determined by the behavior of the user, the nicotine dose obtained from a "chew" of smokeless tobacco is largely controlled by the product (Henningfield et al., 1995). In contrast to delivery from tobacco products, delivery of nicotine from polacrilex (nicotine gum) is slower and takes a great deal of practice and work to achieve even modest nicotine plasma levels. Transdermal nicotine medications (patches) provide slow absorption—so slow that users cannot reliably detect nicotine's effects. The speed of delivery is clearly an important determinant of addictive effects, and the cigarette, like crack cocaine, provides an explosive dose of nicotine.

NICOTINE'S EFFECTS   Nicotine is a fascinating psychoactive drug. It was used to help map the cholinergic nervous system early in the 20th century. Much of receptor theory and many of the methods used to study competitive agonists and antagonists were developed at the turn of the century using nicotine (Langley, 1905).

Nicotine has diverse effects, not only in the brain but also in the adrenals and skeletal muscles. These diverse effects may explain why a smoker reports that on some occasions cigarettes have relaxing effects and on other occasions, stimulating effects. This has been referred to as a paradoxical effect, but it is not paradoxical at all; other drugs generally referred to either as sedatives or stimulants also produce both sedating and stimulating effects (Gilman et al., 1990). Like the effects of these other drugs, nicotine's effects are complicated; they depend on the dose, the time since dosing, how the drug was administered, which responses are being measured, and other factors (Henningfield and Keenan, 1993; Pomerleau and Rosecrans, 1989).

If people with histories of drug abuse are given nicotine, they like the nicotine; that is, liking scale scores increase with greater doses within a certain range of parameters (Henningfield et al., 1985). Among drug abusers, similar findings are reported for morphine and amphetamines but not for drugs that have little psychoactivity (Fischman and Mello, 1989). Such psychoactive effects are predictive of addiction potential and are correlated with the ability of a drug to serve as a reinforcer for animals and humans (Griffiths et al., 1980). Nicotine is psychoactive in humans and is readily discriminated by animals; several forms of nicotine delivery have been shown to serve as reinforcers for animals and humans (U.S. Department of Health and Human Services, 1988).

Physical Dependence and Withdrawal   The cellular and neurological changes that lead to tolerance also lead to physical dependence so that when people abruptly discontinue tobacco use, withdrawal occurs (U.S. Department of Health and Human Services, 1988). Withdrawal onset begins within a few hours of the last cigarette; symptoms include decreased cognitive capabilities and heart rate and increased dysphoria or depressed mood, insomnia, craving, anxiety, irritability, restlessness, appetite, and tendency to smoke (American Psychiatric Association, 1994; Hughes and Hatsukami, 1992). Altered brain electrical potentials and hormonal output are generally opposite in direction of those produced by acute nicotine administration, and decrements in evoked electrical potentials of the brain indicate impaired information processing capabilities (Pickworth et al., 1989; U.S. Department of Health and Human Services, 1988).

Nicotine dependence seems to be mediated primarily by the activation of nicotinic cholinergic receptors in the brain (U.S. Department of Health and Human Services, 1988) and secondarily through the cascading effects of nicotinic systems to modulate levels of hormones such as epinephrine (adrenaline) and cortisol (Pomerleau and Pomerleau, 1984; U.S. Department of Health and Human Services, 1988). The mesolimbic dopaminergic reward system, which mediates the ability of cocaine to produce dependence, also has been implicated in nicotine dependence (Corrigall, 1991; U.S. Department of Health and Human Services, 1988). The cells of this system are located in the ventral tegmental area of the midbrain. Axons project to the limbic system—specifically, to the nucleus accumbens, olfactory tubercle, nuclei of the stria terminalis, and parts of the amygdala. Behaviors followed by such neural activation can become extremely persistent. Cortical effects of nicotine administration include changes in local cerebral metabolism (London and Morgan, 1993) and electroencephalogram results (Jones, 1987). Prominent endocrine effects include release of catecholamines, serotonin, prolactin, growth hormone, arginine vasopressin, beta-endorphin, and adrenocorticotropic hormone (Pomerleau and Pomerleau, 1984; U.S. Department of Health and Human Services, 1988). These effects mediate both the positive nicotine reinforcement sought by smokers and even

117

animals (Corrigall, 1991; Henningfield and Goldberg, 1983; Pomerleau, 1992; U.S. Department of Health and Human Services, 1988) and the negative reinforcement of withdrawal symptoms that also fuel the compulsion to smoke (Hughes and Hatsukami, 1992; Pomerleau and Pomerleau, 1984). Nicotine also produces increased expression of brain nicotinic receptors in humans and animals (U.S. Department of Health and Human Services, 1988). Taken together, these physiologic effects confirm that nicotine exposure alters the structure and function of the nervous system and leads to modification of behavior. Thus, there are physiological factors that drive smokers to sustain continued nicotine intake across changing delivery systems.

Smokers may report that they feel impaired and distracted after only a few hours of abstinence, and their performance on various cognitive and psychomotor tasks can decline within approximately 4 hours (Heishman et al., 1994). Symptoms are rapidly reversed with resumed smoking or nicotine replacement, thus providing a potentially powerful source of reinforcement for continued smoking. The degree of reversal is generally proportional to the percentage of plasma nicotine that is replaced (Pickworth et al., 1989; U.S. Department of Health and Human Services, 1988).

Data from a performance study indicated that when patients abstained from cigarettes and used placebo gum, they made more errors and took longer to complete a task than during their smoking baseline. When they were given 2 mg gum, their performance returned to baseline. With 4 mg gum, they did not do significantly better than at baseline, but 4 mg appeared to produce somewhat more reliable clinical effects than 2 mg (Snyder and Henningfield, 1989).

The same pattern of effects occurs with theta power, a measure of brain function (Pickworth et al., 1989). This nicotine-withdrawal-induced deficit can be completely reversed with nicotine replacement. When other volunteers resumed smoking, electrocortical potentials recovered quickly in all volunteers. Interestingly, these people did not like the gum, and they were not trying to quit smoking. The lesson is that nicotine replacement can maintain physiological function and cognitive performance. The conclusion relating to performance is not that nicotine makes the user perform better, faster, or more intelligently but that nicotine deprivation results in impairments that are quickly and dose-dependently reversed by nicotine readministration (Heishman et al., 1994).

The nicotine-withdrawal-induced decline in performance has practical ramifications in policy decisions. Currently, the Federal Aviation Administration is examining its policies on smoking by pilots in the flight decks of commercial airlines. Because of the time course of nicotine withdrawal, if smoking were eliminated in the flight deck, acutely deprived pilots might suffer withdrawal-induced performance declines on flights longer than approximately 4 hours. Thus, the nicotine withdrawal syndrome poses a potential safety hazard if it is not rationally addressed by appropriate strategies to detoxify pilots safely and treat their withdrawal symptoms with nicotine replacement medications.

The duration of the nicotine withdrawal syndrome varies across individuals, but on average, the acute physical syndrome is worst during the first month. Gross and Stitzer (1989) studied the time course of the nicotine withdrawal syndrome in detail. In their study, people quit smoking and received either active or placebo nicotine gum. People who received active gum chewed an average of 6.9 pieces of 2 mg gum per day, which provided less nicotine than they were obtaining by smoking cigarettes. People given placebo gum gradually decreased their intake from 6.8 pieces per day during the first week of treatment to 4.9 pieces per day by the 10th week. The nicotine gum substantially reduced withdrawal symptom severity relative to that observed in placebo subjects.

Nicotine's Beneficial Effects Nicotine provides many effects that cigarette smokers may consider useful. These include weight control, mood control, and preventing withdrawal symptoms (U.S. Department of Health and Human Services, 1988). The issue of whether nicotine would provide substantial cognitive enhancement in healthy persons who had never been nicotine dependent is controversial. In nonsmokers, nicotine administration can increase finger-tapping rate and slightly (but significantly in some studies) attenuate the deterioration in attention that occurs during protracted testing (Heishman et al., 1994). However, complex cognitive performance may be impaired by nicotine in cigarette smokers as well as nonsmokers (Heishman et al., 1994). On the other hand, there is no question that nicotine intake restores withdrawal-induced deficits (Snyder and Henningfield, 1989). Nicotine intake also may provide some level of cognitive enhancement in persons who are cognitively impaired by Alzheimer's disease (Heishman et al., 1994; Sahakian et al., 1989; Newhouse and Hughes, 1991).

One of the Brown and Williamson Tobacco Corporation (B&W) documents made available for the National Cancer Institute conference on the FTC cigarette test method also supported the conclusion that nicotine's central nervous system effects contribute to the strong motivation to use tobacco products. The document concluded that

> to understand smoking, just as any other behavior, it is necessary to consider it as a process embedded within everyday life . . . . It is apparent that nicotine largely underpins these contributions through its role as a generator of central physiological arousal effects which express themselves as changes in human performance and psychological well being. (Brown and Williamson, 1984)

SMOKING AND NICOTINE DOSE Nicotine dosage is an important factor in smoking behavior. Currently available cigarettes allow people to fairly easily administer the nicotine dose they need or desire (Henningfield et al., 1994). This was true of a low-content cigarette, NEXT, that was marketed a few years ago and removed from the market following poor sales, even though taste and draw characteristics were similar to conventional cigarettes. With that cigarette, the nicotine content was so low that no amount of compensatory puffing and inhaling could result in the extraction of substantial amounts of nicotine (Butschky et al., 1995).

Compensatory Behavior

Compensation is nicely described in the B&W documents (Brown and Williamson, 1984) as "the tendency for a smoker to obtain similar delivery, intake and uptake of smoke constituents on a daily basis from a variety of products with different standard (machine-smoked) deliveries."

As the B&W researchers noted, if smokers are dependent, then the nicotine they receive from cigarettes can be supplemented by other forms, and this will reduce smoking. Likewise, cigarettes of different strengths are smoked differently; that is, smokers given low-delivery cigarettes smoke them more intensively and vice versa.

In fact, this is what has been found in many studies (U.S. Department of Health and Human Services, 1988). Cigarette consumption increases in response to reduced nicotine, and most compensation occurs at the individual cigarette level, not by cigarettes per day. Whereas people given cigarettes of lower nicotine yield also may smoke a few more cigarettes per day, they smoke each of the cigarettes more intensely to obtain proportionately more nicotine than the rating of nicotine yield would suggest (Hill and Marquardt, 1980; Russell et al., 1980; Benowitz et al., 1983; Robinson et al., 1983).

When people are given nicotine gum and their smoking is measured, smoking decreases as the nicotine gum dose increases (Nemeth-Coslett and Henningfield, 1986). When mecamylamine is administered to antagonize nicotine's effects, people smoke more cigarettes, take more puffs per cigarette, and take in more total smoke, as can be seen by increased carbon monoxide level (Nemeth-Coslett et al., 1986; Rose et al., 1989). Taste and other sensory factors are also important modulators of human smoking behavior (Butschky et al., 1995; Rose and Behm, 1987; U.S. Department of Health and Human Services, 1988).

This finding addresses why the nicotine dependence issue is relevant to why the FTC method of measuring tobacco smoke constituents is seriously flawed. Simply put, the FTC method uses machines that do not change their behavior to self-administer a preferred nicotine dose or in response to the taste of the smoke, as human smokers do. It may be an accurate predictor of what smoking machines obtain under specifically programmed conditions, but it is not an accurate predictor of what people get from cigarettes.

The dose-response relationship between FTC ratings and plasma nicotine levels is weak, except at low doses (Russell et al., 1980 and 1986; Rickert and Robinson, 1981; Benowitz et al., 1983 and 1986b; Robinson et al., 1983; Gori and Lynch, 1985; Maron and Fortmann, 1987; Coultas et al., 1993). The relationship between cigarette dosage ratings and plasma nicotine levels may be better in studies using research cigarettes where nicotine content varies. With other drugs, compensation can be diminished when the cost of compensation increases. That is, if a drug becomes too costly in terms of expense or physical difficulty in sustaining intake, users may not compensate as effectively and will not administer as much of the drug as they did when the cost was lower (U.S. Department of Health and Human Services, 1988; Lemaire and Meisch, 1985; Bickel et al., 1993). Thus, if cigarettes have low enough nicotine contents, smokers would be expected to adjust over time to lower nicotine levels rather than spend the time and money necessary to maintain constant dose intake. Conversely, most smokers probably would not smoke 160 to 200 low-nicotine-content cigarettes per day to continue to receive the intake that they previously obtained from conventional cigarettes.

Measurement of Smoking and Nicotine Intake   The role of dependence is assumed by the authors and the tobacco industry to be important determinants of nicotine intake. Brown and Williamson (1983) noted

> the basic assumption is that nicotine, which is almost certainly the key smoke component for satisfaction, is fully released to the body system before exhalation takes place. It is essential, therefore, to quantify the change in chemical composition between inhaled and exhaled smoke under different smoking conditions.

Cigarette dose determination is indeed complicated, and some may suggest that it is so complex that use of the flawed FTC method might as well continue simply because it has been used for nearly 30 years. However, such a conclusion contradicts the enormous research advances made over the past 30 years. This research can be used to devise a better method. Furthermore, the complexity of dose determination is not unique to cigarettes. The Food and Drug Administration (FDA) faces this issue routinely whenever a manufacturer submits a new drug. Unless the drug is injected into a vein, determination of dosing is complicated. If the drug is delivered by an inhaler or oral capsule, many factors must be and are considered so that consumers are provided with realistic estimates of what they will get. In particular, they are provided with information relevant to the maximal doses that they are likely to receive from a drug-delivering product.

To provide accurate dosing information for drug delivery systems, FDA uses different methods as indicated by the chemical and its delivery system; moreover, verification of dosing estimates is accomplished in human bioavailability testing studies because, in the final analysis, we care about the dose that people receive, not the machine-derived dose. Also, if there are factors that produce major changes in bioavailability, such as whether the drug is taken with food or on an empty stomach, this can be indicated in the labeling.

A PROPOSAL FOR MORE MEANINGFUL CIGARETTE LABELING   One approach to more meaningful cigarette labeling is that described by Henningfield and colleagues (1994). This approach was adapted from that used by FDA to label food products with constituents of health-related relevance. One issue that FDA addressed in food labeling was serving size. In the case of cigarettes, research has indicated the need for larger and more intense puffs from the machine to more closely parallel smokers' behavior (U.S. Department of Health and Human Services, 1988). A second issue for cigarette labeling is the need to use biologically meaningful categories. For example, labels might specify "no nicotine" or "low nicotine" instead of including numerical values that imply that differences of a few percentage points have practical meaning and provide the consumer with the illusion that she or he will obtain different doses from different cigarettes. Similarly, terms such as "light" should be banned altogether because they imply health benefits; these terms are permitted with foods only if the food type provides a health benefit relative to the conventional type of food in a given category. Actual nicotine content of the cigarettes also should be provided to consumers because the content determines the absolute limit of nicotine that could be extracted.

Nicotine delivery ratings also could be linked to other factors having health effects, for example, tar. Thus, a low-nicotine-delivering cigarette could not be labeled "low nicotine" unless it was also low in tar and carbon monoxide delivery. A comparable situation in food labeling is that a label may not use the phrase "fat free" if a product contains cholesterol. Finally, nicotine yield estimates from standardized machine tests should be validated with bioavailability testing, as is done with other drugs, because what is of interest is the dose obtained by smokers.

This approach would not in itself solve the health problem posed by tobacco use, but it would at least provide consumers with what they have come to expect in the United States, namely, honest labeling that gives them the information on which to make decisions about the products they use. Three decades of research on cigarette smoking, nicotine dependence, and measurement of tobacco constituent intake have provided the means to give consumers such information.

QUESTION-AND-ANSWER SESSION

DR. DEBETHIZY: Dr. Henningfield, you really did not speak very much to the FTC method, but I think it is important to point out that the FTC method was never intended to measure nicotine uptake.

I also agree with you. I think we can do better in terms of measuring nicotine uptake when we want to do that. I think the methods that have been used in the past are estimates. I think the study that I will tell you about a little bit later is a step in that direction, and I will be looking forward to sharing that with you.

I would like to make a point about your proposal to measure content. I have heard that a number of times today, and we have to remember that people do not eat cigarettes; they smoke cigarettes. And there is no indication that people obtain the amount of nicotine that is contained in a cigarette.

DR. HENNINGFIELD: On content, I think that the most important thing is bioavailability tests. Again, that is the gold standard: what people are likely to get and generally under maximum conditions. The importance of content, though, is that content limits the amount of nicotine that you can get. If it is not there, you cannot get it.

DR. DEBETHIZY: I think the important thing is the FTC method is set up to provide relative ranking, so that consumers can get an idea of what different cigarettes will yield. It was not intended to measure uptake.

Now, if you want to measure uptake and evaluate the FTC method, that is a different activity, and I think that we need to make sure that we distinguish those two activities. One is to provide a relative ranking. The FTC method has done an excellent job of that over the years.

DR. HENNINGFIELD: I am not addressing the method, but I think it is pretty clear that it has not done a good job of telling people what they will have in their bloodstream. And that is what I am addressing: that what people get in their bloodstream does not bear much relation to the FTC yields. So, I am not sure how much use that has been.

DR. HARRIS: I see the dispute as distinguishing between an ordinal ranking and a cardinal ranking. An ordinal ranking merely says one brand, to some degree, delivers more or less nicotine than another; whereas, a cardinal ranking would say, this brand delivers one-fifth as much or five times as much.

And what I understand the dispute to be about is that the FTC ranking actually may preserve an ordinal ranking in the roughest sense, but it does not preserve the cardinal ranking. From what I can gather, a 10-percent increase in FTC nicotine corresponds with, at most, about a 2-percent increase in blood nicotine, roughly speaking, and that that is where the problem lies.

DR. HENNINGFIELD: It is not even that good, because if the slope were constant, you could maybe say there is an ordinal ranking. That still may not tell you if it is meaningful if it was so trivial. But what Dr. Benowitz showed was if there is a break.

In other words, at the ultralow end, those cigarettes are in a slightly different category. From the data I have seen, it is not even a meaningful ordinal ranking. It is a pretty flat ranking. The slope is, I would contend until proven otherwise, biologically trivial.

REFERENCES

American Psychiatric Association. *Diagnostic and Statistical Manual of Mental Disorders: Fourth Edition.* Washington, DC: American Psychiatric Press, 1994.

Benowitz, N.L., Hall, S., Herning, R.I., Jacob, P., Jones, R.T., Osman, A.-L. Smokers of low-yield cigarettes do not consume less nicotine. *New England Journal of Medicine* 309: 139-142, 1983.

Benowitz, N.L., Jacob, P., Kozlowski, L.T., Yu, L. Influence of smoking fewer cigarettes on exposure to tar, nicotine, and carbon monoxide. *New England Journal of Medicine* 315: 1310-1313, 1986a.

Benowitz, N.L., Jacob, P., Yu, L., Talcott, R., Hall, S., Jones, R.T. Reduced tar, nicotine, and carbon monoxide exposure while smoking ultralow- but not low-yield cigarettes. *Journal of the American Medical Association* 256: 241-246, 1986b.

Bickel, W.K., DeGrandpre, R.J., Higgins, S.T. Behavioral economics: A novel approach to the study of drug dependence. *Drug and Alcohol Dependence* 33: 173-192, 1993.

Brown and Williamson. "Summary." Tobacco Corporation Research Conference, Rio de Janeiro, Brazil, August 22-26, 1983.

Brown and Williamson. "Proceedings of the Smoking Behaviour-Marketing Conference." Tobacco Corporation Smoking Behaviour-Marketing Conference, Montreal, Quebec, Canada, July 9-12, 1984.

Butschky, M.F., Bailey, D., Henningfield, J.E., Pickworth, W.B. Smoking without nicotine delivery decreases withdrawal in 12-hour abstinent smokers. *Pharmacology, Biochemistry and Behavior* 50(1): 91-96, 1995.

Corrigall, W.A. Regulation of intravenous nicotine self-administration—dopamine mechanisms. In: *Effects of Nicotine on Biological Systems, Advances in Pharmacological Sciences*, F. Adlkofer and K. Thurau (Editors). Boston: Berkhauser Verlag, 1991, pp. 423-432.

Coultas, D.B., Stidley, C.A., Samet, J.M. Cigarette yields of tar and nicotine and markers of exposure to tobacco smoke. *American Review of Respiratory Disease* 148: 435-440, 1993.

Cummings, S.R., Richard, R.J. Optimum cutoff points for biochemical validation of smoking status. *American Journal of Public Health* 78: 574-575, 1988.

Djordjevic, M.V., Hoffmann, D., Glynn, T., Connolly, G.N. U.S. commercial brands of moist snuff, 1994. Assessment of nicotine, moisture, and pH. *Tobacco Control* 4(1): 62-66, 1995.

Fiore, M.C. Trends in cigarette smoking in the United States. The epidemiology of tobacco use. *Medical Clinics of North America* 76: 289-303, 1992.

Fischman, M.W., Mello, N.K. (Editors). *Testing for Abuse Liability of Drugs in Humans.* National Institute on Drug Abuse Research Monograph 92. DHHS Publication No. 89-1613. Washington, DC: Supt. of Docs., U.S. Govt. Print. Off., 1989.

Gilman, A.G., Rall, T.W., Nies, A.S., Taylor, P. (Editors). *Goodman and Gilman's The Pharmacological Basis of Therapeutics.* New York: Pergamon Press, 1990.

Gori, G.B., Lynch, C.J. Analytical cigarette yields as predictors of smoke bioavailability. *Regulatory Toxicology and Pharmacology* 5: 314-326, 1985.

Griffiths, R.R., Bigelow, G.E., Henningfield, J.E. Similarities in animal and human behavior. In: *Advances in Substance Abuse: Behavioral and Biological Research, Vol. 1*, N.K. Mello (Editor). Greenwich, CT: JAI Press, 1980, pp. 1-90.

Gross, J., Stitzer, M.L. Nicotine replacement: Ten-week effects on tobacco withdrawal symptoms. *Psychopharmacology* 98: 334-341, 1989.

Heishman, S.J., Taylor, R.C., Henningfield, J.E. Nicotine and smoking: A review of effects on human performance. *Experimental and Clinical Pharmacology* 2: 345-395, 1994.

Henningfield, J.E., Goldberg, S.R. Nicotine as a reinforcer in human subjects and laboratory animals. *Pharmacology, Biochemistry and Behavior* 19: 989-992, 1983.

Henningfield, J.E., Keenan, R.M. Nicotine delivery kinetics and abuse liability. *Journal of Consulting and Clinical Psychology* 61: 1-8, 1993.

Henningfield, J.E., Kozlowski, L.T., Benowitz, N.L. A proposal to develop meaningful labeling for cigarettes. *Journal of the American Medical Association* 272: 312-314, 1994.

Henningfield, J.E., London, E.D., Benowitz, N.L. Arterial-venous differences in plasma concentrations of nicotine after cigarette smoking. *Journal of the American Medical Association* 263: 2049-2050, 1990.

Henningfield, J.E., Miyasato, K., Jasinski, D.R. Abuse liability and pharmacodynamic characteristics of intravenous and inhaled nicotine. *Journal of Pharmacology and Experimental Therapeutics* 234: 1-2, 1985.

Henningfield, J.E., Radzius, A., Cone, E.J. Estimation of available nicotine content of six smokeless tobacco products. *Tobacco Control* 4(1): 57-61, 1995.

Henningfield, J.E., Stapleton, J.M., Benowitz, N.L., Grayson, R.F., London, E.D. Higher levels of nicotine in arterial than in venous blood after cigarette smoking. *Drug and Alcohol Dependence* 33: 23-29, 1993.

Hill, P., Marquardt, H. Plasma and urine changes after smoking different brands of cigarettes. *Clinical Pharmacology and Therapeutics* 27: 652-658, 1980.

Hughes, J.R., Gulliver, S.B., Fenwick, J.W., Valliere, W.A., Cruser, K., Pepper, S., Shea, P., Solomon, L.J., Flynn, B.S. Smoking cessation among self-quitters. *Health Psychology* 11(5): 331-334, 1992.

Hughes, J.R., Hatsukami, D.K. The nicotine withdrawal syndrome: A brief review and update. *International Journal of Smoking Cessation* 1: 21-26, 1992.

Hunt, W.A., Barnett, L.W., Branch, L.G. Relapse rates in addiction programs. *Journal of Clinical Psychology* 27: 455-456, 1971.

Jarvis, M.J. Application of biochemical intake markers to passive smoking measurement and risk estimation. *Mutation Research* 222: 101-110, 1989.

Jarvis, M.J., Tunstall-Pedoe, H., Feyerabend, C., Vesey, C., Saloojee, Y. Comparison of tests used to distinguish smokers from nonsmokers. *American Journal of Public Health* 77: 1435-1438, 1987.

Jones, R.T. Tobacco dependence. In: *Psychopharmacology: The Third Generation of Progress*, H.Y. Meltzer (Editor). New York: Raven Press, 1987, pp. 1589-1595.

Kottke, T.E., Brekke, M.L., Solberg, L.I., Hughes, J.R. A randomized trial to increase smoking intervention by physicians: Doctors helping smokers. Round I. *Journal of the American Medical Association* 261: 2101-2106, 1989.

Kozlowski, L.T. Reduction of tobacco health hazards in continuing users: Individual behavioral and public health approaches. *Journal of Substance Abuse* 1: 345-357, 1989.

Kozlowski, L.T., Wilkinson, A., Skinner, W., Kent, C., Frankin, T., Pope, M.A. Comparing tobacco cigarette dependence with other drug dependencies: Greater or equal "difficulty quitting" and "urges to use" but less pleasure from cigarettes. *Journal of the American Medical Association* 261: 898-901, 1989.

Langley, J.N. On the reaction of cells and of nerve endings to certain poisons, chiefly as regards the reaction of striated muscle to nicotine and to curari. *Journal of Physiology* 33: 374-413, 1905.

Lemaire, G.A., Meisch, R.A. Oral drug self-administration in rhesus monkeys: Interactions between drug amount and fixed-ratio size. *Journal of the Experimental Analysis of Behavior* 44: 377-389, 1985.

London, E.D., Morgan, M.J. Positron emission tomographic studies on the acute effects of psychoactive drugs on brain metabolism and mood. In: *Imaging Drug Action in the Brain*, E.D. London (Editor). Boca Raton, FL: CRC Press, 1993, pp. 265-280.

Maron, D.J., Fortmann, S.P. Nicotine yield and measures of cigarette smoke exposure in a large population: Are lower-yield cigarettes safer? *American Journal of Public Health* 77: 546-549, 1987.

Nemeth-Coslett, R., Henningfield, J.E. Effects of nicotine chewing gum on cigarette smoking and subjective and physiologic effects. *Clinical Pharmacology and Therapeutics* 39: 625-630, 1986.

Nemeth-Coslett, R., Henningfield, J.E., O'Keefe, M.K., Griffiths, R.R. Effects of mecamylamine on human cigarette smoking and subjective ratings. *Psychopharmacology* 88: 420-425, 1986.

Newhouse, P.A., Hughes, J.R. The role of nicotine and nicotinic mechanisms in neuropsychiatric disease. *British Journal of Addiction* 86: 521-526, 1991.

Peto, R., Lopez, A.D., Boreham, J., Thun, M., Heath, C., Jr. *Mortality From Smoking in Developed Countries, 1950-2000: Indirect Estimates From National Vital Statistics*. World Health Organization. Oxford: Oxford University Press, 1994.

Pickworth, W.B., Herning, R.I., Henningfield, J.E. Spontaneous EEG changes during tobacco abstinence and nicotine substitution. *Journal of Pharmacology and Experimental Therapeutics* 251: 976-982, 1989.

Pomerleau, O.F. Nicotine and the central nervous system: Biobehavioral effects of cigarette smoking. *American Journal of Medicine* 93(Suppl 1A): 2S-7S, 1992.

Pomerleau, O.F., Pomerleau, C.S. Neuroregulators and the reinforcement of smoking: Towards a biobehavioral explanation. *Neuroscience and Biobehavioral Reviews* 8: 503-513, 1984.

Pomerleau, O.F., Rosecrans, J. Neuroregulatory effects of nicotine. *Psychoneuroendocrinology* 14: 407-423, 1989.

Rickert, W.S., Robinson, J.C. Estimating the hazards of less hazardous cigarettes. II. Study of cigarette yields of nicotine, carbon monoxide, and hydrogen cyanide in relation to levels of cotinine, carboxyhemoglobin, and thiocyanate in smokers. *Journal of Toxicology and Environmental Health* 7: 391-403, 1981.

Robinson, J.C., Young, J.C., Rickert, W.S., Fey, G., Kozlowski, L.T. A comparative study of the amount of smoke absorbed from low yield ('less hazardous') cigarettes. Part 2: Invasive measures. *British Journal of Addiction* 78: 79-87, 1983.

Rose, J.E., Behm, F. Refined cigarette smoke as a method for reducing nicotine intake. *Pharmacology, Biochemistry and Behavior* 28: 305-310, 1987.

Rose, J.E., Sampson, A., Levin, E.D., Henningfield, J.E. Mecamylamine increases nicotine preference and attenuates nicotine discrimination. *Pharmacology, Biochemistry and Behavior* 32(4): 933-938, 1989.

Russell, M.A., Jarvis, M., Iyer, R., Feyerabend, C. Relation of nicotine yield of cigarettes to blood nicotine concentrations in smokers. *British Medical Journal* 280(6219): 972-976, 1980.

Russell, M.A., Jarvis, M.J., Feyerabend, C., Saloojee, Y. Reduction of tar, nicotine and carbon monoxide intake in low tar smokers. *Journal of Epidemiology and Community Health* 40(1): 80-85, 1986.

Sahakian, B., Jones, G., Levy, R., Gray, J., Warburton, D. The effects of nicotine on attention, information processing, and short-term memory in patients with dementia of the Alzheimer's type. *British Journal of Psychiatry* 154: 797-800, 1989.

Snyder, F.R., Henningfield, J.E. Effects of nicotine administration following 12 h of tobacco deprivation: Assessment on computerized performance tasks. *Psychopharmacology* 97(1): 17-22, 1989.

U.S. Department of Health and Human Services. *The Health Consequences of Smoking: Nicotine Addiction. A Report of the Surgeon General, 1988*. DHHS Publication No. (CDC) 88-8406. Rockville, MD: U.S. Department of Health and Human Services, Public Health Service, Centers for Disease Control, Center for Health Promotion and Education, Office on Smoking and Health, 1988.

Consumer/Smoker Perceptions of Federal Trade Commission Tar Ratings

Joel B. Cohen

INTRODUCTION   A telephone survey among a national probability sample of 1,005 adults (502 men and 503 women) 18 years of age and older was conducted between November 17 and 20, 1994. Data were weighted by age, sex, geographic region, and race so that each respondent was assigned a single weight based on the relationship between the actual population proportions of the listed characteristics and the comparable sample proportions.

The author's estimate of every-day smoking (23 percent) matches current assessments of adult U.S. smoking prevalence (22 percent). When every-day and some-days smokers were combined, the current smoking percentage (28.7 percent) was slightly higher than the Centers for Disease Control and Prevention (CDC) (1994) comparable estimate of 26.5 percent for 1992. This sample reported somewhat higher current smoking percentages for females (29 percent) than did the 1992 CDC surveys (24.6 percent). Total smoking reported by whites (29 percent) was slightly higher than in the 1992 CDC surveys (27.2 percent), whereas total smoking reported by blacks in this sample (27 percent) was virtually identical (27.8 percent). A high percentage of those who report having attended but not graduated from college were some-days smokers. When added to every-day smokers, this total was substantially higher (36 percent) than that reported in the CDC surveys (24 percent) and was closer to the CDC estimate for high school graduates (31 percent). College graduates in this sample were also somewhat more likely to smoke (19 percent compared with 15.5 percent reported in CDC surveys). Age breakdowns were not entirely comparable among the surveys, but the author's sample reported a higher incidence of smoking among 18- to 24-year-olds (32 percent compared with 26.4 percent).

TAR LEVEL OF   Table 1 reports the tar levels of cigarettes last smoked, determined by
CIGARETTES   asking the brand, size, and other characteristics of the cigarette. These answers were compared with actual Federal Trade Commission (FTC) tar ratings. In 15 percent of the cases, respondents could not provide sufficiently detailed product information to make this comparison ("Cannot Determine" respondents). These respondents were likely to come disproportionately from lower tar categories. A four-category designation of tar levels was selected. It allowed for somewhat greater differentiation among lower tar users, had an equal number of rating scale points in each of the low-tar categories, and was consistent with a recently proposed four-category nicotine and tar rating system. Unweighted cell sizes for the five tar categories (including "Cannot Determine") shown in Table 1 were small: 28, 75, 70, 116, and 48 for those smoking cigarettes in the past 2 to 3 years.

Table 1
Tar level (percent) of cigarette last smoked

Smoker Classification (weighted data) (N)	Tar Levels (mg)				
	Very Low 1-5	Low 6-10	Medium 11-15	High 16+	Cannot Determine
Current Smokers					
Some-days smokers (56)	9	34	9	23	25
Every-day smokers (232)	8	22	21	40	10
Recent (2 to 3 years) quitters (36)	11	11	25	28	25
Those Smoking in the Past 2 to 3 Years					
All smokers (325)	9	22	19	35	14
Male (152)	5	24	13	42	17
Female (174)	12	21	25	29	12
White (268)	10	23	21	31	15
Black (28)	0	14	18	64	4
Hispanic (26)	4	15	4	58	19
High school or less education (107)	6	15	21	41	18
At least some college education (146)	12	32	23	30	12
Smokers of regular size cigarettes (145)	5	28	11	40	16
Smokers of longer cigarettes (173)	12	19	27	32	11
Smokers of soft pack cigarettes (180)	13	17	22	33	16
Smokers of hard pack cigarettes (133)	3	29	17	41	9
Smokers of plain cigarettes (223)	9	24	18	35	15
Smokers of menthol cigarettes (101)	8	20	23	38	12

Fifty-eight percent of current smokers smoked a cigarette with 15 mg or less of tar, and 9 percent smoked a cigarette with 1 to 5 mg of tar. Recent quitters tended to come from relatively higher tar categories, consistent with evidence suggesting that switching to the lowest tar cigarettes was a substitute for, rather than a stepping stone to, quitting. High-tar cigarette use was more frequent among males, blacks, and Hispanics and decreased markedly with educational attainment.

KNOWLEDGE OF ADVERTISED TAR NUMBERS Those smoking cigarettes in the past 2 to 3 years were asked to tell the interviewer the tar number of their most recently smoked cigarette. Seventy-nine percent indicated that they did not know. This increased to about 90 percent for those having less than a high school education, smokers ages 55 and older, and black smokers. Respondents answering "do not know" then were asked to come as close as they could, and interviewers were to probe for their "best guess." Fifty-eight percent still reported not knowing.

Initial responses were slightly more likely to be underestimates (9 percent) than correct answers (defined as plus or minus 1 mg from the actual tar level) or overestimates (6 percent in both of the latter two categories). When probed responses were included in the analysis, there was a substantial increase in responses that underestimated tar levels (from 9 to 20 percent); there were only small changes in correct answers or overestimates. When actual tar numbers were regressed against respondents' initial and probed answers, the relationships were weak (r = .26 and .20, respectively).

Smokers of very-low-tar cigarettes had a much greater awareness of their cigarettes' tar numbers. Thirty-nine percent of those who smoked 1- to 5-mg tar cigarettes were correct initially, increasing to 50 percent with probing. These figures stand in marked contrast to responses of smokers of cigarettes with 6 to 10 mg tar, whose comparable percentages of correct responses were 4 and 9 percent, respectively.

To assess "knowledge in practice" (in addition to recall-based knowledge), half the members of the sample were asked whether a 16-mg (or, for the other half, a 5-mg) tar cigarette is lower in tar than most other cigarettes on the market. The correct answers are "no" for the 16-mg tar cigarette and "yes" for the 5-mg tar cigarette. Table 2 shows respondents' answers cross-tabulated by the tar level of their most recently smoked cigarette. Whereas 35 percent of the smokers of 1- to 5-mg tar cigarettes did not know that a 16-mg tar cigarette was *not* lower in tar, between 55 and 66 percent of all other smokers either did not know or gave incorrect responses to this question. For those

Table 2
Interpretation of Federal Trade Commission tar numbers corresponding to lower tar levels

Interpretations	Tar Levels (mg)				
	Very Low 1-5	Low 6-10	Medium 11-15	High 16+	Cannot Determine
Believe That a 16-mg Tar Cigarette Is Lower in Tar Than Most Other Cigarettes (N = 179)	(14)	(36)	(40)	(64)	(25)
% Correct	65	45	44	34	32
% Incorrect	0	10	10	16	12
% Do not know	35	45	46	50	56
Believe That a 5-mg Tar Cigarette Is Lower in Tar Than Most Other Cigarettes (N = 158)	(14)	(39)	(30)	(52)	(23)
% Correct	15	34	44	27	25
% Incorrect	13	10	14	19	16
% Do not know	73	56	42	55	59

smoking cigarettes having more than 5 mg of tar, between 56 and 74 percent either did not know that a 5-mg tar cigarette was lower in tar than most other cigarettes or said that it was not lower (with 10 to 20 percent incorrect).

SMOKERS'
INTERPRETATIONS
OF TAR NUMBERS
Two approaches were used to better understand how smokers interpreted the advertised tar numbers. In the first, half the sample members were asked whether a pack-a-day smoker could significantly lower his or her health risks due to smoking by switching from a 20-mg tar cigarette to a 5-mg tar cigarette; for the other half, the switch was to a 16-mg tar cigarette. In total, 56 percent of smokers thought that a switch to a 5-mg tar cigarette would significantly lower health risks, whereas 28 percent thought that a switch to a 16-mg tar cigarette would significantly lower health risks.

Table 3 cross-tabulates answers to these questions against the actual tar levels of smokers' cigarettes. For the substantive shift to a 5-mg cigarette, light-to-heavy tar cigarette smokers are evenly divided between believing there would be a significant reduction in health risks and either believing this would *not* be the case or being unsure about this. Whereas more than 60 percent of smokers did *not* think switching to a 16-mg tar cigarette would lead to a significant reduction in health risks due to smoking, a sizable proportion of light-to-heavy tar cigarette smokers either thought it would or did not know.

Table 3
Inferences (percent) about health risks as a result of switching to lower tar cigarettes

	Tar Levels (mg)				
Inference	Very Low 1-5	Low 6-10	Medium 11-15	High 16+	Cannot Determine
Switching From a 20-mg to a 5-mg Tar Cigarette Would Significantly Reduce Health Risks	83	49	49	55	60
Switching From a 20-mg to a 5-mg Tar Cigarette Would Not Significantly Reduce Health Risks	13	32	35	25	29
Do Not Know	4	19	15	20	12
Switching From a 20-mg to a 16-mg Tar Cigarette Would Significantly Reduce Health Risks	18	35	28	25	33
Switching From a 20-mg to a 16-mg Tar Cigarette Would Not Significantly Reduce Health Risks	68	61	61	61	37
Do Not Know	14	4	10	14	31
Relative Difference in Health Risks Between Those Asked About Switching to a 5-mg and Those Asked About Switching to a 16-mg Tar Cigarette	65	14	21	30	27

The interpretation of data in Table 3 is complicated by almost certainly differing beliefs of smokers in the four tar categories regarding the risks of smoking a 20-mg tar cigarette and hence about the decrease in risk from any reduction in tar level. Because the belief factor is likely to be a constant in the two versions of this question, it is useful to examine the relative reduction in health risk (i.e., the difference in benefits between switching to the 5-mg tar alternative compared with the 16-mg alternative), shown in the last row of Table 3. Once again, the evidence points to a clear difference between smokers of cigarettes with 1 to 5 mg of tar and all other smokers. These very-low-tar smokers believe that it takes a substantial reduction in tar yields to significantly reduce health risk, whereas this belief does not appear to be held by a substantial number of smokers in other categories. Unfortunately, this belief also may support a judgment that a substantial reduction in tar levels may be a reasonable substitute for quitting.

In the second approach, we examined smokers' understanding of the distinction between tar yield and delivery, together with their willingness to treat the numerical information as if it had ratio-scale properties rather than merely ordinal properties. Many of those supporting the dissemination of tar numbers have assumed that consumers would use these numbers in an ordinal fashion, essentially as if they were simply rank-ordered data. Ordinal scales do not possess the property that each numerical interval is of the same magnitude (i.e., the difference between 1 and 2 being precisely equal to the difference between 10 and 11). The FTC method may produce tar ratings that have this interval scale property for tar yields, but it cannot be said to do so for actual deliveries of tar because smokers' inhalation patterns seem to vary as they move lower on the scale. A ratio scale has the further property of having a genuine zero point so that it is proper to regard a scale score of 10 as being twice as high as a scale score of 5.

Respondents were asked to assume that a person switched from a 10-mg tar cigarette to a 1-mg tar cigarette. Then the three statements shown in Table 4 were read twice, and respondents were asked to decide which of these came closest to their opinion. Primacy and recency effects were controlled by rotating the order of the first and third statements. The first answer is the correct choice, whereas the second answer suggests some reluctance to rely on the absolute numerical values when thinking about such tradeoffs.

The general conclusion to be drawn from these data is that at least one-quarter of smokers (i.e., those selecting the third interpretation) clearly have been misled about the meaning of the tar yield numbers. Interestingly, this increases to 44 percent for smokers of very-low-tar cigarettes, in line with other evidence presented here; it also increases concern about the safety reassurances that such very-low-tar cigarettes appear to provide.

Table 4
Inferences (percent) about tradeoffs between tar deliveries and number of cigarettes smoked

Inference (relative to a 10-mg tar cigarette)	Tar Levels (mg)				
	Very Low 1-5	Low 6-10	Medium 11-15	High 16+	Cannot Determine
Person Probably Could Smoke More Than One, but These Numbers Cannot Tell You How Much Less Tar the Person Would Take in From the 1-mg Tar Cigarette	28	33	31	40	39
Person Could Smoke More Than 1 or 2 but Less Than 9 or 10 of the 1-mg Tar Cigarettes Without Taking in More Tar	18	33	22	25	22
Person Could Smoke About 10 of the 1-mg Tar Cigarettes Without Taking in More Tar	44	25	31	21	21
None of These/Do Not Know	10	10	16	14	18

SMOKERS' USE OF ADVERTISED TAR NUMBERS The final issue under study in this survey was whether smokers reported having used these tar numbers to make judgments about the relative safety of different brands of cigarettes. In answering this question, only 14 percent of the sample indicated doing so. Once again, the smokers of 1- to 5-mg tar cigarettes were different: 56 percent of them reported using advertised tar numbers to make judgments about the relative safety of various cigarettes.

CONCLUSIONS This study demonstrates inherent difficulties in using advertised tar yield numbers to communicate meaningful information to consumers. Most smokers do not seem to pay careful attention to the numerical values per se, even to the extent of having a strong sense of the range of numerical values. Smokers of cigarettes with low- to high-tar content had considerable uncertainty about the health implications of switching to lower tar cigarettes. However, very-low-tar numbers seem to have a strong appeal to a particular group of smokers and may convey a message of absolute safety.

QUESTION-AND-ANSWER SESSION

DR. TOWNSEND: Dr. Cohen, can you tell me if you also asked the subjects the category of cigarettes that they smoked; for example, was it regular or lights or ultralights?

DR. COHEN: We did not ask them their perception of their cigarette. We asked them exactly what they smoked in terms of the size and whether their cigarettes were menthol or plain and hard pack or soft pack—but we did not ask them their perception.

DR. TOWNSEND: I am not speaking about their perception. I am speaking about the advertising associated with the cigarettes that smokers purchase. For example, if you go into a store to buy cigarettes, you can buy Winston regulars, Winston Lights, or Winston Ultra Lights. And of course, those relative categories are based on FTC tar numbers. So, you did not ask them a question like that?

DR. COHEN: No, we didn't ask that specific question.

DR. TOWNSEND: My experience, in talking with a lot of consumers, is that they do know, very clearly, the category of cigarettes that they are smoking, even though some of them do not know the accurate numbers of the cigarettes that they are smoking.

DR. COHEN: I would not disagree with you.

DR. TOWNSEND: And that ranking of categories is based on the FTC numbers. So, I think that your conclusion that the numbers are useless, I certainly do not agree with.

I think another example of that is in my recent purchase of a hot water heater. I certainly used the energy efficiency ratings in making that choice. I cannot tell you today what the energy efficiency rating actually is.

DR. COHEN: If we are here looking at the utility of the FTC tar numbers in advertising, then I think it is fair to ask if people are taking away this information. The assertion is made that this information has value to people. I am examining that assertion.

Now, if you are saying, well, it is not the numbers they care about; it is the categories, then you can present information that says they are done in four categories.

DR. TOWNSEND: In addition to that, you also said that there is at least one category where a high percentage of those smokers do look at those numbers very carefully. So, I think your conclusion that the FTC numbers are useless is certainly not true.

DR. COHEN: I do not know that I went that far; I stopped a little short of that.

DR. TOWNSEND: And I think another very practical example of the utility of the FTC relative numbers is, in fact, what has happened to the industry over the past 40 years. We have reduced the level of tar delivery, by the FTC method, from about 38 mg down to about 12 mg. I think Dr. Hoffmann spoke to that very clearly.

What has happened to cause that dramatic a change is that people trade off taste. The lower tar cigarettes generally have—or always have—fewer taste characteristics. And people find that more acceptable. So, they are making this tradeoff in the marketplace of taste and something else.

DR. COHEN: I appreciate your position, though I think we are talking about different issues here. I am talking about the utility of this information presented in this form as numbers. I am not talking about the utility of providing information about tar.

MS. WILKENFELD: I do want to add one thing to the mix to make it more complicated. You said they had to tell you the name of the cigarette they were smoking. And in order to get the actual tar number, they would have had to report specifically about the category, for example, Marlboro and Marlboro Lights. So, they may have reported correctly.

DR. KOZLOWSKI: I have found out that a lot of people in the United States who do not smoke somehow have the impression that tar and nicotine ratings are printed on the packs of cigarettes. They are in some places, for example, in Canada, but not in the United States. I think the one notable exception is the ultralow-tar cigarettes. You know, when you test Carlton as low as 1 mg tar, they are right on the pack.

If it is not on packs, if a brand is not advertised, or a person does not see an ad, how in the world would they know what the tar and nicotine yields were?

DR. COHEN: I think there is a fundamental problem. I do not think the scale has integrity. We had a scale that goes from 1 to 27. People don't care about tar; they don't know what it is. They care about harmfulness; they care about smoking risk.

If you don't present information to people along a dimension that they care about, they are not going to pay as much attention to it. And if you don't present information to people in a way so that they know how to use it, where the numbers have some meaningful quality, they will not pay attention to it. Then people are not going to be able to do as much with it.

I think there is a fundamental problem with providing information. It may be the wrong information presented the wrong way. Other than that, it is OK.

REFERENCE

Centers for Disease Control and Prevention. Cigarette smoking among adults—United States, 1992, and changes in the definition of current cigarette smoking. *MMWR. Morbidity and Mortality Weekly Report* 43(19): 342-346, 1994.

Sensitivity of the Federal Trade Commission Test Method to Analytical Parameters

Michael R. Guerin

INTRODUCTION   The Federal Trade Commission (FTC) test method for determining the tar, nicotine, and carbon monoxide yields of commercial cigarettes was designed to characterize and compare brands. Relevance to human smoking was a consideration in choosing the test method, but the principal objective was to select a method that provided the most accurate and reproducible result. Relevance to human smoking was addressed by using intermittent puffing and by choosing puff volume, puff duration, puff frequency, and butt length based on observations of human smokers. Accuracy and reproducibility were addressed by selecting a single set of smoking conditions, demanding narrow tolerances for variation in the conditions, and standardizing everything from cigarette selection, to the smoking environment, to the laboratory analytical chemical methods.

Requirements associated with producing a standard method tend to conflict with those associated with maximizing relevance to the human situation. Bradford and colleagues (1936) recognized from the beginning that humans smoke cigarettes in different and varying ways, but a standardized procedure requires that variables be set and controlled. For practical purposes, only one set of conditions could be selected.

At least two factors have led to an increased concern about the relevance of the FTC test procedure. First, FTC results increasingly have been viewed as a measure of human exposure and therefore health risk. The problem is compounded by the assumption that even a small difference in FTC results signifies a meaningful difference in human exposure. Second, a much greater variety of cigarettes is available today. They range from nonfilter and filter cigarettes similar to those available when the method was adopted, to increasingly popular products with very low FTC yields. Behavioral research has demonstrated that low-yield products are consistently smoked differently than are higher yield products (Kozlowski et al., 1989).

This chapter reviews the nature of the FTC test procedure and the influence of changes in its specifications on yields. Smoking parameters likely to be different for humans from FTC machine smoking are emphasized.

STANDARD MACHINE SMOKING   The quantities of tar, nicotine, carbon monoxide, and other constituents in cigarette smoke are measured using smoking machines. One or more cigarettes are smoked by a machine, the constituents of interest are collected in a suitable trap, and the contents of the trap are chemically analyzed. The quantity in the trap is divided by the number of cigarettes smoked to compute a yield (or delivery) per cigarette. In the case of the FTC procedure, the particle phase of the smoke is collected on glass fiber (Cambridge) filters, and the gas phase (passing through the filter) is collected in gas sampling bags. Carbon monoxide is measured in the gas sampling bags. The filter is weighed to yield a measure of total particulate matter (TPM) and is analyzed for nicotine and water content. Tar (or nicotine-free dry particulate matter) is computed by subtracting the weights of nicotine and water from the weight of TPM.

The principal reason for using smoking machines is to maximize the reproducibility of results (DeBardeleben et al., 1991). This is particularly important for quality control and product comparison and is essential for interlaboratory comparisons. However, machine smoking is limited in that it provides results accurate only for the specific set of smoking conditions employed by the machine.

Smoking parameters used in the FTC procedure are based largely on empirical observations of smokers reported by Bradford and colleagues (1936). They suggested a nominal 35-mL ("mL" is used interchangeably in the literature with "cc") puff volume of a 2-second duration taken once per minute to a 23-mm butt length. Current FTC smoking conditions (Federal Trade Commission, 1994) specify a puff volume of 35 ± 0.5 mL, a puff duration of 2.0 ± 0.2 seconds, and a puff frequency of 1 per 60 ± 1 second. Butt length is specified as 23 mm for nonfilter cigarettes and the length of filter overwrap plus 3 mm for filtered cigarettes. The international standard method (Thomsen, 1992) ISO 3308 currently uses the same conditions but requires more stringent tolerances. Puff volume is 35 ± 0.25 mL, puff duration is 2.0 ± 0.05 second, and puff frequency is 1 per 60 ± 0.5 second.

Machine-smoking parameters are only one of several conditions that have been specified to constitute standard FTC testing. Other conditions include the number and manner of selection of cigarettes to be tested, cigarette conditioning (see below), the smoking environment, and the methods and instrumentation used. FTC testing specifies the analysis of 100 cigarettes selected at random from two packages purchased at each of 50 geographical locations throughout the United States. Cigarettes must be conditioned at 60 percent relative humidity and 24 °C for at least 48 hours before smoking and must be smoked in a room maintained under the same conditions. Smoking is performed using a Phipps and Bird 20-port linear smoking machine, thus specifying by default that "restricted" rather than "free" (butt end closed rather than open to the atmosphere between puffs) smoking be performed. Finally, the air flow across the cigarettes must be reproducible and controlled to control the rate at which the cigarette burns between puffs.

The introduction of cigarettes with ventilated filters has made it necessary to pay additional attention to the depth to which the cigarette is inserted into the holder. The cigarette must be inserted sufficiently deep to hold it firmly for the smoking process but not so deep as to occlude the ventilation holes.

Standardization has produced a remarkably reproducible procedure given that the process involves the combustion of highly processed and packaged plant material. This is illustrated by the data shown in Table 1. Individual laboratories typically generate results with a precision of ±5 percent (relative standard deviation) or better for tar, nicotine, and carbon monoxide yields of high-tar products. Interlaboratory agreement is generally within 4 and 8 percent of the mean, depending on the constituents and number of cigarettes considered. Precision and interlaboratory agreement as a percentage of the mean are poorer for very-low-delivery (e.g., 1 mg tar) products, but the absolute error is similar. The procedure is sufficiently reproducible to allow rounding of FTC results for tar and carbon monoxide to the nearest whole milligram based on a difference between brands of only 0.1 mg (0.4 mg or less reported as <1 mg or below detection limit of the method, 0.5 mg or more rounded up to 1 mg, 1.04 mg rounded down to 1 mg, etc.). Results for nicotine are rounded to the nearest tenth mg. Those with 0.05 mg or greater are rounded up, whereas those with 0.04 mg or less are rounded down, as above.

INFLUENCE OF SMOKING PARAMETERS Each parameter specified in the FTC testing procedure influences the yields of tar, nicotine, and carbon monoxide. Restrictive tolerances specified for acceptable puff volume, puff duration, and so forth are required to allow comparison of similar products and to allow interlaboratory comparability. Parameters such as cigarette conditioning prior to smoking are specified to accommodate the realities of laboratory measurements: in this case, that the cigarettes are likely to be analyzed after long periods of cold storage. Minor variations in any of these parameters can result in detectable differences in yields. Realistic (comparable with human smoking practices) variations also can result in large differences in yields.

Darrall (1988) has reported a systematic study of the influence of smoking parameters on yields of tar, nicotine, and carbon monoxide. Puff durations of 1.6 seconds and 2.3 seconds produced essentially the same yields for very-low-tar (≤4 mg) cigarettes and almost indistinguishable yields for higher tar products (Table 2). No clear trend toward increasing or decreasing yields was noted. Changing puff volume from 35 to 40 mL produced a small but generally consistent increase in tar and nicotine (Table 3). Low-tar products yielded 1 to 3 mg more tar and 0.1 to 0.3 mg more nicotine at 40-mL puff volumes than at 35-mL puff volumes. Higher tar products increased yield by 2 to 5 mg of tar and 0.1 to 0.5 mg of nicotine. The increases, although small, still may be larger than would be found using the standard FTC method because the investigator in Darrall's study (1988) smoked at 2 puffs per minute, thus increasing the number of puffs per cigarette. Larger changes in puff volume produce larger changes in yields. Browne and colleagues (1980) reported that particulate matter yield increased from 29 mg to 55 mg for a U.S. blend experimental cigarette when the puff volume was changed from 17.5 mL to 50 mL under otherwise standard conditions. Carbon monoxide yields were 9 mg and 20 mg for puff volumes of 17.5 mL and 50 mL, respectively.

Table 1
Collaborative study of tar, nicotine, and carbon monoxide yields of 2R1[a], A-2[b], and A-3[b] cigarettes

Cigarette	Laboratory	Cigarettes/Port	Number of Ports	Yield (mg/cigarette), Average ± Standard Deviation		
				Tar	Nicotine	Carbon Monoxide
2R1	1	4	24	36.6 ± 0.7	2.41 ± 0.06	23.1 ± 0.8
	2	5	16	35.0 ± 1.2	2.42 ± 0.07	24.9 ± 1.6
	3	4	5	36.5 ± 1.6	2.12 ± 0.14	23.5 ± 0.9
	4	5	20	35.6 ± 0.6	2.49 ± 0.14	—
A-2	1	4	16	12.5 ± 0.2	0.92 ± 0.02	15.3 ± 0.3
	2	5	16	12.9 ± 0.8	0.96 ± 0.02	16.3 ± 1.0
	3	5	5	12.9 ± 0.5	0.89 ± 0.03	17.0 ± 0.4
	4	5	20	13.0 ± 0.7	0.97 ± 0.07	—
A-3	1	6	8	1.3 ± 0.1	0.11 ± 0.01	2.3 ± 0.1
	2	5	16	1.3 ± 0.2	0.21 ± 0.03	2.4 ± 0.5
	3	5	5	1.4 ± 0.2	0.19 ± 0.01	2.3 ± 0.3
	4	5	20	1.6 ± 0.3	0.17 ± 0.04	—

[a] *University of Kentucky reference nonfilter cigarette.*
[b] *National Cancer Institute "Nicotine Series" experimental nonfilter cigarette.*

Table 2
Influence of puff duration on machine yields

| Brand (FTC tar) | Yield (mg/cigarette)[a] | | | | | |
| | Tar | | Nicotine | | Carbon Monoxide | |
	1.6 Seconds	2.3 Seconds	1.6 Seconds	2.3 Seconds	1.6 Seconds	2.3 Seconds
B (1 mg)	2	2	0.3	0.3	1	1
D (4 mg)	8	7	0.8	0.7	10	8
E (6 mg)	12	10	0.8	0.8	15	12
G (9 mg)	15	14	1.4	1.3	15	12
K (13 mg)	23	22	2.1	2.1	19	17
T (15 mg)	25	27	2.2	2.4	27	24
X (25 mg)	38	39	3.6	3.7	22	20

[a] 35-mL puff, 30-second interval.

Source: Darrall, 1988.

Table 3
Influence of puff volume on machine yields

| Brand (FTC tar) | Yield (mg/cigarette)[a] | | | | | |
| | Tar | | Nicotine | | Carbon Monoxide | |
	35 mL	40 mL	35 mL	40 mL	35 mL	40 mL
(B) KS-UM-V (1 mg)	2	3	0.3	0.4	1	1
(D) KS-EM-V (4 mg)	7	10	0.7	1.0	8	11
(G) KS-V (9 mg)	14	16	1.3	1.7	12	15
(H) Regular-V (12 mg)	21	21	0.9	1.0	25	25
(K) KS-V (13 mg)	22	24	2.1	2.2	17	17
(O) KS-NV (14 mg)	22	24	2.0	2.3	21	22
(P) KS-NV (14 mg)	24	28	1.6	2.4	18	24
(W) Regular-NF (16 mg)	27	26	2.1	2.4	16	14
(X) Regular-NF (25 mg)	39	44	3.7	4.2	20	21

[a] 2.3-second duration, 30-second frequency.

Key: KS = king size; UM = ultramild (< 4 mg tar); V = ventilated; EM = extra mild (4 to 7 mg tar); NV = nonventilated; NF = nonfilter.

Source: Darrall, 1988.

Puff frequency (Table 4) and filter ventilation (Table 5) were found to have the greatest effect on yields. Decreasing the puff interval from 60 to 40 seconds increased the deliveries of tar, nicotine, and carbon monoxide by 20 to 50 percent on a per-cigarette basis. Using a puff interval of 30 seconds increased deliveries by 40 to 90 percent. Blocking the ventilation system of ventilated filter cigarettes has similar effects for products using a low degree of ventilation and a much greater effect for highly ventilated products. This is particularly important for very-low-delivery (e.g., ≤1 mg tar) products because they typically use highly ventilated filters. Darrall (1988) reported that complete blockage of the filter ventilation of a nominally 4.0-mg tar product resulted in a tar yield of 10 mg (Table 5); nicotine increased from 0.5 to 0.8 mg, and carbon monoxide rose from 4 to 13 mg. Lower yield products employ more highly ventilated filters than in Darrall's (1988) example, and the influence of filter blockage would be expected to be greater for such products.

The importance of filter ventilation to FTC testing is illustrated by the results summarized in Figure 1. Nonfilter, filter (F), and ventilated filter (VF) commercial cigarettes were smoked (see next section, "Influence of Human Smoking Practices") under standard FTC conditions and again under standard conditions but with 23 mm of the butt end taped (FTC+). All cigarettes,

Table 4
Influence of puff frequency on machine yields

| | Percentage Increase Over Standard Federal Trade Commission Method | | | | | | | |
| | 40 Seconds | | | | 30 Seconds | | | |
	Puffs	Tar	Nicotine	Carbon Monoxide	Puffs	Tar	Nicotine	Carbon Monoxide
Regular (M-H)	28	31	29	26	62	60	49	38
Regular (M-H)	24	33	32	23	52	69	54	42
KS-UM-V (L)	47	55	24	43	90	154	47	67
KS-EM-V (L)	27	31	32	32	52	94	60	64
KS-EM-V (L)	30	21	19	27	69	84	48	79
KS (L)	38	19	19	24	76	54	38	43
KS-NV (L-M)	31	44	35	33	57	62	61	39
KS-NV (M)	26	26	16	16	60	60	32	32
IS-NV (L-M)	38	46	42	39	70	62	58	46

Key: M-H = middle to high tar (23 to 28 mg); KS = king size; UM = ultramild (<4 mg tar); V = ventilated; L = low tar (0 to 10 mg); EM = extra mild (4 to 7 mg tar); NV = nonventilated; L-M = low to middle tar (11 to 16 mg); M = middle tar (17 to 22 mg); IS = international size.

Source: Darrall, 1988.

Table 5
Influence of ventilation on machine yields

Brand (ventilation)	Constituents	Yield per Cigarette (mg)		
		Percent Blockage		
		0	50	100
A (55%)	Tar	3.8	5.9	10.0
	Nicotine	0.46	0.55	0.82
	Carbon monoxide	3.8	6.0	12.7
B (35%)	Tar	9.2	10.6	12.8
	Nicotine	0.90	0.90	0.98
	Carbon monoxide	9.2	10.9	15.2

Source: Darrall, 1988.

including nonfilter, were taped. Nonfilter cigarettes and filter cigarettes with little or no ventilation were seen to be only slightly affected by the tape. Some effect would be expected for nonfilter cigarettes because taping blocks air flow through the cigarette paper, but the changes observed were barely statistically significant for the experimental design used. The effect on ventilated filter cigarettes (VF-A to VF-F in Figure 1) was significant and major. Products rated as FTC 1 mg tar yielded 5 mg or more of tar when the ventilation was completely occluded. Products rated at 2 to 4 mg of tar delivered up to 10 mg of tar. In the case of brand F-F, the substantial increase in delivery when cigarettes were taped suggested that the filter incorporated ventilation even though it was not obvious from visual inspection. Trends for nicotine and carbon monoxide yields were generally parallel to those for tar.

INFLUENCE OF HUMAN SMOKING PRACTICES   Standardized machine smoking was developed to ensure that differences in yields among cigarettes were caused by the nature of the cigarettes and not by differences in the measurement method. The FTC adopted standardized machine smoking to maximize its ability to discriminate accurately among brands. The FTC test has been successful for this purpose but is accurate only where cigarettes are smoked as prescribed by the method.

The relevance of the FTC test parameters to human smoking practices has been called into question as FTC ratings have increasingly been viewed as a measure of human exposure. This concern is heightened by the increasing popularity of low-tar and ultralow-tar products relying largely on filter ventilation and by a better understanding of compensatory smoking practices. Observation of more recent smoking practice showed that filter ventilation was commonly compromised, puff volume was somewhat greater

Figure 1

Tar yields using standard (FTC) smoking conditions and FTC smoking conditions with tips taped (FTC+)

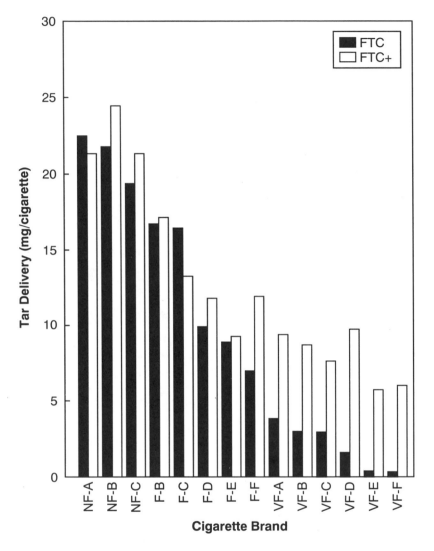

Key: *NF = nonfilter; F = filter; VF = ventilated filter.*

Source: *Jenkins et al., 1982.*

than the standard 35 mL, and a puff frequency of 2 to 3 per minute was more common than was 1 per minute (U.S. Department of Health and Human Services, 1988).

Jenkins and colleagues (1982) surveyed the influence of major changes in smoking parameters on the yields of tar, nicotine, and carbon monoxide by commercial cigarettes. Results are given in Tables 6 through 8.

Table 6
Effect of smoking conditions on tar yield

Brand	FTC Rate	Low 17 mL, 1 Sec 1 Puff/Min	FTC 35 mL, 2 Sec 1 Puff/Min	FTC+ Tip Taped 35 mL, 2 Sec 1 Puff/Min	Average 45 mL, 2 Sec 2 Puffs/Min	High 75 mL, 3 Sec 3 Puffs/Min	High+ Tip Taped 75 mL, 3 Sec 3 Puffs/Min
				Yield (mg/cigarette ± one standard deviation)			
VF-A	6.3	1.7 ± 0.3	3.8 ± 0.5	9.4 ± 0.9	11.2 ± 1.3	18.7 ± 3.9	38.2 ± 3.4
VF-B	2.3	0.3 ± 0.3	3.0 ± 0.7	8.7 ± 1.2	7.7 ± 1.4	12.8 ± 2.0	38.3 ± 5.4
VF-C	2.9	0.4 ± 0.4	2.9 ± 0.6	7.6 ± 0.9	8.8 ± 0.6	15.2 ± 1.8	26.4 ± 1.8
VF-D	1.1	.04 ± 0.14	1.6 ± 0.2	9.7 ± 0.8	2.6 ± 0.4	10.4 ± 3.2	35.5 ± 2.8
VF-E	[a]	.03 ± 0.12	0.4 ± 0.4	5.7 ± 0.7	1.5 ± 0.5	0.9 ± 0.9	24.5 ± 2.8
VF-F	[a]	−0.1 ± 0.2	0.3 ± 0.3	6.0 ± 0.5	3.0 ± 0.8	7.5 ± 2.0	23.5 ± 1.8
F-A	16.0	8.4 ± 0.6	18.5 ± 1.2	[b]	33.6 ± 4.3	53.9 ± 2.7	56.6 ± 3.5
F-B	15.4	7.7 ± 0.8	16.7 ± 0.8	17.1 ± 2.0	35.4 ± 3.2	53.3 ± 2.3	55.5 ± 3.1
F-C	16.3	7.9 ± 0.8	16.4 ± 1.4	13.2 ± 0.6	32.9 ± 1.6	44.9 ± 4.5	46.5 ± 7.6
F-D	8.3	3.8 ± 0.5	9.9 ± 0.8	11.7 ± 1.3	17.2 ± 1.5	31.7 ± 1.3	41.7 ± 2.3
F-E	7.3	3.4 ± 0.6	8.9 ± 1.0	9.2 ± 1.0	17.7 ± 1.3	30.9 ± 1.8	39.4 ± 6.9
F-F	7.0	2.6 ± 0.3	7.0 ± 0.6	11.9 ± 2.1	20.3 ± 3.4	28.7 ± 1.7	41.7 ± 5.2
NF-A	20.6	10.1 ± 1.4	22.5 ± 1.0	21.3 ± 1.5	36.2 ± 2.8	60.7 ± 2.2	60.0 ± 3.2
NF-B	24.3	12.6 ± 0.7	21.8 ± 2.6	24.4 ± 3.2	43.9 ± 2.3	65.0 ± 2.1	71.5 ± 4.4
NF-C	24.8	10.7 ± 0.6	19.4 ± 1.1	21.3 ± 1.0	43.7 ± 1.5	65.7 ± 7.6	63.3 ± 4.5

[a] Below reporting limit.
[b] Not determined.

Key: VF = ventilated filter; F = filter; NF = nonfilter.

Table 7
Effect of smoking conditions on nicotine yield

				Yield (mg/cigarette ± one standard deviation)			
Brand	FTC Rate	Low 17 mL, 1 Sec 1 Puff/Min	FTC 35 mL, 2 Sec 1 Puff/Min	FTC+ Tip Taped 35 mL, 2 Sec 1 Puff/Min	Average 45 mL, 2 Sec 2 Puffs/Min	High 75 mL, 3 Sec 3 Puffs/Min	High+ Tip Taped 75 mL, 3 Sec 3 Puffs/Min
VF-A	.54	.13 ± .01	.40 ± .05	.72 ± .05	1.05 ± .10	1.08 ± .18	2.02 ± .19
VF-B	.32	.10 ± .04	.35 ± .03	.62 ± .07	.68 ± .15	1.11 ± .16	2.04 ± .24
VF-C	.31	.07 ± .03	.25 ± .04	.45 ± .03	.62 ± .10	.82 ± .04	1.23 ± .12
VF-D	.19	.05 ± .01	.19 ± .05	.62 ± .07	.52 ± .05	.84 ± .15	1.53 ± .12
VF-E	.11	.01 ± .01	.05 ± .01	.37 ± .08	.21 ± .03	.42 ± .03	1.08 ± .18
VF-F	.11	.02 ± .01	.06 ± .02	.31 ± .03	.28 ± .08	.52 ± .11	.83 ± .13
F-A	1.04	.56 ± .10	1.09 ± .07	a	1.99 ± .17	2.20 ± .18	2.47 ± .17
F-B	1.10	.50 ± .01	.99 ± .02	.80 ± .06	1.92 ± .09	2.16 ± .16	2.29 ± .08
F-C	1.24	.53 ± .05	.94 ± .02	.71 ± .06	1.56 ± .39	2.31 ± .16	2.20 ± .20
F-D	.72	.25 ± .05	.61 ± .02	.68 ± .10	1.15 ± .07	1.81 ± .33	1.90 ± .15
F-E	.71	.31 ± .03	.77 ± .07	.81 ± .09	1.56 ± .22	1.92 ± .05	2.00 ± .12
F-F	.51	.19 ± .04	.40 ± .03	.56 ± .03	1.13 ± .06	1.29 ± .06	1.42 ± .08
NF-A	1.42	.69 ± .05	1.14 ± .05	1.37 ± .07	1.89 ± .16	2.68 ± .21	2.54 ± .20
NF-B	1.52	.70 ± .03	1.04 ± .11	1.16 ± .08	2.62 ± .27	3.61 ± .16	2.75 ± .22
NF-C	1.66	.74 ± .08	1.13 ± .13	1.60 ± .23	3.19 ± .33	3.29 ± .28	3.46 ± .24

[a] Not determined.

Key: VF = ventilated filter; F = filter; NF = nonfilter.

Table 8
Effect of smoking conditions on carbon monoxide yield

Brand	FTC Rate	Low 17 mL, 1 Sec 1 Puff/Min	FTC 35 mL, 2 Sec 1 Puff/Min	FTC+ Tip Taped 35 mL, 2 Sec 1 Puff/Min	Average 45 mL, 2 Sec 2 Puffs/Min	High 75 mL, 3 Sec 3 Puffs/Min	High+ Tip Taped 75 mL, 3 Sec 3 Puffs/Min
				Yield (mg/cigarette ± one standard deviation)			
VF-A	9.0	1.2 ± 0.3	4.1 ± 0.7	12.3 ± 1.5	11.2 ± 0.8	18.8 ± 1.7	34.5 ± 4.7
VF-B	2.9	1.8 ± 0.5	2.1 ± 0.5	8.8 ± 1.6	6.2 ± 1.9	12.9 ± 1.9	26.2 ± 3.2
VF-C	4.8	0.7 ± 0.2	2.1 ± 0.2	8.7 ± 1.2	9.9 ± 1.5	18.7 ± 4.0	27.5 ± 2.0
VF-D	1.2	.06 ± 0.0	1.0 ± 0.1	10.7 ± 0.4	5.0 ± 0.7	6.0 ± 1.7	28.7 ± 2.8
VF-E	1.1	.08 ± .03	0.6 ± .1	10.8 ± 1.4	2.3 ± 0.2	6.2 ± 0.4	21.5 ± 1.6
VF-F	1.3	0.1 ± 0.6	0.7 ± 0.3	8.8 ± 1.1	3.4 ± 0.7	8.3 ± 1.4	23.6 ± 2.1
F-A	14.5	5.8 ± 0.5	15.7 ± 1.8	[a]	25.3 ± 2.4	35.8 ± 2.6	35.5 ± 2.2
F-B	15.5	5.6 ± 1.1	17.6 ± 0.9	16.2 ± 1.0	24.2 ± 1.5	29.8 ± 5.7	33.4 ± 2.2
F-C	16.3	6.9 ± 0.5	13.4 ± 1.2	17.9 ± 1.2	24.2 ± 2.6	29.1 ± 3.2	29.2 ± 3.4
F-D	10.6	3.5 ± 0.5	8.5 ± 0.3	11.5 ± 0.7	13.5 ± 1.7	23.4 ± 2.2	33.3 ± 2.6
F-E	8.1	2.6 ± 0.5	8.8 ± 1.0	10.1 ± 1.7	17.6 ± 1.3	25.1 ± 2.2	25.1 ± 2.4
F-F	10.4	2.5 ± 0.9	9.9 ± 1.2	12.1 ± 1.6	14.6 ± 2.2	22.6 ± 1.7	27.8 ± 3.2
NF-A	12.5	4.5 ± 0.4	11.3 ± 1.0	12.8 ± 2.7	17.6 ± 1.4	25.6 ± 1.0	28.4 ± 1.2
NF-B	16.7	5.9 ± 0.7	12.3 ± 0.8	14.5 ± 1.6	21.7 ± 0.5	30.3 ± 3.1	34.8 ± 0.9
NF-C	16.1	4.6 ± 0.6	11.3 ± 1.2	12.9 ± 0.8	22.9 ± 1.6	31.8 ± 2.7	28.5 ± 5.7

[a] Not determined.

Key: VF = ventilated filter; F = filter; NF = nonfilter.

Smoking parameters were chosen to represent less intense smoking (17-mL, 1-second puffs, once per minute), conditions considered to be "average" smoking (45-mL, 2-second puffs, twice per minute) at the time, and extreme ("high") smoking (75-mL, 3-second puffs, three times per minute) conditions. These results were compared with results generated using the standard FTC conditions, FTC conditions with 23 mm of the butt end of each cigarette taped to completely occlude tip ventilation (FTC+), and the extreme conditions with the tips taped (high+). Yields under high+ conditions were viewed as the maximum practical yields of the cigarettes.

The cigarettes chosen for analysis were selected by weight and pressure drop (the differential pressure from end to end when air is drawn through a cigarette at a rate of 1,050 mL per minute [equivalent to a 35-mL puff taken over a 2-second period]) from two cartons purchased locally; they were conditioned and smoked under FTC-specified environmental conditions. The smoke was trapped and analyzed using FTC methods except that carbon monoxide was determined using gas chromatography (Horton and Guerin, 1974) rather than nondispersive infrared spectroscopy. A single-port and a linear four-port Filimatic smoking machine were used rather than the standard 20-port machine, and one to six cigarettes were smoked per port depending on the smoking conditions used. At least four ports of cigarettes were smoked per brand or condition, but the precision of the results remained 2 to 3 times poorer than would be expected using the standard 20-port protocol.

Results for tar deliveries are diagramed in Figure 2. Results for nicotine and carbon monoxide generally parallel those for tar (although carbon monoxide yields are more scattered and less systematically varied). Several observations are apparent. First, the trend toward decreasing yields generally parallels the decrease in FTC yields regardless of the conditions used for most products. Second, products with barely detectable yields of tar measured by the FTC method produce readily detectable quantities of tar when smoked under reasonable conditions. Third, even the lowest FTC tar products can yield 10 to 20 mg of tar under sufficiently aggressive smoking conditions. Products with very low FTC tar yields that depend largely on filter ventilation are those most subject to underestimation of practical yields by the FTC method.

Several investigators have reported on the influence of more relevant combinations of smoking conditions on the yields of tar and nicotine. Table 9 summarizes some of these observations for tar. Rickert and colleagues (1983) reported that increasing the puff volume to 48 mL and decreasing the puff interval to 44 seconds resulted in an increase of approximately 40 to 90 percent in the yield of tar over that found using standard FTC conditions. Using the same conditions but also occluding 50 percent of the filter ventilation resulted in an increase of from 70 to 500 percent depending on the product. Percentage increase in yield tended to correlate inversely with yield of FTC tar; that is, the lower the FTC yield, the greater the percentage increase.

Figure 2
Influence of smoking parameters on constituent yield

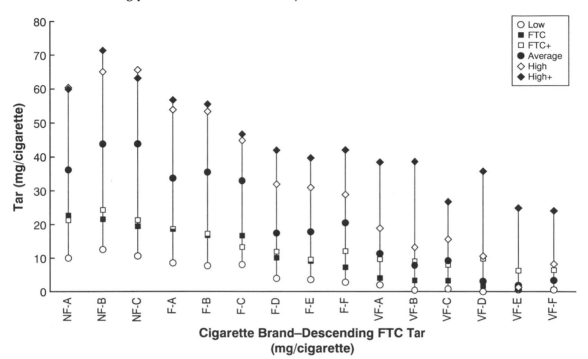

Key: *low = 17-mL puff volume, 1-second duration, 1 puff/minute; FTC = 35-mL puff volume, 2-second duration, 1 puff/minute; FTC+ = same as FTC plus butt end taped; average = 45-mL puff volume, 2-second duration, 2 puffs/minute; high = 75-mL puff volume, 3-second duration, 3 puffs/minute; high+ = same as high plus butt end taped; NF = nonfilter; F = filter; VF = ventilated filter.*

Source: Jenkins et al., 1982.

The Rickert and colleagues (1983), Darrall (1988), and Jenkins and colleagues (1982) studies all considered the effect of increasing the puff frequency from one per minute to two per minute. Puff volumes varied from 40 to 48 mL across the studies, but the results were similar. Smoking at two puffs per minute approximately doubled the tar yield for most products tested.

Filter ventilation also has been considered. The Jenkins and colleagues (1982) data illustrated that 100 percent ventilation blockage increased the tar delivery by a factor of 10 to 20 for very low (< 1 mg) FTC tar products if all other smoking parameters were kept constant. Kozlowski and coworkers (1982) reported increases of a factor of 20 to 40 using conditions of 100 percent blockage, a 47-mL puff volume, and a 44-second puff interval for products rated as <1 mg FTC tar. The influence of ventilation blockage was smaller but still important for products rated as 1 to 6 mg FTC tar (2 to 6 times increased delivery compared with that measured using the FTC method without ventilation blockage), was readily detectable for products

Table 9
Influence of "more relevant" smoking parameters on tar yields

FTC Tar mg/Cigarette	Ratio: Experimental/Standard Tar						
	Rickert et al., 1983	Rickert et al., 1983	Rickert et al., 1983	Darrall, 1988	Jenkins et al., 1982	Kozlowski et al., 1982	Jenkins et al., 1982
<1	1.6, 2.0	5.2, 5.6	—	—	3.8, 10.0	19 - 39	14, 20
1 - 3	1.6 - 1.9	2.8 - 4.3	—	3.0, 3.0	1.6 - 3.0	—	2.6 - 6.1
4 - 6	1.4 - 1.7	2.1 - 2.9	—	2.0 - 2.7	2.9	—	2.5
7 - 10	1.4 - 1.9	2.0 - 2.6	—	1.8, 1.9	1.7 - 2.9	—	1.0 - 1.7
11 - 15	1.4 - 1.9	1.7 - 2.4	2.1 - 2.3	1.7 - 2.0	—	1.5	—
16 - 20	1.6, 1.7	—	2.0, 2.1	1.6 - 1.9	1.8 - 2.2	—	0.8 - 1.1
>20	—	—	—	1.8	1.6, 2.0	—	1.1, 1.1
NV	—	—	2.0 - 2.3	1.7 - 2.0	1.6 - 2.2	—	0.9 - 1.1
Experimental Conditions							
Puff Volume (mL)	48	48	48	40	45	47	35
Puff Duration (sec)	2.4	2.4	2.4	2.3	2.0	2.4	2.0
Puff Interval (sec)	44	44	31	30	30	44	58
Ventilation Block (%)	0	50	0	0	0	100	100

Key: NV = nonventilated.

rated up to 10 mg FTC tar, and became insignificant for products rated as 15 mg FTC tar and higher. It is conceivable that a higher tar (e.g., > 10 mg) product exists that incorporates a highly ventilated filter. Such a product would be affected by ventilation blockage similar to the way lower tar products are affected.

CONCLUSIONS   The FTC procedure for measuring the tar, nicotine, and carbon monoxide yields of cigarettes provides an accurate measure of yield for cigarettes smoked in the specified manner. It serves the purpose of comparing the yields of brands smoked under the same (specified) conditions. The utility of the procedure for measuring human exposure is doubtful because it is unlikely that all brands are smoked in the same way. This is especially the case given the wide variety of products currently available. Results using realistic combinations of puff volume, puff frequency, and filter ventilation blockage suggest that human smoking conditions can produce from two times (nonfilter and standard filter brands) to ten times (low-tar and very-low-tar ventilated filter brands) the yields of tar that are measured by the FTC test. Nicotine and carbon monoxide yields vary similarly.

The current FTC test procedure must continue to be used if there is a need to compare current products with those of the past. New or additional sets of smoking parameters must be adopted if a more accurate measure of human exposure is desired.

QUESTION-AND-ANSWER SESSION

DR. RICKERT: There was a question I had asked earlier today and I wonder if you could answer it. It looks as though you have some information about interlaboratory variation, plus within-lab variation, plus variation over time. If you measure, for example, a 12-mg cigarette—how different would another brand have to be before you would be comfortable in calling it truly different?

DR. GUERIN: Certainly it would have to be more than 10 percent different. I think that it is more like, at that range, about 2 mg different.

DR. RICKERT: So, you would say that, for example, 10 mg would be considered different from one that was 14; but other than that, there would be virtually no difference.

DR. GUERIN: Right.

REFERENCES

Bradford, J.A., Harlan, W.R., Hanmer, H.R. Nature of cigaret smoke. Technic of experimental smoking. *Industrial and Engineering Chemistry* 28(7): 836-839, 1936.

Browne, C.L., Keith, C.H., Allen, R.E. The effect of filter ventilation on the yield and composition of mainstream and sidestream smokes. *Beitrage zur Tabakforschung International* 10: 81-90, 1980.

Darrall, K.G. Smoking machine parameters and cigarette smoke yields. *Science of the Total Environment* 74: 263-278, 1988.

DeBardeleben, M.Z., Wickham, J.E., Kuhn, W.F. The determination of tar and nicotine in cigarette smoke from an historical perspective. *Recent Advances in Tobacco Science* 17: 115-149, 1991.

Federal Trade Commission. "Tar, Nicotine, and Carbon Monoxide of the Smoke of 933 Varieties of Domestic Cigarettes." Internal report prepared for the National Cancer Institute. Washington, DC: Federal Trade Commission, 1994.

Horton, A.D., Guerin, M.R. Gas-solid chromatographic determination of carbon monoxide and carbon dioxide in cigarette smoke. *Journal - Association of Official Analytical Chemists* 57: 1-7, 1974.

Jenkins, R.A., Pair, D.D., Guerin, M.R. "Deliveries of Tar, Nicotine, and Carbon Monoxide of Selected U.S. Commercial Cigarettes Smoked Under 'More Relevant' Smoking Parameters." Oak Ridge National Laboratory (ORNL) Project Topical Report No. 120. Unpublished report, available from the authors. Oak Ridge, TN, 1982, 13 pp.

Kozlowski, L.T., Heatherton, T.F., Frecker, R.C., Nolte, H.E. Self-selected blocking of vents on low-yield cigarettes. *Pharmacology, Biochemistry and Behavior* 33(4): 815-819, 1989.

Kozlowski, L.T., Rickert, W.S., Pope, M.A., Robinson, J.C., Frecker, R.C. Estimating the yield to smokers of tar, nicotine, and carbon monoxide for the "lowest yield" ventilated filter cigarettes. *British Journal of Addiction* 77: 159-165, 1982.

Rickert, W.S., Robinson, J.C., Young, J.C., Collishaw, N.E., Bray, D.F. A comparison of the yields of tar, nicotine, and carbon monoxide of 36 brands of Canadian cigarettes tested under three conditions. *Preventive Medicine* 12: 682-694, 1983.

Thomsen, H.V. International reference method for the smoking of cigarettes. *Recent Advances in Tobacco Science* 18: 69-94, 1992.

U.S. Department of Health and Human Services. *The Health Consequences of Smoking: Nicotine Addiction: A Report of the Surgeon General, 1988.* DHHS Publication No. (CDC) 88-8406. Rockville, MD: U.S. Department of Health and Human Services, Public Health Service, Centers for Disease Control, Center for Health Promotion and Education, Office on Smoking and Health, 1988.

ACKNOWLEDGMENTS   This is to thank Ms. Andi Palausky of our group for the graphic summaries of data from the Jenkins and colleagues (1982) study. This work was sponsored by the National Cancer Institute under Interagency Agreement DOE No. 0485-FO53-A1 under U.S. Department of Energy contract DE-AC05-84OR21400 with Martin Marietta Energy Systems, Inc.

Human Smoking Patterns

James P. Zacny and Maxine L. Stitzer

INTRODUCTION It has been established that human exposure to tobacco smoke constituents does not reflect package yield characteristics of cigarettes as determined by Federal Trade Commission (FTC) smoking machine methods. This chapter describes some reasons for this discrepancy by examining features of human smoking behavior and how smoking behavior interacts with cigarette yield characteristics. The chapter is divided into four sections. The first section describes the topography of cigarette smoking; the second identifies the parameters of smoking topography that influence smoke exposure; the third shows that human smoking patterns are dynamic rather than static; and the fourth draws conclusions about the relevance of the FTC methodology to human smoking patterns.

HOW DO HUMANS SMOKE? The first behavioral aspect of smoking involves holding the cigarette. When smoking low-yield cigarettes (nicotine yield < 0.9 mg), smokers may knowingly or unknowingly block some or all the filter vents with their fingers or lips. Blockage of these vents increases the density of mainstream smoke that enters the mouth from the cigarette rod because the opportunity for air to be drawn into the smoke stream via the vents is reduced. Vent blocking essentially can turn a low-yield cigarette into a high-yield cigarette. Over the past 10 years, Dr. Lynn Kozlowski has performed a series of studies in which cigarette butts were assessed for vent blocking. He obtained these butts from public access places such as shopping malls. From his butt analyses, he estimated the extent to which smokers in the United States engage in vent blocking. In one study (Kozlowski et al., 1988), the incidence of partial or complete vent blocking of ultralow-yield cigarettes (0.1 to 0.4 mg of nicotine) was 58 percent. In a more recent study, Kozlowski and colleagues (1994) collected butts of so-called "light" cigarettes (0.5 to 0.8 mg of nicotine yield) and found that 53 percent of the butts showed evidence of some degree of vent blocking. Vent blocking can be detected by looking at the filter stain: Cigarettes that are not vent blocked have a dark stain in the middle of the filter toe with a visible white ring surrounding the stain (i.e., "bulls-eye" pattern); cigarettes that are vent blocked have filter stains that encompass to varying degrees not only the middle of the filter toe but also the periphery.

What are other features of smoking behavior? The smoker draws on the cigarette, inhales the smoke into the lungs, then exhales. Drawing or puffing parameters that can be measured include the size of the puff (puff volume), the duration of the puff, and the interval between puffs. Inhalation parameters that can be measured include the amount of air that is mixed with the smoke as it is inhaled into the lungs (inhalation volume, also referred to as inhalation depth), the duration to peak inhalation, and any breath holding that occurs. Exhalation parameters include exhalation volume and duration. These smoking parameters can now be measured with technologies that have been developed over the past 20 years. Puffing parameters can be measured with a plastic flowmeter, which is attached to a pressure transducer; this system measures pressure differences between two points in the flowmeter as the cigarette is puffed. Respiratory parameters can be measured with noninvasive respiratory inductive plethysmography. Essentially, the degree of movement of the chest and abdomen after calibration procedures is directly proportional to volumes of smoky air inhaled and exhaled. Thus, smoking is a complex behavior with a number of discrete, measurable elements.

WHICH HUMAN SMOKING BEHAVIORS DETERMINE SMOKE EXPOSURE?

It is important to identify which specific elements of smoking behavior influence smoke exposure to focus on relevant parameters of the FTC testing procedures vs. human smoking comparison. Stitzer, Zacny, and other colleagues over the past several years have conducted three studies (Zacny et al., 1986 and 1987; Weinhold and Stitzer, 1989) that have examined the relative importance of various smoking topography parameters in determining smoke exposure. Smoke exposure is measured by determining the amount of carbon monoxide (CO) and nicotine absorbed from smoking a single cigarette—these parameters are called CO boost and nicotine boost, respectively.

In these studies, smokers were trained to puff and inhale the cigarette in a standardized fashion. The procedure of the standardization is simple: The computer involved in the measurement of smoking topography parameters can be programmed to beep when a specified level of a smoking parameter has been reached. The investigator programs the computer to give the smoker feedback as to when to (1) stop puffing (this controls puff volume), (2) stop inhaling (this controls inhalation volume), and (3) start exhaling (this controls breath-hold duration). After practice with this biofeedback system, the smoker is able to reproduce a given smoking pattern that includes a fixed puff volume, inhalation volume, and breath-hold duration.

In the first study (Zacny et al., 1986), an ultralow-yield cigarette was smoked in this standardized fashion, and the number of vents that were blocked was varied. In this way, the effect of vent blocking on smoke exposure could be determined, as measured by CO boost. Either no vents were blocked with tape, 50 percent of vents were blocked, or 100 percent of the vents were blocked. Smokers took eight fixed-volume puffs (60 mL) from the cigarette, inhaled to a certain volume (25 percent of vital capacity), held the breath for a certain duration (10 seconds), and then exhaled. Any differences in CO boost could be attributed to manipulation of vent blocking because other smoking topography parameters were controlled. The authors found a systematic increase in CO boost as a function of number of vents blocked. In a second study, Weinhold and Stitzer (1989) varied the number of puffs (from 8 to 16) taken from a cigarette. CO boost again increased in a linear fashion as a function of number of puffs taken. In a third study

(Zacny et al., 1987), three parameters were systematically manipulated: puff volume (15, 30, 45, and 60 mL), inhalation volume (0, 20, 40, and 60 percent of vital capacity, respectively), and breath-hold duration (0, 4, 8, and 16 seconds, respectively). As puff volume increased, the amount of nicotine and CO absorbed from a cigarette increased in a systematic fashion. However, varying the amount of air mixed with the smoke as it was inhaled (inhalation volume) did not affect nicotine or CO boost; exposure was as great with a shallow inhalation as with a deep inhalation. Breath-hold duration increased CO boost but had no effect on nicotine boost. In summary, the smoking topography parameters that appear to have the larger effect on smoke exposure are vent blocking of low-yield cigarettes and the number and size of puffs taken from any cigarette.

ARE HUMAN SMOKING PATTERNS DYNAMIC OR STATIC? Much literature indicates that human smoking patterns are dynamic and different from the static FTC smoking method. Puffing parameters change during the course of smoking a single cigarette. Initially, smokers take larger and longer puffs from the cigarette, but as they smoke down the rod, the puffs get shorter and smaller. Interpuff intervals are shortest at the beginning of the cigarette and longest near the end of the cigarette. Smokers engage in activities that can have an influence on smoking topography. Hatsukami and colleagues (1990) developed a portable device that measures number of puffs, interpuff intervals, and puff durations and assessed these parameters in a smoker's natural environment. They found that variables, including mood of the smokers (relaxed vs. stressed) and activities of the smoker (working vs. socializing), influenced smoking topographies. Psychoactive drugs other than tobacco (e.g., stimulants, alcohol, opioids) also can influence smoking topographies. Several investigators have noted changes in smoking topography as a function of alcohol. Keenan and associates (1990) studied smoking topography in alcoholic and nonalcoholic smokers: Alcoholic smokers took more puffs from their cigarettes than did the nonalcoholic smokers, indicating more intensive smoking and suggesting higher exposure levels per cigarette.

Two other examples demonstrate that smoking is a dynamic process. In the first example, Fant and associates (1995) studied smoking deprivation. The number of cigarettes that subjects were permitted to smoke varied from 0 to 11 during a 6-hour period. The number of puffs taken was directly related to the interval between cigarettes and inversely related to the number of cigarettes smoked. In the second example, the authors reviewed studies over the past 15 years that examined smoking topography as a function of cigarette yield. We included only those studies that assessed the smoking of commercially available, as opposed to research, cigarettes. We also arbitrarily defined high-yield cigarettes as having nonventilated filters and an FTC nicotine yield of 0.8 mg or more and low-yield cigarettes as having ventilated filters and an FTC nicotine yield of 0.6 mg or less. Table 1 summarizes the seven studies that fit these criteria. A consistent finding in these studies is that puff volume and puff number are both larger when low-yield compared with high-yield cigarettes were smoked. Overall, it is clear that smoking

Table 1

Studies that assessed smoking topography across different cigarette yields, using commercially available cigarettes

Reference	Number	Low-High Nicotine Yield (mg)	Puff Volume			Puff Number		
			Low Yield	High Yield	*p* Value	Low Yield	High Yield	*p* Value
Bridges et al., 1986	5 vs. 65[a]	0.3-1.1	85.4	52.2	0.05	13.2	10.6	ns
Woodman et al., 1987	10	0.6-1.4	59.5	43.6	0.05	14.0	12.1	ns
Zacny and Stitzer, 1988	10	0.1-1.1	64.7	52.4	0.05	11.3	12.9	ns
Nil and Battig, 1989	15	0.5-0.8	25.7	26.6	ns	17.5	13.7	0.05
Hofer et al., 1991	36[a]	0.1-1.2	44.5	36.8	0.05	15.6	11.1	0.05
Kolonen et al., 1991	10	0.4-0.9	76.9	64.6	0.05	18.7	14.4	ns
Kolonen et al., 1992	8	0.3-1.0	35.6	29.5	0.05	18.5	12.9	0.05
Mean			56.0	43.7		15.5	12.5	
Range			25.7-85.4	26.6-64.6		11.3-18.7	10.6-14.4	

[a] *Cross-sectional study; the sample size in these studies represents each group of smokers studied within a yield category.*

Note: All studies were conducted with filtered, commercial brand cigarettes; low-yield brands were all ventilated and ranged in nicotine yield from 0.1 to 0.6 mg, and high-yield brands were all unventilated and ranged in nicotine yield from 0.8 to 1.4 mg.

Key: ns = not significant.

topography is dynamic and changes in response to several factors, including yield characteristics of the cigarette.

DOES THE FTC METHOD ACCURATELY REFLECT HUMAN SMOKING PATTERNS?   The FTC machine takes 2-second, 35-mL puffs every minute until a certain point has been reached along the length of the cigarette (i.e., filter overwrap plus 3 mm). The length of the cigarette plays a large role in how many puffs are taken by the smoking machine, although porosity of the cigarette paper and tobacco burn rate also play roles. How does the FTC method of smoking compare with how humans smoke cigarettes? A table in the 1988 Surgeon General's Report on smoking (U.S. Department of Health and Human Services, 1988) summarizes results from 32 studies that assessed ad libitum human smoking topography. Table 2 lists the average values, along with the range of puffing parameters observed in each study. Average puff duration across the 32 studies was 1.8 seconds, which is fairly close to the smoking machine value. Human puff volumes tend to be larger than the 35 mL used in standard FTC smoking machine assays. The biggest difference between human and FTC machine smoking parameters was in the rate of puffing. The average interpuff interval in the human studies was 34 seconds, whereas FTC testing used a 60-second interval. Thus, humans took puffs at nearly twice the rate of smoking

Table 2
Published values of common measures of smoking

Reference	Number of Subjects	Puffs/ Cigarette	Interpuff Interval (seconds)	Puff Duration (seconds)	Puff Volume (mL)
Rawbone et al., 1978	12	10	41	1.8	
Rawbone et al., 1978	9	10	35	2.1	43
Woodman et al., 1986	9	13	18	1.9	49
Nemeth-Coslett et al., 1986a	8	8	64	1.8	
Nemeth-Coslett et al., 1986b	8	8	47	1.4	
Nil et al., 1986a	132	13	28	2.2	30
Jarvik et al., 1978	9	10			
Russell et al., 1980	10	11	35		
Ashton et al., 1978	14		24	1.5	
Schulz and Seehofer, 1978	100	11	50	1.4	
Schulz and Seehofer, 1978	218	12	42	1.3	
Henningfield and Griffiths, 1981	8	10	39	1.0	
Stepney, 1981	19	13			38
Bättig et al., 1982	110	13	26	2.1	40
Epstein et al., 1982	63	13		2.4	21
Russell et al., 1982	12	15	26	2.3	40
Gritz et al., 1983	8	9	47	2.2	66
Ossip-Klein et al., 1983	9	8		1.4	
Ossip-Klein et al., 1983	9	12		1.9	
Guillerm and Radziszewski, 1978	8	12	41	1.9	39
Gust et al., 1983	8	9	48	1.6	44
Adams et al., 1983	10		26	1.9	44
Moody, 1980	517	9	26	2.1	44
Nil et al., 1984	20	15	26	1.6	40
McBride et al., 1984	9	16	25	2.1	42
Medici et al., 1985	17	14	19	2.2	43
Burling et al., 1985	24	12	28	1.7	
Nil et al., 1986b	117	13	22	2.1	42
Hughes et al., 1986	46	11		1.6	
Bridges et al., 1986	108	11			56
Puustinen et al., 1986	11	13	22	2.3	44
Hilding, 1956	27	10			
Mean		11	34	1.8	43
Range		8-16	18-64	1.0-2.4	21-66

Note: Data were taken from the baseline phase (or placebo treatment) of studies involving an experimental manipulation with at least eight subjects. Values are rounded off to the nearest unit and, in some cases, were calculated from other variables or estimated from data presented in figures; missing values indicate that the variable was not measured or was not presented in the published study.

Source: U.S. Department of Health and Human Services, 1988.

machine rates used in standardized testing. Across the 32 studies, there appears to be a large degree of variability in the values (as shown by the range of values listed at the bottom of the table) that is not reflected in the FTC method. The average number of puffs taken per cigarette by human smokers was 11; FTC does not publish the number of puffs taken from a cigarette by the machine. Differences in puffing rates suggest that the FTC method probably underestimates the number of puffs taken from a cigarette by humans.

It is possible to estimate the number of puffs used to determine FTC cigarette yield by having cigarettes machine-smoked in a research laboratory. The authors had a low-yield cigarette brand, Now, smoked according to the FTC method at the Tobacco and Health Research Institute in Lexington, Kentucky. Two hundred cigarettes were smoked; the average number of puffs taken per cigarette was 6.8. This same procedure was repeated with a high-yield cigarette, Camel, and an average of 8.3 puffs was taken. Thus, the machine took more puffs from the high-yield than from the low-yield cigarette, which is at odds with the human data presented in Table 1 in which the opposite occurs. Therefore, there appears to be a discrepancy between the FTC method of smoking and the way humans smoke different-yield cigarettes: Machines tend to puff *less* smoke from low-yield than from high-yield cigarettes, and humans tend to compensate for air dilution by puffing *more* smoke from low-yield than from high-yield cigarettes. Thus, humans smoke low-yield cigarettes in a manner that attenuates machine-determined yield differences.

SUMMARY   In conclusion, we have shown that the number and size of puffs are key factors that determine per-cigarette smoke exposure. Vent blocking is another important smoking behavior that can occur with low-yield cigarettes. Human smoking behavior is dynamic, not static. There is between-smoker variability in smoking topography, and there are dynamic changes in response to smoking deprivation, cigarette characteristics, other drugs, and situational determinants. The evidence suggests that the FTC method does not accurately reflect human smoking patterns. The FTC method takes smaller, fewer, and more widely spaced puffs than do humans, on average. The underestimation of puff volume is exaggerated with low-yield cigarettes because people tend to increase both the size and number of puffs drawn from lower, as compared with higher, yield cigarettes, whereas smoking machines decrease the number of puffs drawn while holding puff size constant. In addition, the FTC method does not take into account the important behavior of vent blocking of low-yield cigarettes. Thus, there are important differences between FTC and human smoking that result in the machines underestimating the amount of smoke drawn by humans from low-yield as compared with high-yield cigarettes.

QUESTION-AND-ANSWER SESSION

DR. HOFFMANN: How did you cover half of the ventilation holes?

DR. ZACNY: We did not tape half of the cigarette. We put little pieces of square tape all the way around it, so that approximately half the holes were unblocked.

DR. HARRIS: Why is it that it is not how big a puff they took once it was in their mouths, but how deeply they drag that puff into the lungs?

DR. STITZER: I think the explanation is that the dose of nicotine that is drawn in with the puff is the critical determinant. The amount of air that is breathed in along with it, which is what determines the depth, is how much additional volume of air was breathed in with the smoke. That does not seem to be relevant with nicotine.

DR. ZACNY: Even with a shallow inhalation, the surface volume of the lungs is pretty huge.

DR. HARRIS: I understand. It is all in that 1.8-second drag on the cigarette.

DR. STITZER: Yes.

DR. HARRIS: Once the smoke is in your mouth, then you can jump up and down; it does not matter.

DR. STITZER: No, once it is in your lungs. Once you have made that inhalation maneuver, because if you just hold it in your mouth, that was the zero inhalation condition.

DR. HARRIS: So, as long as you inhale it, it does not matter how much air goes in with it.

DR. RICKERT: One important point is that you haven't looked at tar. Tar may react differently. Depth of inhalation and volume of inhalation might be more important. Deposition of tar is not nearly as efficient as for water-soluble vapors and gases. In one of the documents that we received from the tobacco industry, there is a study that has been cited by Stitzer, which says that, on 1,631 cigarette butts, only .1 percent were completely blocked. The information that you have provided today suggests that it is somewhere between 53 and 58 percent. What is the reason for the discrepancy?

DR. ZACNY: The reason for the discrepancy is that those 1,600 butts are from only 10 subjects. We had them smoke the ultralow cigarettes for a week and save the butts. We then analyzed the stain patterns.

We were looking at the acute effects of smoking these ultralow cigarettes in the field, and there may be a lower incidence of blocking than what you see when Lynn Kozlowski does his cross-sectional studies—when people have been normally smoking these cigarettes for a long time. Plus, our data were from only 10 subjects.

DR. RICKERT: Do you feel that this blocking is something that we should be concerned about?

DR. ZACNY: Yes.

DR. SHIFFMAN: One of the issues that you raised that we have not discussed much is variability within a given smoker, due to brand switching, for example. Can you give us some quantitative estimates of the degree of variability?

DR. ZACNY: I believe Dr. Stitzer would be the best person to answer this question.

DR. STITZER: In one example, it was shown for deprivation to be 10 to 15 puffs. And that makes quite a big difference when you multiply it by the puff volumes, leading to a substantial difference in cumulative puff volume.

DR. HATSUKAMI: Also, one subject after meals typically took about eight puffs per cigarette, whereas on the telephone, they would take about five puffs from the cigarette.

DR. TOWNSEND: Dr. Zacny, I am a bit confused about the whole blockage question. Is the measure that you used to determine hole blockage just the staining at the mouth end of the filter?

DR. ZACNY: Yes. Different cigarettes have different types of what we call tipping and different types of perforations. The perforations differ largely in the number of holes and the size of those holes.

Those parameters of ventilation, in fact, determine to a large degree the staining pattern in the first place. So, it is possible to make a highly air-diluted cigarette with many ventilation holes that are very small and, in fact, see relatively uniform staining patterns right at the mouth end of the cigarette.

If you are interpreting that as vent blocking, then I think that is probably an incorrect conclusion, because of the design of that specific filter. Filters with large though very few holes will tend to force the smoke to the center of the filter, and you will see that bullet shape right at the mouth end that was shown in one of the slides.

The concern is that not all cigarettes are built in the same way and so that it is probably a bit premature to conclude that there is vent blocking solely on the basis of filter observation.

DR. STITZER: The data that were presented in this talk showed what happened to smoke *exposure* when the vents were experimentally blocked with tape. Dr. Townsend is asking a different kind of question about measurement of blocking in the natural environment.

DR. TOWNSEND: So, these were not with actual subjects, then?

DR. STITZER: They were with natural subjects, but we blocked the vents.

DR. ZACNY: You were talking about the first study when we looked at 50 and 100 percent of hole blocking.

DR. TOWNSEND: I understand. I would like to talk with you some more about this, because we have some data at R.J. Reynolds where we have gone directly to an inhydrin staining test where the saliva on the filter, in fact, stains with inhydrin; therefore, we can visually see how much saliva has gotten up to the vents.

What we have seen in a study with a number of subjects is that the spent butts show some blockage, but it is a very infrequent phenomenon. So, I would like to talk to you further about that. Perhaps we can propose doing some additional studies.

REFERENCES

Adams, L., Lee, C., Rawbone, R., Guz, A. Patterns of smoking: Measurement and variability in asymptomatic smokers. *Clinical Science* 65(4): 383-392, 1983.

Ashton, H., Stepney, R., Thompson, J.W. Smoking behaviour and nicotine intake in smokers presented with a "two-thirds" cigarette. In: *Smoking Behaviour. Physiological and Psychological Influences*, R.E. Thornton (Editor). Edinburgh: Churchill Livingstone, 1978, pp. 315-329.

Bättig, K., Buzzi, R., Nil, R. Smoke yield of cigarettes and puffing behavior in men and women. *Psychopharmacology* 76: 139-148, 1982.

Bridges, R.B., Humble, J.W., Turbek, J.A., Rehm, S.R. Smoking history, cigarette yield and smoking behavior as determinants of smoke exposure. *European Journal of Respiratory Diseases* 69[Suppl 146]: 129-137, 1986.

Burling, T.A., Stitzer, M.L., Bigelow, G.E., Mead, A.M. Smoking topography and carbon monoxide levels in smokers. *Addictive Behaviors* 10: 319-323, 1985.

Epstein, L.H., Dickson, B.E., Ossip, D.J., Stiller, R., Russell, P.O., Winter, K. Relationships among measures of smoking topography. *Addictive Behaviors* 7: 307-310, 1982.

Fant, R.V., Schuh, C.J., Stitzer, M.L. Response to smoking as a function of prior smoking amounts. *Psychopharmacology* 119: 385-390, 1995.

Gritz, E.R., Rose, J.E., Jarvik, M.E. Regulation of tobacco smoke intake with paced cigarette presentation. *Pharmacology, Biochemistry and Behavior* 18(3): 457-462, 1983.

Guillerm, R., Radziszewski, E. Analysis of smoking pattern including intake of carbon monoxide and influences of changes in cigarette design. In: *Smoking Behaviour. Physiological and Psychological Influences*, R.E. Thornton (Editor). Edinburgh: Churchill Livingstone, 1978, pp. 361-370.

Gust, S.W., Pickens, R.W., Pechacek, T.F. Relation of puff volume to other topographical measures of smoking. *Addictive Behaviors* 8(2): 115-119, 1983.

Hatsukami, D.K., Morgan, S.F., Pickens, R.W., Champagne, S.E. Situational factors in cigarette smoking. *Addictive Behaviors* 15(1): 1-12, 1990.

Henningfield, J.E., Griffiths, R.R. Cigarette smoking and subjective response: Effects of d-amphetamine. *Clinical Pharmacology and Therapeutics* 30(4): 497-505, 1981.

Hilding, A.C. On cigarette smoking, bronchial carcinoma and ciliary action. I. Smoking habits and measurement of smoke intake. *New England Journal of Medicine* 254(17): 775-781, 1956.

Hofer, I., Nil, R., Bättig, K. Nicotine yield as determinant of smoke exposure indicators and puffing behavior. *Pharmacology, Biochemistry and Behavior* 40: 139-149, 1991.

Hughes, J.R., Pickens, R.W., Gust, S.W., Hatsukami, D.K., Svikis, D.S. Smoking behavior of Type A and Type B smokers. *Addictive Behaviors* 11: 115-118, 1986.

Jarvik, M.E., Popek, P., Schneider, N.G., Baer-Weiss, V., Gritz, E.R. Can cigarette size and nicotine content influence smoking and puffing rates? *Psychopharmacology* 58(3): 303-306, 1978.

Keenan, R.M., Hatsukami, D.K., Pickens, R.W., Gust, S.W., Strelow, L.J. The relationship between chronic ethanol exposure and cigarette smoking in the laboratory and the natural environment. *Psychopharmacology* 100: 77-83, 1990.

Kolonen, S., Tuomisto, J., Puustinen, P., Airaksinen, M.M. Smoking behavior in low-yield cigarette smokers and switchers in the natural environment. *Pharmacology, Biochemistry and Behavior* 40: 177-180, 1991.

Kolonen, S., Tuomisto, J., Puustinen, P., Airaksinen, M.M. Effects of smoking abstinence and chain-smoking on puffing topography and diurnal nicotine exposure. *Pharmacology, Biochemistry and Behavior* 42: 327-332, 1992.

Kozlowski, L.T., Pillitteri, J.L., Sweeney, C.T. Misuse of "light" cigarettes by means of vent blocking. *Journal of Substance Abuse* 6: 333-336, 1994.

Kozlowski, L.T., Pope, M.A., Lux, J.E. Prevalence of the misuse of ultra-low-tar cigarettes by blocking filter vents. *American Journal of Public Health* 78: 694-695, 1988.

McBride, M.J., Guyatt, A.R., Kirkham, A.J.T., Cumming, G. Assessment of smoking behaviour and ventilation with cigarettes of differing nicotine yields. *Clinical Science* 67(6): 619-631, 1984.

Medici, T.C., Unger, S., Rüegger, M. Smoking pattern of smokers with and without tobacco-smoke-related lung diseases. *American Review of Respiratory Disease* 131(3): 385-388, 1985.

Moody, P.M. The relationships of qualified human smoking behavior and demographic variables. *Social Science and Medicine* 14A(1): 49-54, 1980.

Nemeth-Coslett, R., Henningfield, J.E., O'Keefe, M.K., Griffiths, R.R. Effects of mecamylamine on human cigarette smoking and subjective ratings. *Psychopharmacology* 88(4): 420-425, 1986a.

Nemeth-Coslett, R., Henningfield, J.E., O'Keefe, M.K., Griffiths, R.R. Effects of marijuana smoking on subjective ratings and tobacco smoking. *Pharmacology, Biochemistry and Behavior* 25(3): 659-665, 1986b.

Nil, R., Bättig, K. Separate effects of cigarette smoke yield and smoke taste on smoking behavior. *Psychopharmacology* 99: 54-59, 1989.

Nil, R., Buzzi, R., Bättig, K. Effects of single doses of alcohol and caffeine on cigarette smoke puffing behavior. *Pharmacology, Biochemistry and Behavior* 20(4): 583-590, 1984.

Nil, R., Buzzi, R., Bättig, K. Effects of different cigarette smoke yields on puffing and inhalation: Is the measurement of inhalation volumes relevant for smoke absorption? *Pharmacology, Biochemistry and Behavior* 24(3): 587-595, 1986b.

Nil, R., Woodson, P.P., Bättig, K. Smoking behavior and personality patterns of smokers with low and high CO absorption. *Clinical Science* 71(5): 595-603, 1986a.

Ossip-Klein, D.J., Martin, J.E., Lomax, B.D., Prue, D.M., Davis, C.J. Assessment of smoking topography generalization across laboratory, clinical, and naturalistic settings. *Addictive Behaviors* 8(1): 11-17, 1983.

Puustinen, P., Olkkonen, H., Kolonen, S., Tuomisto, J. Microcomputer-assisted measurement of inhalation parameters during smoking. *Archives of Toxicology* [Suppl 9]: 111-114, 1986.

Rawbone, R.G., Murphy, K., Tate, M.E., Kane, S.J. The analysis of smoking parameters: Inhalation and absorption of tobacco smoke in studies of human smoking behaviour. In: *Smoking Behaviour. Physiological and Psychological Influences*, R.E. Thornton (Editor). Edinburgh: Churchill Livingstone, 1978, pp. 171-194.

Russell, M.A.H., Sutton, S.R., Feyerabend, C., Saloojee, Y. Smoker's response to shortened cigarettes: Dose reduction without dilution of tobacco smoke. *Clinical Pharmacology and Therapeutics* 27(2): 210-218, 1980.

Russell, M.A.H., Sutton, S.R., Iyer, R., Feyerabend, C., Vesey, C.J. Long-term switching to low-tar low-nicotine cigarettes. *British Journal of Addiction* 77(2): 145-158, 1982.

Schulz, W., Seehofer, F. Smoking behaviour in Germany—the analysis of cigarette butts (KIPA). In: *Smoking Behaviour. Physiological and Psychological Influences*, R.E. Thornton (Editor). Edinburgh: Churchill Livingstone, 1978, pp. 259-276.

Stepney, R. Would a medium-nicotine, low-tar cigarette be less hazardous to health? *British Medical Journal* 283(6302): 1292-1303, 1981.

U.S. Department of Health and Human Services. *The Health Consequences of Smoking: Nicotine Addiction. A Report of the Surgeon General, 1988.* DHHS Publication No. (CDC) 88-8406. Rockville, MD: U.S. Department of Health and Human Services, Public Health Service, Centers for Disease Control, Center for Health Promotion and Education, Office on Smoking and Health, 1988.

Weinhold, L.L., Stitzer, M.L. Effects of puff number and puff spacing on carbon monoxide exposure from commercial brand cigarettes. *Pharmacology, Biochemistry and Behavior* 33: 853-858, 1989.

Woodman, G., Newman, S.P., Pavia, D., Clarke, S.W. Inhaled smoke volume, puffing indices and carbon monoxide uptake in asymptomatic cigarette smokers. *Clinical Science* 71(4): 421-427, 1986.

Woodman, G., Newman, S.P., Pavia, D., Clarke, S.W. Response and acclimatization of symptomless smokers on changing to a low tar, low nicotine cigarette. *Thorax* 42: 336-341, 1987.

Zacny, J.P., Stitzer, M.L. Cigarette brand-switching: Effects on smoke exposure and smoking behavior. *Journal of Pharmacology and Experimental Therapeutics* 246: 619-627, 1988.

Zacny, J.P., Stitzer, M.L., Brown, F.J., Griffiths, R.R. Human cigarette smoking: Effects of puff and inhalational parameters on smoke exposure. *Journal of Pharmacology and Experimental Therapeutics* 240: 554-564, 1987.

Zacny, J.P., Stitzer, M.L., Yingling, J.E. Cigarette filter vent blocking: Effects on smoking topography and carbon monoxide exposure. *Pharmacology, Biochemistry and Behavior* 25: 1245-1252, 1986.

Compensation for Nicotine by Smokers of Lower Yield Cigarettes

Lynn T. Kozlowski and Janine L. Pillitteri

BACKGROUND   The question has been asked whether brand-switching smokers oversmoke lower nicotine cigarettes. The Federal Trade Commission (FTC) testing method is a *per-cigarette* test and should be judged as such. (Forty truly low-calorie candy bars together could be high calorie and still, individually, be low calorie.) The FTC test cannot be blamed because smokers smoke more cigarettes when they switch to those having a lower yield. Therefore, for this review compensation data were adjusted to per-cigarette values. However, such per-cigarette adjustments only approximate what would happen if the number of cigarettes were fixed for smokers. If smokers have already compensated by smoking many more cigarettes, then presumably they would have less need to smoke more of each cigarette. In the five studies included in the authors' main review, the compensatory percentage change in cigarettes per day averaged 15 percent (±6, 95-percent confidence interval). No studies showed a decreased number of cigarettes smoked with a lower yield brand of cigarettes.

Experimental brand-switching studies offering measures of nicotine and cotinine were reviewed. An index of compensation was calculated using a sequence of formulas developed by Russell and colleagues (1982). Calculation of these formulas first requires information on the machine-smoked nicotine yields of cigarettes to calculate (a) the percentage change in nicotine yields. Information on the measured level of nicotine (or cotinine) in body fluids is then used to calculate (b) the percentage change in nicotine (or cotinine) intake. Finally, three consecutive formulas are used to calculate (c) the actual compensatory increase in smoke intake [(b/a − 1) × 100]; (d) the increase in smoke intake necessary for complete compensation [(1− a)/a × 100]; and (e) using the values obtained in (c) and (d) above, the degree of compensation [(c/d) − 100].

CIGARETTE BRAND SWITCHING IN EXPERIMENTAL RESEARCH   Research on brand switching makes use of repeated-measures designs. With these designs, the same smokers get different cigarettes. This controls for individual differences in drug metabolism (Benowitz et al., 1982) and for important biases in brand selection, which usually are not controlled for in cross-sectional research. This issue has been discussed by others (e.g., Giovino et al. [this volume]; Cohen [this volume]). Wynder and coworkers (1984) explored the demographics of smokers of the low-yield cigarettes and showed that age, sex, race, education, and religion were strongly related to the selection of low-tar cigarettes. Wynder and colleagues (1984) reported that education is negatively associated with tar for males, but not for females. (Tar and nicotine are highly correlated across the full range of tar and nicotine yields.) People who smoke low- and ultralow-yield cigarettes may be more health conscious, have better diets, and be interested in smoking less. A random sample of persons does not select ultralow-yield cigarettes.

Despite their advantages, experimental brand-switching studies have important limitations. Outside of laboratories, smokers select their own brands. There is a free market for most purchases of cigarettes. An unsatisfying brand is likely to be rejected for a satisfying brand. Persons trying an ultralow-yield cigarette may feel that they are puffing on air, so they decide not to smoke these cigarettes and probably will not buy more than one pack. Some compensatory smoking techniques (e.g., vent blocking [Kozlowski et al., 1980 and 1989]) may take time to be learned by trial and error. Short-term studies (i.e., less than 1 week of exposure on lower yield brands) do not provide an adequate indication of the nature of compensatory smoking in self-selected smokers. All reviewed studies involved brand manipulations (change of "treatment" or brand in experimental study) of more than 7 days.

Studies of brand switching also have biased samples. Who does and does not volunteer for these studies? One of the five studies reviewed (Guyatt et al., 1989) showed a dramatic number of dropouts following informed consent. Of the people who went to at least one session in this study, 81 percent dropped out. Another study on brand switching (Benowitz et al., 1986a) required that participants be hospitalized for 14 days. Some smokers, knowing that they were going to get ultralow-yield cigarettes, either might not have wanted to smoke them or spend 14 days in the hospital. One must wonder who would be available to participate in a 14-day study requiring confinement to a hospital room. Most studies of brand switching also have small samples (mean = 22 subjects). As for demographic differences, there is no way to represent the complexities of age, sex, race, and education adequately in a sample of 22 participants.

According to the boundary model of drug regulation, plasma nicotine levels are not precisely regulated (Kozlowski and Herman, 1984); there are aversive upper and lower limits or boundaries on intake for dependent smokers. At the upper limit, when people are smoking a great deal, it is difficult for them to smoke more due to overdose or toxic effects of nicotine. When they are smoking a little, it is hard for them to smoke less than the lower limit because of insufficient nicotine intake. However, within these broad limits or boundaries, psychosocial factors primarily (i.e., the presence of others smoking) determine nicotine ingestion, and dose manipulations tend to have a smaller effect on smoking behavior (Kozlowski and Herman, 1984; Kozlowski, 1989) and how smokers feel (Benowitz et al., 1986b).

RESEARCH   Table 1 shows the five studies reviewed and gives a summary of their results.   The following studies were not included in the review because they were either too short term or used cigarette holders, which could interfere with natural smoking behavior: Benowitz and colleagues (1986a), Kolonen

Table 1
Summary of five experimental brand-switching studies demonstrating changes in cigarette yields due to compensation

Study	Number of Subjects	% Change in Nicotine Yield in Low- vs. Usual-Yield Cigarettes (Low vs. Usual in mg)	% Change in Plasma Nicotine in Low- vs. Usual-Yield Cigarettes (Low vs. Usual in ng/mL)	% Change in Plasma Cotinine of Low- vs. Usual-Yield Cigarettes (Low vs. Usual in ng/mL)	% Compensation
Ashton et al. (1979)	6 men 6 women	43 (0.6 vs. 1.4)	71 (83.8 vs. 117.3)	—	49
Guyatt et al. (1989)	10 men 18 women	67 (0.91 vs. 1.36)	—	71 (10.8 vs. 15.2)	12
Robinson et al. (1983), Stage 1[a]	16 treatment 6 control	67 (0.64 vs. 0.96)	—	78 (9.0 vs. 11.5)	33
Robinson et al. (1983), Stage 2[a]	16 treatment 6 control	40 (0.38 vs. 0.96)	—	77 (8.8 vs. 11.5)	62
Russell et al. (1982)	4 men 8 women	54 (0.7 vs. 1.3)	70 (22.8 vs. 32.4)	—	35
West et al. (1984)	12 treatment 12 control	8 (0.1 vs. 1.3)	41 (9.4 vs. 22.8)	—	36

[a] *This is a two-part study that allows for two different comparisons.*

Note: Five studies gave six comparisons between low- and usual-yield cigarettes. Formulas used to calculate compensatory change in cigarette yields are reported in Russell and colleagues (1982), p. 153. Per-cigarette adjustments have been made so that all results are on the same scale.

and colleagues (1991), Russell and colleagues (1975), and Zacny and Stitzer (1988).

Figure 1 shows the pattern of results across the five studies. The solid line summarizes results from the studies after adjusting for changes in the number of cigarettes smoked. As nicotine yields go below the usual "normal" levels (1.0 to 1.4 mg nicotine), more compensation takes place until the lowest yield is reached. At this point, too much work may be required of smokers to achieve substantial compensation. This kind of dose-response pattern is consistent with that for other reinforcers. It may not be important to compensate for a 0.9-mg nicotine cigarette; it easily provides adequate levels of nicotine. The dashed line shows what happens when there is no adjustment for changes in the number of cigarettes smoked. This shows that compensation also is supported by an increase in cigarettes per day in these brand-switching studies (the 0.4-mg nicotine cigarette now shows close to 80 percent compensation).

Figure 1

Pattern of results illustrating percentage compensation across the five reviewed studies, unadjusted (dashed line) and adjusted (solid line) for number of cigarettes

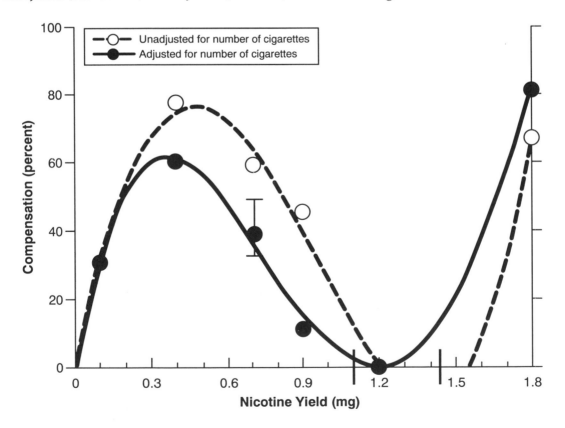

The short-term study by Zacny and Stitzer (1988) (not included in our review) examined smokers who had been given three different lower yield brands (i.e., 0.1 mg, 0.4 mg, 0.7 mg nicotine). This study produced a pattern of compensation similar to that in Figure 1.

For consumers, the *average* percentage compensation may be less important than the likelihood of substantial compensation. If 1 in 2, 1 in 5, 1 in 10, 1 in 50, or even 1 in 100 smokers shows compensation of 25, 33, 55, or 75 percent, then a problem exists. If automobile brakes failed at a rate of even 1 in 1,000, this rate would be of great concern to manufacturers, consumers, and regulatory agencies.

ONE REPEATED-MEASURES STUDY OF SELF-SELECTED BRAND SWITCHING

Lynch and Benowitz (1987) conducted a self-selected brand-switching study of participants who spontaneously switched cigarette brands. The study included 62 people who had lowered their standard yield. When they had been studied earlier, they had had plasma measures taken, and they were recontacted 3 to 6 years later. In this group, the low-yield cigarette was 62 percent of the former usual cigarette yield of nicotine (.68 mg versus 1.09 mg). Plasma cotinine per cigarette was unchanged: 10.3 ng per mL for the low-yield cigarette versus 10.2 ng per mL for the former usual cigarette. This represents a compensation of 103 percent!

SMOKERS CAN GET HIGH YIELDS FROM THE LOWEST OF THE LOW-YIELD CIGARETTES: MORE ON THE ISSUE OF VENT BLOCKING

Some points should be made about vent blocking and the possibility of getting high yields from ultralow-yield brands. In one study, 14 people were smoking ultralow-yield cigarettes (Kozlowski et al., 1989), and half the smokers were vent blockers. Two of the seven vent blockers smoked about 25 cigarettes per day and each blocker showed carbon monoxide scores of 37 parts per million, which are very high. Salivary cotinine levels of 303 and 385 ng per mL, from a nominally .01-mg nicotine cigarette, are also very high. Therefore, there were high exposures from a very-low-yield cigarette, clear evidence that some smokers—if only two—were able to get substantial levels from the lowest of the low-yield cigarettes.

Some submissions from the cigarette industry have indicated that vent blocking is not a substantial problem. In contrast, four laboratories have produced eight peer-reviewed studies that found evidence of vent blocking (Hofer et al., 1991; Kozlowski et al., 1982a, 1988, 1989, and 1994; Lombardo et al., 1983; Robinson et al., 1983; Zacny and Stitzer, 1988). In these studies, the prevalence of "extreme" vent blocking ranged from 1 to 210 per 1,000 (median = 19 percent), and the prevalence of "at least some blocking" ranged from 61 to 580 per 1,000 (median = 50 percent).

One submission from the cigarette industry notes that ventilation has changed a great deal recently. However, invisible laser ventilation has been available for at least a decade. From a consumer's point of view, it is unclear why invisible ventilation techniques should be viewed as appropriate.

Smokers can block the vents inadvertently if they do not know where the vents are and what they do. If smokers know where the vents are located, they can decide to avoid blocking the vents. There are real questions about who is most advantaged by laser techniques and invisible perforations.

Marlboro Lights, Winston Lights, Camel Lights, and Newport Lights ("lights" in general) are ventilated-filter cigarettes. Much of the focus of research has been on the ultralight cigarettes of 5 mg of tar or less. Unlike the ultralights, these light cigarettes are best sellers, but like the ultralights, they are ventilated-filter cigarettes. Therefore, the principle of informing the consumer that these are ventilated cigarettes, discussing how the vents work, and warning about blocking the vents with the fingers or lips is relevant to lights as well as ultralights.

Anyone who is skeptical about vent blocking of ultralow-yield cigarettes should take the lowest tar challenge: Light a 1-mg tar cigarette, placing your lips on the filter as close to the smoker end as possible. Keep your fingers off the filter so your fingers do not get in the way (i.e., do not block the vents with your fingers) and take a puff. Consider its taste, temperature, and feel. Now put your lips at least three-quarters of the way to the tobacco column (i.e., block the vents with your lips) and take another puff of similar size. (In our butt collection studies [Kozlowski et al., 1988 and 1994], we regularly have found lipstick stains beyond the filter vents, on the filter end of the cigarette, showing how far the cigarette had been put into the mouth.) Compare the second puff to the first. See for yourself how easy it is to block the vents and how much difference it makes to real tobacco pleasure by doing this. Those onlookers who prefer not to take a puff of cigarette smoke can usually see the difference in the smoke that is exhaled by someone else because blocked vents produce a "juicy" mouthful of smoke that billows out from a noninhaled puff of smoke. With unblocked vents, onlookers will see only a little smoke exhaled.

GRAPHIC INFORMATION ON TAR AND NICOTINE YIELDS: THE COLOR-MATCHING TECHNIQUE

In 1982, a study was published on a color-matching technique to provide better information on tar and nicotine yields to smokers (Kozlowski et al., 1982b). The color-matching technique can be used to estimate the number of puffs taken on a cigarette, and thus tar and nicotine yields, by comparing the color intensity of the end of a spent cigarette filter with a color scale. The study demonstrated a strong relationship between the "darkness" of color of the filter and the tar and nicotine yield of the cigarette. Figure 2 illustrates a modified version of the color-matching scale that the authors incorporated on a cigarette package. Three different color papers (meant to represent tar stains of low, standard, and high yields) developed by the authors from the Pantone by Letraset Color-Matching System are used to compare the filter stain colors from spent cigarettes. The low (Pantone 127U), standard (Pantone 117U), and high (Pantone 139U) colors are mounted on the scale at points 2, 5, and 8, respectively. Smokers rated the filter stain color on the 0-to-10 scale, moving from the lower to the higher intensity color blocks. They decided "whether the filter looked lighter,

Figure 2

The color-matching technique scale shown on a cigarette package. (Pantone-colored papers representing low, standard, and high yields at scale locations 2, 5, and 8, respectively.) The appearance of an unblocked vented filter is shown in the bull's-eye stain; the uniform stain on the filter end indicates extreme vent blocking.

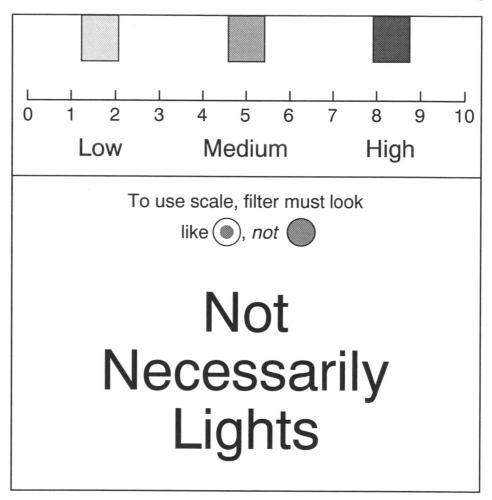

darker, or about the same as each of the colored blocks, and then selected the most appropriate scale number" (Kozlowski et al., 1982b).

Figure 2 also shows how stain patterns on spent filters can be used to indicate whether vent blocking has taken place on a conventional ventilated filter cigarette (Kozlowski et al., 1980). The bull's-eye tar stain on the left indicates no vent blocking. (Diluting air rather than smoke has been drawn through the periphery of the filter.) The uniform tar stain on the right indicates extreme vent blocking. On ventilated-filter cigarettes, vent blocking decreases filter efficiency so that the amount of stain left in the filter *underestimates* the amount of smoke that has gone through the filter;

in other words, the color-matching technique requires the assumption that vents remain unblocked. Because vent blocking alters yields dramatically, the graphic reminder not to block vents also may be useful in its own right.

The color-matching technique is a tool that can be used in future studies on compensation. Figure 2 also demonstrates how the color-matching technique and the stain-pattern technique could be included on cigarette packaging for consumer use. Color-matching information may better reflect the actual cigarette yields to smokers than the alternative FTC method. The FTC machine estimates of tar and nicotine yields can be unreliable given the variability among smokers and the various methods of compensation.

Further developmental work is needed on this color-matching technique. In the land of a largely blind FTC testing method, even a one-eyed color-matching technique could be king (Kozlowski and Rickert, 1984). It is not necessary to be perfect in providing the consumer with better information about the tar and nicotine yields of cigarettes to improve on the current standard method. A color scale attached to cigarettes can emphasize to the consumer that the yields from a cigarette depend on how the cigarette is smoked. Graphically, a color scale helps smokers see that yields are not captured by any one tar or nicotine number, and thus smokers can get a sense of where they stand in relation to the standard.

SUMMARY   Our review of brand-switching studies indicated that smokers increase nicotine intake from lower yield cigarettes by compensatory behavior, including filter-vent blocking. This behavior is a neglected issue for smokers of light and ultralight cigarettes. The current FTC testing method used to estimate average tar and nicotine yields of cigarettes is compromised by compensatory smoking behavior and individual variability among smokers. Graphic techniques (e.g., the color-matching technique and the stain-pattern technique) also need to be explored as ways to provide estimates of tar and nicotine yields to smokers of lower yield cigarettes. Simple graphic materials may help these smokers realize that a low-yield cigarette can provide high yields when smoked in certain ways.

QUESTION-AND-ANSWER SESSION

DR. BENOWITZ: Lynn, you said that in one study about half the people were vent blockers. My work and the Gori study suggest that people are taking in, on average, about .7 mg of nicotine per cigarette, which is tremendously more than would be possible taking more puffs. So, I think virtually everyone who smokes ultralow-tar cigarettes must be blocking. And how many of the holes do these ultralow-tar cigarette smokers block?

DR. KOZLOWSKI: The story I like is the student of mine in class who said his aunt, who smokes an ultralow-tar cigarette, keeps a roll of transparent tape on her coffee table. When offering a cigarette to a friend she will say, "Do you want that taped or untaped?" Bizarre as that might be; it happens.

It illustrates that people do not understand what ventilation does to their cigarette. I had a call years ago from an angry executive as a result of some media exposure about the results of some of these studies. He said, "I have a 1-mg tar cigarette, and yes, I block the vents on that cigarette, and yes, it makes it taste better and it is easier to light, but I thought it was a 1-mg tar cigarette; it says so right on the pack."

Ventilation is not the only manufacturing technique that contributes to an ultralow-yield cigarette. There can be other differences that mean that, even with blocking, the smoker will not necessarily get the same really high levels that you might with some other cigarettes. But it is clear that it is a major factor; it is clear that smokers can subvert it completely or even partially.

Lombardo did a study years ago with people staining their fingers with printer's ink. And he found that, as the cigarette coal burns down, and your fingers are getting away from it, they start to get in the way of the vent holes. It is also interesting that those last few puffs are the richest, and if you were to block those holes, that would be a particularly good time to do that to get higher yields.

DR. TOWNSEND: Dr. Kozlowski, how did you measure the vent blockage?

DR. KOZLOWSKI: We have done it a few ways. Most of the time it is a stain pattern method.

DR. TOWNSEND: On the mouth end of the filter?

DR. KOZLOWSKI: Yes.

DR. TOWNSEND: What I do not understand about something you just said is that people will purposefully tape holes closed. I think my experience with consumers is that they clearly know the tradeoffs between tar delivery of a cigarette and taste characteristics.

It would really surprise me that consumers would make that purposeful change to the design of a cigarette and not understand that they are increasing tar. Besides, they have the choice to go out into the market and buy a higher tar product if that is what they choose; so I do not understand the rationale or the psychology here.

DR. KOZLOWSKI: I think it is something to be surprised about.

DR. TOWNSEND: About the compensation issue, there is another answer that I do not completely understand.

Let's assume that compensation occurs to a very large degree, and people get essentially the same deliveries from a low-tar cigarette that they get from a higher tar cigarette. Then, why do consumers complain to us that the taste of low-tar cigarettes is weaker, milder, less strong, and less acceptable?

Again, their perception is that tar and taste go together. As a smoker, I can fairly accurately estimate the tar yield of a cigarette by smoking it, and I can get within a couple of milligrams.

I think many smokers, while they may not be as accurate in estimating FTC tar yields, still can rank cigarettes by tar. Now, how could they possibly do that if compensation were extensive?

DR. KOZLOWSKI: I think you do not want to think of compensation as something that influences everybody's smoking behavior. What we found in the *Pharmacology, Biochemistry and Behavior* study, half of the people block vents quite a lot, and the other half did not block them at all.

And if you looked further at those who did not block, you found that they did not smoke as many cigarettes per day. If you did taste ratings and how they liked the taste of the cigarette, they seemed to be consumers who were after a really low-yield smoke. They weren't blocking the holes. Not everybody smoking a low-yield cigarette blocks the vents. But this gets back to the issue of subject self-selection biases. We have to expect that there are individual differences in how much nicotine a person might want and also to the extent that a person is smoking for nicotine.

So, half of those subjects who were smoking ultralow-yield cigarettes in the long term were not blocking vent holes; they did not smoke many cigarettes per day; and they had low CO levels. The other half smoked a lot more cigarettes a day, smoked earlier in the morning, and got higher nicotine levels. You average them, and you get the kind of figures that are commonly described as "intermediate." Some people were showing a lot of compensation; some were showing very little; and that figure of mean compensation can be misleading.

DR. DEBETHIZY: I think you have pointed out an important fact: No machine-smoking method can predict individual behavior. This method was never intended to predict individual behavior, and it does not. I think people use different strategies when they smoke cigarettes, and it is rather obvious in the data you presented today.

DR. COHEN: Is it your intuition that a great many people who compensate are just following classic learning theory and do not even know they are doing it?

DR. KOZLOWSKI: Some people are not aware they are doing it; that is clear. They are not aware they are blocking the holes. I think that some people find the cigarettes relatively difficult to light. You push it a bit further in your mouth and it is a lot easier to light. Blocking could get started in a number of ways.

DR. SHIFFMAN: We have all been struggling with the issue of variability within a given product or products of equal FTC yield, I think, in talking about compensation and in the difference between the machine yield and the human biological exposure.

Now, with this issue of color matching, you are introducing something that I think has to do with true exposure rather than FTC yield. I wonder what you could tell us about the prospects of using a system like this to estimate exposure, the differences that might be due to things other than number of puffs, and all the kinds of things we think a compensating smoker might do.

DR. KOZLOWSKI: I think Dr. Rickert might be able to comment intelligently on that.

DR. RICKERT: One of the things that we have done is to look at the yield of a cigarette in relationship to the color of the filter itself. We have established that there is an extremely good regression between the measured color characteristic of the filter and the FTC yield. We have done that on the smoking machine and for the actual filter on cigarettes. We have looked at yields under 87 different conditions to cover a wide range of potential behavioral conditions. And we have looked at the yields under those conditions and have looked at the relationship between that and color. And color of the filter is a very good predictor of yields under a wide variety of conditions.

DR. HENNINGFIELD: I would just like to point out that the kinds of compensation that you see are consistent with what Dr. Zacny was talking about, the dynamic smoker, what I was talking about, the addicted and behavior-modified smoker. But it is also very similar to what you see in the animal laboratory, with addictive drugs like alcohol, sedatives, and opiates.

What you see is that as you push the dose up, you get some downward compensation. As you decrease the dose, you get some upward. But it is within a boundary. It is rarely perfect, because as you increase the dose, the animals tend to get a little more drug. If you decrease the dose to a certain point, the behavior can kind of just fall apart and get very erratic. It just struck me how similar it was, what we see with animals and addictive drugs, and what you are seeing.

DR. KOZLOWSKI: I agree.

DR. HENNINGFIELD: It looks like a basic biological phenomenon, in other words.

REFERENCES

Ashton, H., Stepney, R., Thompson, J.W. Self-titration by cigarette smokers. *British Medical Journal* 2: 357-360, 1979.

Benowitz, N.L., Jacob, P., Jones, R.T., Rosenberg, J. Interindividual variability in the metabolism and cardiovascular effects of nicotine in man. *Journal of Pharmacology and Experimental Therapeutics* 221: 368-372, 1982.

Benowitz, N.L., Jacob, P., Kozlowski, L.T., Yu, L. Influence of smoking fewer cigarettes on exposure to tar, nicotine, and carbon monoxide. *New England Journal of Medicine* 315: 1310-1313, 1986b.

Benowitz, N.L., Jacob, P., Yu, L., Talcott, R., Hall, S., Jones, R.T. Reduced tar, nicotine, and carbon monoxide exposure while smoking ultralow- but not low-yield cigarettes. *Journal of the American Medical Association* 256: 241-246, 1986a.

Guyatt, A.R., Kirkham, A.J.T., Mariner, D.C., Baldry, A.G., Cumming, G. Long-term effects of switching to cigarettes with lower tar and nicotine yields. *Psychopharmacology* 99: 80-86, 1989.

Hofer, I., Nil, R., Battig, K. Ultralow-yield cigarettes and type of ventilation: The role of ventilation blocking. *Pharmacology, Biochemistry and Behavior* 40: 907-914, 1991.

Kolonen, S., Tuomisto, J., Puustinen, P., Airaksinen, M.M. Smoking behavior in low-yield cigarette smokers and switchers in the natural environment. *Pharmacology, Biochemistry and Behavior* 40: 177-180, 1991.

Kozlowski, L.T. Reduction of tobacco health hazards in continuing users: Individual behavioral and public health approaches. *Journal of Substance Abuse* 1: 345-357, 1989.

Kozlowski, L.T., Frecker, R.C., Khouw, V., Pope, M. The misuse of "less-hazardous" cigarettes and its detection: Hole-blocking of ventilated filters. *American Journal of Public Health* 70: 1202-1203, 1980.

Kozlowski, L.T., Heatherton, T.F., Frecker, R.C., Nolte, H.E. Self-selected blocking of vents on low-yield cigarettes. *Pharmacology, Biochemistry and Behavior* 33: 815-819, 1989.

Kozlowski, L.T., Herman, C.P. The interaction of psychosocial and biological determinants of tobacco use: More on the boundary model. *Journal of Applied Social Psychology* 14: 244-256, 1984.

Kozlowski, L.T., Pillitteri, J.L., Sweeney, C.T. Misuse of "light" cigarettes by means of vent blocking. *Journal of Substance Abuse* 6: 333-336, 1994.

Kozlowski, L.T., Pope, M.A., Lux, J.E. Prevalence of the misuse of ultra-low-tar cigarettes by blocking filter vents. *American Journal of Public Health* 78: 694-695, 1988.

Kozlowski, L.T., Rickert, W.S. Kozlowski, Rickert reply. *American Journal of Public Health* 74: 391, 1984.

Kozlowski, L.T., Rickert, W.S., Pope, M.A., Robinson, J.C. A color-matching technique for monitoring tar/nicotine yields to smokers. *American Journal of Public Health* 72: 597-599, 1982b.

Kozlowski, L.T., Rickert, W.S., Pope, M.A., Robinson, J.C., Frecker, R.C. Estimating the yield to smokers of tar, nicotine, and carbon monoxide from the "lowest yield" ventilated filter-cigarettes. *British Journal of Addiction* 77(2): 159-165, 1982a.

Lombardo, T., Davis, C.J., Prue, D.M. When low tar cigarettes yield high tar: Cigarette filter ventilation hole blocking and its detection. *Addictive Behaviors* 8: 67-69, 1983.

Lynch, C.J., Benowitz, N.L. Spontaneous cigarette brand switching: Consequences for nicotine and carbon monoxide exposure. *American Journal of Public Health* 78: 1191-1194, 1987.

Robinson, J.C., Young, J.C., Rickert, W.S., Fey, G., Kozlowski, L.T. A comparative study of the amount of smoke absorbed from low yield ("less hazardous") cigarettes. Part 2: Invasive measures. *British Journal of Addiction* 78: 79-87, 1983.

Russell, M.A.H., Sutton, S.R., Iyer, R., Feyerabend, C., Vesey, C.J. Long-term switching to low-tar low-nicotine cigarettes. *British Journal of Addiction* 77: 145-158, 1982.

Russell, M.A.H., Wilson, C., Patel, U.A., Feyerabend, C., Cole, P.V. Plasma nicotine levels after smoking cigarettes with high, medium, and low nicotine yields. *British Medical Journal* 2: 414-416, 1975.

West, R.J., Russell, M.A.H., Jarvis, M.J., Feyerabend, C. Does switching to an ultra-low nicotine cigarette induce nicotine withdrawal effects? *Psychopharmacology* 84: 120-123, 1984.

Wynder, E.L., Goodman, M.T., Hoffmann, D. Demographic aspects of the low-yield cigarette: Considerations in the evaluation of health risk. *Journal of the National Cancer Institute* 72: 817-822, 1984.

Zacny, J.P., Stitzer, M.L. Cigarette brand-switching: Effects on smoke exposure and smoking behavior. *Journal of Pharmacology and Experimental Therapeutics* 246(2): 619-627, 1988.

Cigarette Design Technologies Reduce Smoke Yield and Expand Consumer Choices: The Role and Utility of the FTC Test Method

David E. Townsend

BACKGROUND   The Federal Trade Commission (FTC) test method for measuring tar and nicotine yields of cigarettes provides accurate and reliable information. Comparison of yields of various brands is a key factor consumers use to make objective choices in the marketplace. Another key factor is the taste of the cigarette, which in most cases is related to the tar and nicotine yield.

Calls for reduced tar yields from cigarettes came from the popular press, the scientific literature, and the public health community beginning in the late 1950's. Many of these included statements that tar reduction would reduce the relative risks for certain diseases.

The implementation of FTC testing for tar and nicotine in 1967 was an important step for cigarette manufacturers to communicate information on lower tar products to consumers for them to use to make informed decisions in the marketplace.

Even at that time, FTC understood the limitations of standardized machine smoking and recognized that no standard method would be able to take into account the wide range in human smoking behavior:

> No two human smokers smoke in the same way. No individual smoker smokes in the same fashion. The speed at which one smokes varies both among smokers, and usually also varies with the same individual under different circumstances even within the same day. Some take long puffs (or draws); some take short puffs. That variation affects the "tar" and nicotine quantity in the smoke generated (Federal Trade Commission, 1967).

The FTC also recognized that the FTC method could not predict the absolute smoke yield any individual smoker might receive from a particular cigarette:

> No test can precisely duplicate conditions of actual human smoking and, within fairly wide limits, no one method can be said to be either "right" or "wrong." The Commission considers it most important that the test results be based on a reasonable standardized method and that they be capable of being presented to the public in a manner that is readily understandable (Federal Trade Commission, 1967).

Daniel Oliver, chairman of FTC, confirmed FTC's position on cigarette testing in a statement before a congressional committee:

> As a general matter, I believe that advertisements that accurately convey information on "tar" and nicotine content can be a valuable source of information to consumers. Advertising that provides comparative information on different "tar" and nicotine levels can be especially useful (Oliver, 1988).

CIGARETTE DESIGN AND CHANGES IN THE CIGARETTE MARKET

The cigarette industry response to the public demand for reduced tar and nicotine cigarettes is evident in the dramatic decline in sales-weighted average tar yields over the past 40 years (Figure 1). In the early 1950's the average tar yield of cigarettes was around 38 mg per cigarette. Today that average is about 12 mg per cigarette. Nicotine yields also have been reduced in a similar fashion, although to a slightly different degree because the available techniques reduce tar and nicotine yields with slightly different efficiencies.

The techniques to reduce tar over the years include filtration, more efficient filtration (through different filter materials, fiber type and density, and filter length), filter ventilation, expanded tobacco, tobacco weight reduction, increased paper porosity or permeability, reconstituted tobacco, faster burning cigarette papers, and reduction of cigarette circumference.

Figure 1
Sales-weighted average tar and nicotine yields, 1954-1993

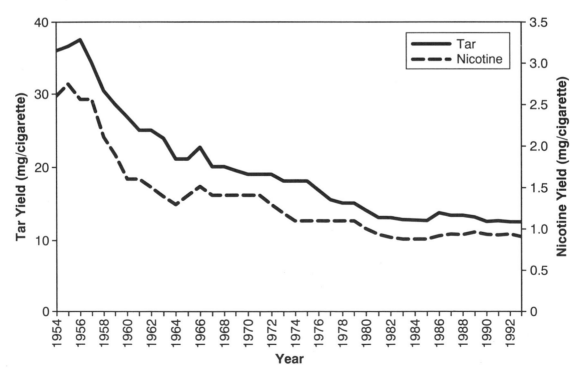

The physics and chemistry of a burning cigarette are exceedingly complex. For example, filter ventilation involves two mechanisms. In the first, fresh air from the outside is admitted to the filter and mixes with the smoke. As a result of this ventilation, a smaller effective puff is drawn on the burning end of the cigarette and less tobacco is then consumed during the puff. In addition, the smoke velocity in the cigarette is dramatically reduced, and the filter efficiency upstream of the ventilation holes increases. Similarly, in the second, a higher paper porosity also allows more outside air to enter the smokestream, also reducing the effective puff volume at the fire cone. The various cigarette design parameters result in many interactive effects on the performance of the cigarette.

The changes in cigarette design to reduce tar and nicotine yields have not been limited to low-tar and ultralow-tar products. Even today's nonfiltered cigarettes, the so-called high-tar brands, have about half the tar yield of their 1950's counterparts.

As a result, consumers today have a much wider range of choices in tar and nicotine than they did previously, and all cigarettes are substantially lower in tar yields than they were in past years (Figure 2). Cigarette design changes have resulted in an overall major reduction in smoke yields.

Figure 2
R.J. Reynolds Tobacco Company offers smokers a range of tar levels (1955-1993, in 5-year intervals)

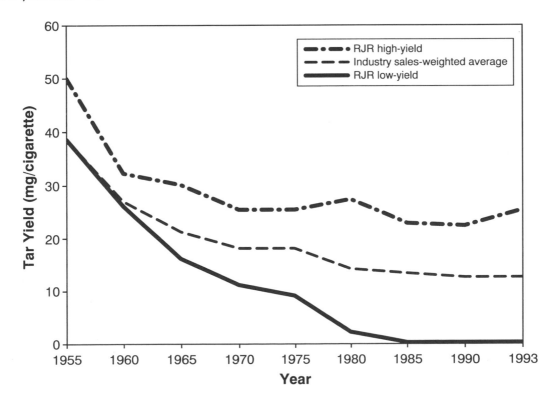

UTILITY OF
THE FTC TEST
METHOD

Although it has been clear that humans do not smoke like machines, it is also clear that changes in the FTC smoking conditions do not alter the relative ranking of cigarettes. The FTC conditions include a 35-cc puff of 2 seconds duration, taken once per minute. If the puffing conditions are changed, the relative ranking or yields of the cigarettes are preserved.

For example, Figure 3 shows tar yield as a function of puff volume. In this chapter, puff volumes of 35 cc, 45 cc, and 55 cc were chosen for comparison of four cigarette products, one each from the lowest tar, ultralight, full-flavor light, full-flavor categories. The 35-cc puff is the FTC condition and is not intended to represent the lowest smoker puff volume; the other two conditions were arbitrarily chosen. As the puff volume increases, tar yield of the product in each category increases. However, the ranking of the categories is preserved. For example, the tar yield of an ultralow-tar product at a 55-cc puff volume is lower than the tar yield of a low-tar product at the same puff volume.

Changing the puff frequency from one puff per minute to one puff every 45 seconds or one puff every 30 seconds also increases the tar yield in each category, yet the ranking of the cigarettes is intact (Figure 4). Puff duration has little, if any, effect on the actual yields (Figure 5).

Figure 3
Effect of puff volume on observed tar yields

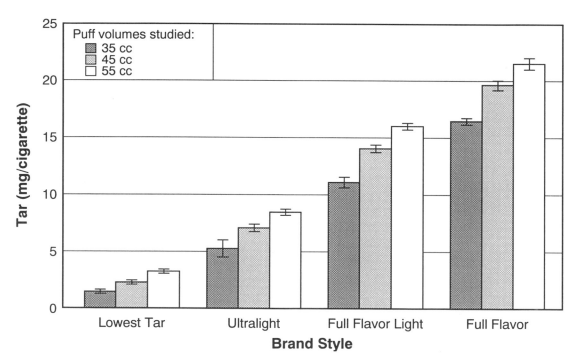

Note: *The puff duration for this experiment was 2 seconds; the puff frequency was one every 60 seconds.*

Figure 4
Effect of puff frequency on observed tar yields

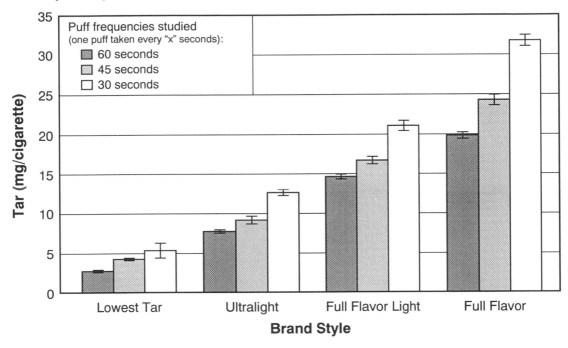

Note: The puff volume for this experiment was 45 cc; the puff duration was 1.7 seconds.

Figure 5
Effect of puff duration on observed tar yields

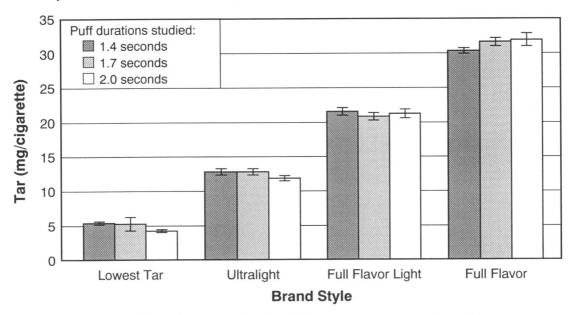

Note: The puff volume for this experiment was 45 cc; the puff frequency was one every 30 seconds.

Figures 6 through 8 show smoke nicotine yields for the same set of cigarettes; however, the smoking machine puffing conditions are different for each figure. Like tar yield, the nicotine yield goes up with increased puff volume and increased puff frequency, and the relative yields among the categories remain ordered. Puff duration also has little if any effect on nicotine yields.

Standard methods are used to provide information to consumers for products other than cigarettes. A classic example is the estimated Environmental Protection Agency (EPA) gas mileage ratings for vehicles. Depending on driving habits, conditions, maintenance, and fuel type, a vehicle may get more or less mileage than indicated by the EPA estimate. Although few drivers will achieve the actual mileage listed for a vehicle, the mileage ratings do provide a means of relative comparison among vehicles. A potential buyer can use the information to determine if a particular vehicle would fit into his or her particular transportation and economic needs.

Similarly, smokers have two primary considerations in making their choices in the cigarette marketplace. The FTC method provides comparative smoke yield information that is an essential part of that process. The second factor of taste is an individual preference that is made with the comparative information in mind.

Figure 6
Effect of puff volume on observed nicotine yields

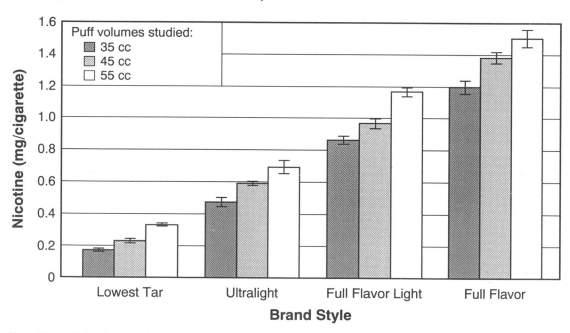

Note: The puff duration for this experiment was 2 seconds; the puff frequency was one every 60 seconds.

Figure 7
Effect of puff frequency on observed nicotine yields

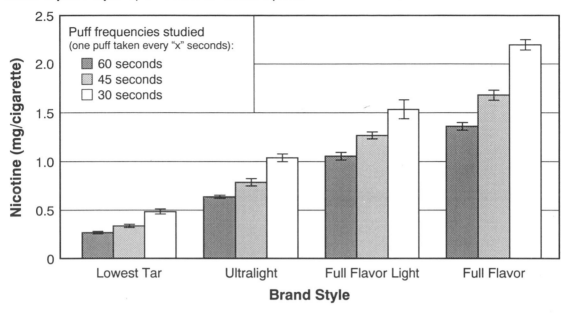

Note: *The puff volume for this experiment was 45 cc; the puff duration was 1.7 seconds.*

Figure 8
Effect of puff duration on observed nicotine yields

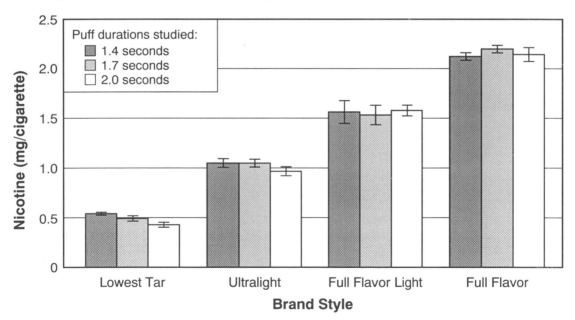

Note: *The puff volume for this experiment was 45 cc; the puff frequency was one every 30 seconds.*

QUESTION-AND-ANSWER SESSION

DR. BENOWITZ: How do you reconcile the differences between your data and other data that show when you get down to very low yields of nicotine, you are getting to a cotinine level of 225 vs. maybe 325 or so at the higher levels, in over 2,000 people. Do you think that is less accurate than your data in 33 subjects?

DR. DEBETHIZY: I think that the method of measuring plasma cotinine is a less accurate measure of nicotine uptake.

DR. BENOWITZ: What bias do you think there is in cotinine that could explain the tremendous difference in findings?

DR. DEBETHIZY: I do believe the data that we have. And I am surprised at them, based on what I know about the cotinine data in the field studies. Now, that does not mean that the data we have are wrong; it may be that at lower yielding products, that what people do over the course of an entire 24-hour period is different from what would be measured, say, at either 9:00 o'clock in the morning or 3:00 o'clock in the afternoon, depending on where people are measuring those plasma samples. So, I would say that, yes, the number is much larger for those plasma cotinine studies. But the point is that, even with those studies, compensation is incomplete. People smoking lower yielding cigarettes absorb less nicotine. Now, I would conclude the same thing from both data sets.

DR. BENOWITZ: I want to go back to your statement when you said the FTC method is accurately reflecting intake, because I think that is patently wrong. It is not whether there is some reduction; it is whether you can look at those cotinine levels, which would indicate that, when you get below 1 mg nicotine, that the FTC method is underestimating consistently based on cotinine levels in a couple of thousand people.

What I am arguing about is, is it reasonable to generalize from your 33 subjects and say that is more valid than the 2,000?

Cotinine levels, as you know, vary throughout the day, but not more than 10 or 15 percent if you are smoking regularly. So, there is no way that 10 or 15 percent can explain the difference, even if there were the worst bias that you can imagine.

DR. DEBETHIZY: I think that we can generalize from the data. I do not think we can give those data the weight that 10 years of analysis has provided us with. But I think that if we look at the plasma cotinine data, people smoking lower yielding cigarettes absorb less nicotine. Those data clearly show that.

They do not show that people get the same amount of material from all the wide range of nicotine-yielding cigarettes; would you agree with that?

DR. BENOWITZ: There is a slope such that there is not 100 percent compensation, although it may be close in some studies. But I would agree that there is a slope.

DR. DEBETHIZY: And I think that what we have done is taken things to the next step, what Dr. Henningfield called for earlier in his talk, which is to apply a technique that is used for other materials.

If you were asking what the amount absorbed of a pharmaceutical product in a 24-hour period would be, you would measure the total amount excreted and sum it up. That is all we have done, and I think that the data deserve consideration. I think that additional work will determine whether that slope will stay as steep as it is now.

I think you will notice that there were people above and below that, so there is wide variation. But the point is that people smoking lower yielding products are absorbing less. How much less, I do not know, and I suspect, even with our own data, we see some evidence that at the lowest yields, they are absorbing more than FTC would predict.

DR. RICKERT: First of all, in looking at your data on the FTC yield and the nicotine, one is impressed by the fact that it looks like there are basically two points on that regression. One is at the very low .1 mg and the other one is up at 1.4.

It seems to me that, for the bulk of the data, there is no relationship, that it is really a two-pronged display, with one at the bottom and one at the top and in the middle.

DR. DEBETHIZY: And I think that what you are looking at is the fact that the two center groupings are very close in nicotine and tar yield, but of course there is a full range of products out there on the market, and that is what we wanted to address with that.

DR. RICKERT: In reading the industry documents, it has been stated time and time again that consumers understand the FTC tar numbers. And my reading of the literature and what I have heard today suggest that is not so. And I was wondering whether there is industry information that supports the hypothesis that consumers, indeed, understand FTC numbers of tar and nicotine?

DR. TOWNSEND: How could the industry have changed so dramatically over the years and people traded taste, if tar levels were not a consideration in their choice?

People tell us, in focus groups and in other ways, "Yes, I am concerned about what I believe are health risks in smoking." They have been told that for 40 years, and they respond by looking at the tar levels of the products that they choose in the marketplace.

DR. RICKERT: I guess the question I am asking is, How do you reconcile that point of view with the information that has been provided here today, which suggests that the majority of smokers do not understand FTC numbers?

DR. TOWNSEND: I am convinced that they understand tar ratings as a relative comparison, the same as I think we understand EPA gas mileage. When you go buy a new car, EPA gas mileage estimates are determined by a number of factors, including the type of engine, how you drive, how properly you inflate the tires, how well you maintain it, how good your mechanic is, and even maybe the region of the country in which you live, because gasoline engines are more efficient in certain climates than others.

I do not take EPA gas mileage ratings to mean that is what I am going to get. The same as I was referring to earlier, I do not think I am necessarily getting the same efficiency on my hot water heater as it is rated.

I think these ratings are for comparison purposes. And I think that is what most consumers look for in the marketplace, and I think that is the way they interpret the FTC numbers.

DR. RICKERT: Let's assume for a moment that the FTC numbers are a perfect predictor of the amount of nicotine that is obtained from a cigarette. How do you think that relates to the other components that may be of concern? There are a whole host of chemicals that are related to various disease phenomena. How do you think the blood nicotine levels will act as a predictor of the absorption of these other constituents?

DR. DEBETHIZY: I think that one of the things about nicotine as a marker is that nicotine represents probably the upper limit for a particular phase for constituents. But one thing that I want to remind everybody is that the FTC method was never intended to measure or assist people with the actual uptake. It is to provide a relative ranking of cigarettes. And I think it has reliably done that for a long time.

It also gives us a way that we can standardize the analysis of cigarette smoking, so that we can compare work done in our laboratory with work done in your laboratory. And it has done that very well for a long time.

DR. HARRIS: I wondered if you could show, once again, one of your slides showing the trends in the sales-weighted tar and nicotine averages over time. And also, you might put up the one of unfiltered Camels also, if you have it. It is not essential which one, and I think Dr. Hoffmann even had one.

Dr. Hoffmann showed a similar slide, although the axes were labeled somewhat differently. And I have also looked at data on sales-weighted average nicotine, using the FTC numbers, at least those that were provided at various times to the Federal Trade Commission.

And I have been led to the general conclusion that, while the FTC-based numbers declined substantially during the 1950's and continued to decline, to some degree, during the 1960's, in the last 10 years, there has been basically no change in the sales-weighted average, whether you measure it by the distribution of tars with a percentage of brands under 15 mg or by the sales-weighted average nicotine.

And in fact, data for 1992, and what I can estimate myself from 1993 and 1994, are a slight upturn in the sales-weighted average nicotine.

If you show your slide on Camel nonfilters, the graph ends in 1982 at a tar level of 20.6. It would be interesting to have the data for after 1982.

DR. TOWNSEND: The tar delivery for Camel nonfilter is virtually flat from 1982 to the present. This is a chart that I prepared for something else, not this.

DR. HARRIS: And my question is really, What, if any, observations you might want to make about what appears to be progress in the decline in FTC yields during the last 30 years, a progress of which is really confined to the preceding two decades, with no change in the last decade?

If this had been a meeting on mileage in the car industry, somebody would be waving a finger and saying, "What have you guys done in the last 10 years with your car model?"

DR. TOWNSEND: My response to your question, first, is that I believe this clearly points out to me the need for the industry to respond with low-tar products that have improved taste characteristics. Clearly that is what consumers have told me: "I trade in tar for what I perceive as a possible benefit, and what I get is less taste." The concept of low tar, great taste, does not wash with consumers.

There are taste deficiencies in the lowest end. Some people choose to make that trade because, again, they weigh both factors in the marketplace: taste and tar levels.

But I think both factors are important in their choice, because there are many, many smokers who do buy products in the lowest category; again, back to the need for some useful and valid comparative information on tar levels, and that is already in the market. The FTC test method provides valid and reliable information.

First, beginning in 1981 or 1982, the price of cigarettes in the United States began to rise much faster than the rate of inflation. And at the same time, we saw a dramatic increase in generic and branded discount cigarettes.

To some degree, the apparent stagnation in tar and nicotine levels may reflect smokers choosing to go from branded to discount and generic cigarettes. In fact, from what data I have seen, the major source of brand switching in the last 10 years has been to the discount and generic segment of the market, which, as you know, is about 35 percent of the market in 1993.

Another possibility that has been raised by some is whether some brands have had their nicotine levels and tar levels actually reconstituted upward slightly.

A third is the changing demographics of the market. As some people quit and other people start, the average smoker is a different person who would intend, on average, to smoke a higher tar or higher nicotine cigarette.

Finally, there is the question of whether or not, in fact, there is a limit that smokers are willing to tolerate, given the current cigarette array of choices.

How does your hypothesis relate to the question at hand: What is the meaningfulness of the FTC test, and is it useful in the market?

DR. HARRIS: There are several points you make. One is whether the test is useful, but also whether the industry has accomplished anything in reducing tar and nicotine levels. And I think that, since that was a preamble of both talks and it is certainly an issue that I have been puzzling over, I thought it was important to wrestle with the question of why have tar and nicotine levels not fallen in the last 10 years, and is there anything that can be done about it.

DR. SHIFFMAN: You have very much emphasized the issue of consumer choice and consumers making a choice based on accurate information. I take it, then, that if consumers could be provided with better, more accurate information about yields, that is something that you would favor.

DR. TOWNSEND: I believe that what the consumer needs is there. The FTC method provides reliable comparative information.

DR. SHIFFMAN: You do not want them to have better information?

DR. TOWNSEND: Convince me that there is better information. I am not convinced that there is.

DR. SHIFFMAN: I am asking it as a hypothetical question.

DR. TOWNSEND: If there is important information that the consumer needs to make choices in the marketplace, then I want to know it.

DR. SHIFFMAN: We have seen individual variability around the trend line, and if we were able to provide individuals with information about where they stood on that, then would that be an improvement that you might be able to support?

DR. DEBETHIZY: That is a tall order for any sort of standardized method.

DR. PETITTI: Your talk, Dr. deBethizy, referenced the historical context of the development of the FTC measures. And the historical context was the claim that these measures would significantly reduce the risk of disease. Do you think that the data so far support a claim that these FTC measures predict or are meaningfully related to disease risk?

DR. DEBETHIZY: Personally, I do not know. But what I would say is that the data that I saw Dr. Samet present today, which were largely taken from the 1981 Surgeon General's report, their conclusion was that people smoking lower yielding products have reduced relative risk for lung cancer.

DR. PETITTI: I think that you saw the quotes from Dr. Wynder and some of the earlier commentators. They mentioned 40-percent reductions in tar might lead to large reductions in lung cancer. I just want to get a sense of the magnitude in the reduction of disease risk with differences in tar levels over the range we are talking about.

I just want to make the point that adjustment is the problem; when you adjust, you assume people smoke the same number of cigarettes, whether they smoke high yield or low yield. And it is very difficult to handle statistically and is, I think, one of the problems in the original data that were published in the 1981 report.

DR. DEBETHIZY: But you know, on average, that people smoking lower yielding products do not smoke more cigarettes.

DR. BOCK: I am having a little bit of a problem. You had mentioned some observations with staining of saliva regarding ventilation and hole blockage. It seems to be the opposite from what was reported. Can you give me some details of how you know you got saliva on the area covered by the lips in every case, or most cases?

DR. TOWNSEND: What I can do is give you detailed information on the whole experiment. And I will have to do that privately, because I don't have the information with me today.

What I said earlier is the case. We saw infrequent hole blockage, but there was hole blockage in some cases, and we determined that by an inhydrin staining process. And I cannot recall the details and the numbers, because I really was not responsible for that experiment. I would be happy to follow up with you on that, if you are interested.

DR. COHEN: Let me quickly state what I think the premises are of your presentation, Dr. Townsend, and see if you disagree with where I disagree.

Suppose we accept the premise that the FTC system provides useful ranking information, everyone understanding the difference between ranking and other kinds of information. Let's say the system does that. Suppose we also accept the premise that truly individual smoking characteristics are beyond the scope of such a rating system.

Now, you have established that there are product design features—type of paper, type of tobacco, etc., that lead to different yields because of smoking parameters that vary with such product design elements, such as puff rate, puff volume, etc.

Doesn't this mean that a numerical scale—say, from 1 to 27—is necessarily misleading and that a categorical rating system would be a more valid way to report such information? You had four categories, I believe, and you showed variance. What I am saying is, I was following that, and it looked to me like you were about to recommend a four-category system.

DR. TOWNSEND: The whole idea of a categorical system, or so-called banded system, has been put on the table by a number of people in the past.

Conceivably, that accomplishes the same endpoint with one exception, I believe. The same endpoint, of course, is that it provides a comparative ranking for consumers. The flaw in that approach, if that is the only ranking, and discrete numbers are not also included, is that, of course, you would expect products to come up against the ceiling of each band.

DR. COHEN: I thought you established, with your own analysis, that individual numbers were inherently misleading?

DR. TOWNSEND: I did not say that individual numbers were misleading. In fact, I believe individual numbers—a numerical rating system—is, in fact, the best and that is what the FTC test method is.

With those data, then, manufacturers have advertised their products as light or ultralight, to fit some range of tar numbers.

DR. COHEN: I think you missed my point.

DR. TOWNSEND: The FTC method is the method that provides the useful comparative information for the smoker.

DR. COHEN: I thought you established with your charts that there was variance due to what is technically an interaction between product design characteristics and smokers' adaptations to them. Is that correct?

DR. TOWNSEND: Okay, you are confusing me. Let me put the chart back up. Standard deviation for replicate measures of that particular product. Different particular puff frequencies. Puff frequency of 60 seconds happens to be blue bars, 45 seconds is the red bars, 30 seconds is the yellow bars. So, the ultralight product that was smoked at 30-second frequency—in fact, this is the variability we saw in 10 replicate measures of that one cigarette.

DR. COHEN: Okay, then I did misunderstand that, but a lot of the presentations today have essentially suggested that smokers respond to product design characteristics by modifying behavior. And I am not talking about idiosyncratic behavior, but standard ways that you put up—puff frequencies, puff duration, number of puffs.

That creates variance around a point estimate. And would it not be more valid to acknowledge that those variances exist when you provide this information to consumers? Ranking is the least informative scale.

DR. TOWNSEND: You are talking about something like the EPA gas mileage ranking, where you have highway and city.

DR. COHEN: Ranking information has only an ordinal property. The absolute numbers have no significance, nor do the units of measurements between—like 16, 17, 18, 19. In a ranking system, you never assume those units are equal.

In this system, presented to consumers, consumers have a right to assume equal appearing units—16, 17, 18, 19. It goes beyond a ranking system. If you just want a ranking system, then there are ways to do that, to build on this kind of variance.

So, if all you want is a ranking system, the one that is in place now attempts to do more than that, and I thought your evidence indicated that it did not do it with great validity.

DR. TOWNSEND: What variance are you speaking of?

DR. COHEN: The interaction of human smoking topography and cigarettes having different design features.

DR. TOWNSEND: Have you quantified that?

DR. COHEN: I have not done it. I think we have discussed it today. I am not a technical expert on it. I am asking from the standpoint of consumer usefulness.

If a ranking system could be preserved to meet your objectives that you set out and, at the same time, it would have more validity because it wouldn't represent units that do not exist because there is too much variance around them; it is only a ranking system.

DR. DEBETHIZY: It sounds like you have put a proposal on the table, and my impression is that is what we will do tomorrow.

DR. COHEN: It sounded like you were saying, "Well, if it achieves its purpose as a ranking system and leaves consumers to know which brands are lower and which are higher, and that is fine."

DR. DEBETHIZY: And we think that the current method does that. So, I will be looking forward to the discussion tomorrow about alternative methods.

DR. HENNINGFIELD: This is actually a nice introduction to my point. Compensation is one of the reasons that you get a good correlation with machines and a lousy correlation with humans. It is not validated that the FTC method predicts what humans get.

But you have seemed concerned that compensation was not perfect, as though the fact that it was not imperfect rejected the notion of compensation.

DR. DEBETHIZY: I think what I was doing was challenging the notion that people get the same amount from every cigarette on the market.

DR. HENNINGFIELD: Do you know of any drug study with humans with addictive drugs where you do get perfect compensation?

DR. DEBETHIZY: I just do not even see a reason to address that question because smoking is a habit that people engage in, and people enjoy smoking. I think we have a situation where people enjoy smoking; they have a wide range of products to choose from; they can choose lower yielding products. The data—whether it is plasma cotinine or total urinary uptake—show that they get, when they smoke lower yielding cigarettes, less material, on average.

Now, the FTC method was never intended to address that question. It was intended to address the relative ranking of cigarettes.

DR. SHIFFMAN: Actually, what your data show is that within the broad range in which sales are actually concentrated—let's say from .4 to about 1.0, 1.2, FTC nicotine—people are getting, on average, the same, regardless of the nominal yield. So, in fact, your own data, as Dr. Rickert pointed out earlier, suggest that, in fact, the numbers do not track.

DR. SHIFFMAN: What your data show is that people who smoke cigarettes of .1 are very much lower than people smoking 1.4. But if you look at the middle range, we could probably compute the correlation by tomorrow, but I would warrant that it is close to zero.

DR. DEBETHIZY: And the middle range is a very narrow range of tar and nicotine yield.

DR. HENNINGFIELD: Let me just bring closure to my point, because what I see—and I think Dr. Shiffman is pointing out, too—is that what you see with humans with other addictive drugs, and what you see in animals, is compensation that is partial. And that seems to be what we are seeing here: another case of an addictive drug that controls behavior, and you do get compensation, although it is not perfect. That seems to be the biological process going on.

DR. TOWNSEND: And I think you and I fundamentally disagree about that, because it is like coffee drinking. I do not see myself as being, if I drink 1 cup of coffee 1 day and 10 cups of coffee the next day, I do not see that as compensation. I just see that as responding to different situations and choosing to drink coffee under those different environmental conditions. And I see smoking as a very similar activity that people engage in.

DR. KOZLOWSKI: This is a supplement to Fred Bock's question and point. Years ago, in Toronto, we tried to do a saliva test, I think similar to the one you did. We collaborated with the forensic laboratory for the Province of Ontario, and a Ph.D. student in pharmacology worked on it.

And we never published it because we did not find it useful, in part because the lips, in general, were too dry and were not depositing that much saliva and were doing it in a very soggy manner.

We found that a much more straightforward technique would be to take chapstick or lip gloss, and that would stain the filter overwrap. You could then dissect the cigarette and count the holes that have been blocked by that. We tried that technique and abandoned it as unsuccessful.

Just months ago, we published in *Pharmacology, Biochemistry and Behavior* a validation of the stain pattern technique using Marlboro Lights, Winston Lights, Marlboro Ultralights—I am not sure about the four or five other brands. They worked just fine.

Even with ventilated filter cigarettes, which may be ventilated in the 20- to 30-percent range rather than 80 or 90, you can get a team of raters to do reliable judgment.

DR. DEBETHIZY: I think what is important is that some individuals may block holes when they smoke cigarettes. What is important is what happens over the course of their entire smoking day and what happens, on average, with people. And I think there has been an incredible emphasis placed on blocking holes here today, and I think that Dr. Townsend's talk clearly showed that there are many, many other techniques used to lower tar and nicotine, techniques that could not be overcome by the smoking behavior of the individual.

DR. FREEMAN: What I am going to do is say to cut this at this point and maybe we can continue it tomorrow. We were due to be finished about 20 minutes ago. It may be a little hard on these two gentleman, who have been very gracious in answering these questions. We do not want to put them under too much, but we would like to bring you back tomorrow, if you do not mind, for further discussion. But let's have these two questions.

DR. BENOWITZ: There has been some suggestion about providing the consumer with more information, such as making ventilation holes visible so that people can see them and not block them, and give them information about what intense smoking would do, which you could simulate by machines. Are there any negative aspects about doing those things, from your perspective, and why not provide more information like that?

DR. DEBETHIZY: I think Dr. Townsend addressed it earlier when he responded that we would consider any reasonable proposal as long as there were some data to support that proposal.

And I am assuming that is what you all will do, and at least start the process. And you all may conclude that the FTC method is fine as it is, but I certainly do not have any problem with looking at reasonable proposals.

We have a motto at our company that we work for smokers. And if we can be convinced that it is meaningful for the consumer, that might warrant consideration.

DR. TOWNSEND: But you understand that we believe, today, that the FTC test method is useful for the consumer; that its presence has been beneficial for consumers making choices and also for driving the industry to reduce tar and nicotine levels to this great extent that we have.

Then the other point, too, ISO—the International Standards Organization—of course, adopted a standard test method that is used throughout the world, that is essentially the same. And they, in the investigations, particularly in Germany and the UK, had many of the same questions here.

DR. BENOWITZ: But there is no drawback for providing more information.

DR. TOWNSEND: Oh, absolutely. I think we always have to look at new information that is available, and look at it in depth, critique it, and see if anything is there.

DR. HOFFMANN: I am somewhat puzzled. I have seen the tobacco field for decades, and I always found the tobacco industry to be flexible. The pressure from the consumer and from the scientific community led to the industry changing the cigarette. And you have in *Science* the outstanding study by Dr. Benowitz.

We all agree that there is some compensation, and I find that you are inflexible. We have to work on it; there is a way. I am surprised. I have, in all the X years I have been working in this field, I have never seen such an inflexible thing as this, where you stick to the FTC method.

I think we can always improve, and U.S. scientists know this just as well as I.

DR. DEBETHIZY: Let me ask this question. Have you seen a proposal put on the table that seriously would improve on the current method?

DR. HOFFMANN: The advances in the research have been done by both sides—by industry as well as the scientific community. Suddenly, I find that you say, "No, the FTC method is the final word."

DR. DEBETHIZY: I think that clearly what we have said is that, with 30 years in a standardized method that has been incredibly valuable to consumers, the industry, and the scientists that we have not seen any reason to walk away from that. I would just give it back to the group and say, let's see a serious proposal.

DR. TOWNSEND: I am sorry that you are misreading this as being inflexible. I think the fact is that the FTC method has worked for a long time, and it continues to work.

But demonstrate what the proposal is, and how it adds to what we have now, to make things better, or to provide some more information. For example, one of the proposals that was floated this morning included a min and max level. Okay, let's smoke a cigarette at FTC conditions, and then let's go to a more intensive smoking condition, to report min and max.

What is going to happen from that is that you get exactly the same ranking; it is just more numbers, but it is the same ranking. And consumers are making their choices based on ranking.

DR. HOFFMANN: But you have shown here, in your paper, it is very detailed. It is for the low-yielding figure and compensation.

DR. DEBETHIZY: Yes, and you are right about that.

DR. HOFFMANN: So, this is not a reason that we should work together?

DR. DEBETHIZY: And we are quite willing to work with anybody, and that is why we are here today.

DR. FREEMAN: Dr. Townsend, I just want to ask one question, and it may be a little naive. Several times you have mentioned the value of tar in cigarettes because you say it is associated with taste. Even conceding that although it seems to be a thing that is killing people.

But what about nicotine? What it is the value of nicotine and cigarettes, and why could it not be dramatically reduced?

DR. TOWNSEND: Nicotine, of course, is part of the smoking sensation. It does provide a sensation to the smoker. I think one of our competitors found that tobacco that had been treated to remove all the nicotine was not successful in the marketplace.

More than that, just as I cannot look into the components of tar and say, this is a very important, tasteful, and flavorful compound. You know, I am not equipped as a chemist to say nicotine is an important compound for this aspect of taste characteristics.

DR. FREEMAN: We will stop at this point.

REFERENCES

Federal Trade Commission. "FTC To Begin Cigarette Testing." News release. August 1, 1967, p. 2.

Oliver, D. Prepared statement by the Federal Trade Commission chairman before the U.S. House Subcommittee on Transportation, Tourism, and Hazardous Materials, Committee on Energy and Commerce. May 4, 1988, p. 11.

Transcript of Second-Day Discussion

DR. FREEMAN: Good morning, everyone. I would like to welcome all of the speakers and panel members and the audience back to these deliberations. We will continue to deliberate concerning the FTC test method, and we will begin this morning with continuation of the dialog that we were having with Dr. Townsend and Dr. deBethizy, who represent the tobacco industry.

DR. BENOWITZ: I would like to follow up with two questions on why the results from the study of 33 subjects relating the total nicotine recovery vs. the FTC yield from cotinine studies are so different. The first question is, since these results were so different, it would be very interesting to have measured cotinine levels in these smokers, as well as looking at urinary metabolites, and I would like to know if that was done and if we could see those data. The second thing I was wondering was, since this question of yield versus intake has been so important for so many years and since R.J. Reynolds has the capability of doing it, I wonder if they have ever done a study like the ones that I showed where they looked at cotinine levels vs. yields in a large population just to see if their own work would replicate the work of other people, and it seems like a very straightforward study that would be something they might have done.

DR. DEBETHIZY: The answer to your first question is no, we did not measure plasma cotinine in those studies. We were studying nicotine metabolism interindividual variation. That was how we got into that work, and we extended it then to ask the question across the tar categories. In the study that we are currently doing, we are actually measuring salivary cotinine. We made a conscious decision not to measure plasma cotinine because we did not want to interfere by taking a blood sample. So, we are doing salivary cotinine in that study to answer the exact question that you have raised. I think that is a good question to ask. In subjects where we see lower total nicotine output, are the plasma concentrations higher? That is a good question. And your second question was?

DR. BENOWITZ: There were data from Dr. Gori's work that I presented that were supported by Brown and Williamson, I believe. We basically looked at cotinine levels vs. yields for a large population, and I think those data were very important. I was wondering if R.J. Reynolds has ever done such a study, and if any data are available addressing that question?

DR. DEBETHIZY: We have not done a field study. There were so many field studies in the literature already, we just have never done a study like that.

DR. SHIFFMAN: Just to follow up on that study, a couple of us were pointing out that the relationship seemed to be very much driven by the extremes, and I took the liberty of computing what the correlation would be in those same data if one excluded the very extremes. I had to impute the data from the graph, but if you look at the data above .13 and at or below 1.02 FTC yield, the correlation is .16. In other words, except for the extremes in your own data, there is no relationship.

DR. DEBETHIZY: Yes, it is interesting to me. I think what we have done is taken the best available technology, done what Jack Henningfield asked people to do, which is to take a look at things using modern techniques, and we have done a study that I think causes us to stop and think about what the previous data have shown. We can manipulate those data to get them to look like what the other data look like, or we can take them on their own merits, and I think that what we need to do is follow this study up with further work, and that is why we are doing that, and I have encouraged Dr. Benowitz to do the same thing. I have encouraged the Swedish Tobacco Company, which has the capability to do the same thing.

I think rather than doing some data selection on this particular study we should take it on its own merit. It is a 33-person study. It suggests that when smokers can freely do their activities, people consuming lower yielding cigarettes absorb less nicotine. Now, it also suggests that there is large interindividual variation, and I think lots of people have pointed that out.

When you do a study like this, you are going to get extremes because people smoke cigarettes across a wide range, and I think you have to include those people, and I think as we and others fill the data in over time we will find out whether this correlation or the slope of this line is as steep as it is now or whether it is shallower, and I just think we need to continue to do that work. We have worked hard to develop a state-of-the-art technique, and I think it has merit.

DR. SHIFFMAN: I think it has merit, too, and I applaud you for doing it. At the same time we ought to be clear on what the data show, and the data show that people smoking brands above 1.03 are getting more than people smoking brands at about .13 and that in the middle range there is no relationship to the FTC yield.

DR. FREEMAN: Dr. Benowitz, does that answer both of your questions?

DR. BENOWITZ: Yes.

DR. FREEMAN: Dr. Rickert?

DR. RICKERT: In the media recently, the cigarette Eclipse was described, and it is obvious from the media description that the cigarette is going to pose some challenges for the FTC methodology, in particular because it does not burn down to a fixed butt length. There are some other challenges that may be posed by that cigarette to the FTC methodology, and in particular I am wondering about the distribution of nicotine between the gas phase and the particulate phase. That is, in the current FTC methodology when testing the Eclipse cigarette, will the amount of nicotine that is being delivered by that cigarette be trapped using the traditional Cambridge Filter method?

DR. TOWNSEND: I do not think we really know the answer right now to the question of nicotine distribution between the gas and particulate phase. I do think we have confidence that the FTC method can provide useful data for Eclipse. Certainly the FTC method will have to be accommodated for that product in much the same way that the FTC considered accommodating the method for Barclay and the use of different holders. That proposal was certainly up for discussion. The FTC method as it stands with some modification, particularly for the fact that Eclipse does not burn down, can provide useful data for that.

DR. FREEMAN: Dr. Henningfield?

DR. HENNINGFIELD: In dealing with the smokeless tobacco issue, which has no labeling, and I think that is a problem, it struck me yesterday that I am not sure what is worse, having no labeling or having labeling that might be misleading to consumers about relative risks. In trying to deal with the relative risk issue yesterday, you spent a lot of time talking about your technologies that address health concerns and implying that there was some health benefit, and I would like to know what your estimate is as to the number of cancer deaths, for example, caused by standard cigarettes and how many lives, if any, would be saved if people were using cigarettes with these advanced technologies of filtration and so forth that you were talking about yesterday? In other words, how many people die of cancer in your estimation from the higher yield cigarettes, and how many fewer, if any, would die from the lower yield cigarettes?

DR. TOWNSEND: I think what you did was completely mischaracterize what I said yesterday. What I said was that the Surgeon General and the public health community called for the reduction in tar and nicotine yields from cigarettes, and I said that the industry and R.J. Reynolds responded to that consumer demand through major design changes to the product, and we successfully reduced the tar and nicotine yields from the very high 30's, as a sales-weighted average, down to currently about 12 mg.

DR. FREEMAN: To follow up on the question, do you think that fewer people die based on the changes that you have made?

DR. TOWNSEND: I am not an epidemiologist. The Surgeon General in 1981, in his report, did say that reduced-tar products pose a reduced health risk.

DR. HENNINGFIELD: I would like to follow this though because the words "light" and things like that are only used with foods when there is a health benefit. Your industry is using those terms relating them to FTC yields, and I would like to know what your estimate of the health benefit is. To know that, we have to know what your estimate of the death rates are with the different products.

DR. TOWNSEND: I just said that I was not an epidemiologist. I happen to be a chemist. I do know what the Surgeon General and epidemiologists have said. Many smokers have heard the same thing.

DR. FREEMAN: Dr. Hughes?

DR. HUGHES: I would like to ask your opinion about ordinal vs. cardinal scales because I think that was not made clear yesterday. You compared the FTC method to the EPA gas mileage. If I buy a car that has 38 miles per gallon and my sister buys a car with 19, I get twice what she gets. Now, even your own data show that is not true with tar and nicotine yields. When you have a tar yield that is twice another cigarette, you do not get twice the tar. So, I find those numbers misleading. I think the normal consumer when they see a cigarette that says, "1 milligram tar," and they see another cigarette that says, "8," they think they are getting one-eighth the tar, and that is not true. It seems to me if that is the case, and all you want is rankings, that we should do away with the numbers because they are misleading, and I would like to hear your thoughts about that.

DR. TOWNSEND: A relative ranking of cigarette yields is what is essential in the marketplace. To date we believe that the FTC method provides useful information for the consumer. Do you really believe that your car gets 19 miles per gallon when you drive it?

DR. HUGHES: I believe that my car that gets 19 gets half the mileage of somebody else's car that gets 38, and I think most consumers would believe that if they saw the numbers 19 and 38.

DR. DEBETHIZY: But what else is on that label? The other part that is on there is, "Your actual mileage may vary," and that is important because again this particular method was not set up to predict what an individual will get. It was set up for relative ranking, and I think it is really important to stick with that.

DR. HUGHES: I agree, and with relative ranking, when you have rankings and ordinal categories, you do not have numerals attached.

DR. DEBETHIZY: You just gave a good example of that when you gave EPA gas mileage.

DR. HUGHES: EPA gas mileage is a cardinal system. It is not a relative ranking. The EPA gas mileage, 38, cars that have 38 miles per gallon do, in fact, get twice the mileage as cars of 19.

DR. DEBETHIZY: Only if driven under standard conditions.

DR. HUGHES: No. You are confusing variability around the mean with ordinal vs. ranking.

DR. DEBETHIZY: I think I understand the difference, and I think that we could argue about this all day, but I think that the FTC method was intended as a machine-based standardized method to provide relative ranking, no more than that.

DR. FREEMAN: Dr. Henningfield?

DR. HENNINGFIELD: Then if we play by your rules, what is wrong with putting on the cigarettes, "Your intake may vary on a cigarette that is so-called an 'ultralow'" and put right on the cigarette, "You may get up to 3 mg of nicotine and 80 mg of tar from this, depending on how you smoke it"? What would be wrong with that? Wouldn't that just provide honest information to consumers so that they would know? Maybe even giving them a little bit of information that you folks know and we know about what pushes it up there, such as smoking harder and things like that; what is wrong with that?

DR. DEBETHIZY: As I said yesterday, we are quite willing to consider any reasonable proposal, and I suspect, Mr. Chairman, we are going to move into that mode eventually where we will discuss those proposals, and that is a proposal to put on the table and discuss.

DR. HENNINGFIELD: I am not sure that is an issue right now, but so, you would not object to that concept?

DR. DEBETHIZY: I would not object to putting that proposal on the table because my understanding of what this panel is supposed to do is to make recommendations like that for serious study and consideration.

DR. FREEMAN: Dr. Cohen?

DR. COHEN: Let me just say that a lot of the discussion proceeds from what experts know about the FTC method and what it was designed to do. I think the real question is what consumers think the numbers mean. So, the important issue is how do consumers understand these numbers, and I think it would come as a shock to them that these are only to be taken as rankings. That would come as a great shock, and I think we should keep that in mind.

DR. TOWNSEND: That is a point, Dr. Cohen, where we clearly disagree.

DR. COHEN: Do you have any data that show that consumers only think about these numbers as rankings?

DR. TOWNSEND: It is clear to us that consumers look at tar information; they also look at the category of cigarettes they smoke, whether it is a light or an ultralight or regular, and they make decisions in the marketplace. The actual fact is that in the market, sales-weighted tar and nicotine yields have declined dramatically over the years, and people have traded taste to do that.

DR. COHEN: Let me say, in response, that that is perfectly consistent with consumers believing that these are real numbers, not rankings. Your scenario fits a situation in which consumers think that by going down to a very-low-yield cigarette that these are cardinal numbers and real numbers. I am asking you whether your company or any cigarette company has data that indicate that consumers only think about these as rankings. The answer is either yes or no.

DR. TOWNSEND: It is clear to us from talking with consumers that they understand the notion of tar and nicotine yield, that they make choices in the marketplace. I am not about to talk about our consumer information at this point. I am not a marketing expert, but it is clear to us that consumers use the information from the FTC test method in one form or another, and even in your words, some use the numbers, and yes, those people who actually use the quantitative numbers may be more skewed to the ultralight category, but consumers do use the numbers or they use the category rankings of cigarettes, whether it be ultralight or regular.

DR. FREEMAN: Dr. Petitti?

DR. PETITTI: I am intrigued by the EPA mileage analogy and also by the water heater analogy, but I think the difference is one about consumer information. When you drive your 38-miles-per-gallon EPA-rated car, you know as you drive, based on measurements that you can make, whether or not you are, indeed, getting 38 miles per gallon or 19 miles per gallon based on your mileage, the way you actually use that car. Similarly for your water heater, you get your bill every month, and you can tell whether or not you are exceeding or not exceeding the conditions that are printed on your label. How does the cigarette consumer know whether or not they are or are not getting what is on the package?

DR. TOWNSEND: I think the point of the analogy is not exactly where you are coming from. The point of the analogy is that consumers do not expect to get exactly that EPA gas mileage. I know I do not because yes, you are right, I can measure it, and I do not, but I do use the EPA gas mileage numbers to a degree in making choices in the marketplace in helping guide my purchases. I said yesterday that I recently bought a new hot water heater. I used the energy efficiency rating in helping me make that choice, and I actually paid more for a more efficient hot water heater, but that tag also said that the average price or the price you would expect to pay for running this hot water heater is $358 per year. Do I believe that is what it is costing me? No. So, it is a matter of providing me guidance for making choices and in no way do I believe that represents an absolute number that predicts my power bill.

DR. PETITTI: I think you already answered this question, but I do think that both for the EPA mileage example and your water heater, and perhaps also for cigarettes, that it would be useful to the consumer to know the specific range that they might expect under certain specified driving conditions and perhaps we are going to get to that in terms of the proposals that we consider.

DR. TOWNSEND: And I believe that is a question on the table because the FTC test method was not intended to do exactly that.

DR. PETITTI: Can you explain to me just once again your view of what the FTC method was meant to do in the context of health? You keep saying that it was not meant to do that. I am having a hard time understanding your view of what it was meant to do.

DR. TOWNSEND: Consumers responded to the calls for reduced-health-risk products for reduced-tar products that were made by the Surgeon General, Wynder and Hoffmann, and other members of the public health community. Consumers responded to that information, and they demanded of the industry a reduction in tar and nicotine yields from cigarettes. A standardized comparative, accurate, and reliable test method was required to accomplish that, and that was the purpose of the FTC method, to provide those comparative data.

DR. PETITTI: So they could make decisions about health?

DR. TOWNSEND: So they could make decisions about tar yields in the marketplace, which they were told by the public health community were related to health.

DR. KOZLOWSKI: I think there are great concerns about how many consumers are getting the information about tar and nicotine yields as they exist now. I think at the last testing, the Federal Trade Commission reported tar and nicotine yields on upward of 900 cigarettes. According to the rules, the tobacco industry is not required to print tar and nicotine yields on cigarette packs. They are only in ads. What, in fact, is the percentage of cigarettes that are not advertised at all so that there is, in fact, no way for the consumer to know? I think that may, indeed, vary from manufacturer to manufacturer, but also in a related point some data have shown that it is on the ultralow tars that people are most likely to know the yields. It is also the fact that it is on the ultralow tars that the yields themselves are likely to be printed on the packs. Does the FTC know what percentage of brands are unadvertised and therefore consumers have no access to information on yields?

MR. PEELER: We do not have those data, but we can get them for the panel if they like.

DR. FREEMAN: Dr. Shiffman?

DR. SHIFFMAN: I take it in a sense that we have a significant degree of consensus. I have heard the gentlemen from R.J. Reynolds say that they would be sympathetic to proposals that would provide more information for the consumer to make informed choices, and so, accordingly, I suggest that we shift from a mode of asking questions of them to a mode of considering proposals that would accomplish that goal on which we seem to have some consensus.

DR. DEBETHIZY: Mr. Chairman, it might help if Mr. Peeler would clarify what the purpose of the FTC method is. I think there has been some confusion here. I know I have been asked 10 times what the purpose is, and if you do not mind doing that, I think if you could do that concisely, that would help.

MR. PEELER: I would go back to the statement that I started with yesterday, and that is to say that the purpose of the FTC rankings when they were put together was to establish a comparative basis for consumers choosing among cigarettes. The reason the Commission asked the National Cancer Institute to commence this review of the cigarette testing methodology was to review whether that approach is still the correct approach, and obviously we are very interested as an agency in the types of questions that Dr. Cohen's research raises, which is how consumers actually use and view these data.

DR. FREEMAN: Mr. Peeler, is it implied in what you said that the FTC was ultimately interested in what was happening to the American public in terms of health? Is that implied in what you say, or was it separate from that or were you as an agency concerned about what is happening to the American people?

MR. PEELER: If you look at the history of the establishment of the current tar and nicotine testing system, it was clearly driven by concerns about health. It was clearly driven by the Surgeon General's findings that were valid at that time, that lower tar, lower nicotine cigarettes had a health benefit for consumers. So, clearly one of the issues that the Commission asked this panel to address is whether those health considerations are still valid in light of research that has occurred since the 1981 Surgeon General's report reviewed those issues and reported them.

DR. FREEMAN: So, then we would conclude that there is a clear connection in the work of this committee, not only to measure appropriately what cigarettes contain, no matter what method is used, but the end result that we are looking for is how can we help people in America with respect to avoiding disease and death, which means we would have to communicate appropriately to them in order to accomplish that. Is that a fair statement?

MR. PEELER: Most of the data that I have looked at indicate that there is a large group of consumers who are concerned about tar and nicotine ratings because of health reasons. So, clearly if the tar and nicotine ratings are communicating that to consumers, the FTC would want to make sure that these numbers are accurately delivering that benefit to consumers.

DR. TOWNSEND: Mr. Chairman, I think I am confused at this point because what I just heard is different from what I heard in your opening statement, and so I pulled out the copy of your opening statement, which says, "The primary purpose of this meeting is not to redesign the FTC testing protocol but rather to examine the protocol and make suggestions for improvements, if warranted." Your opening statement does not really go to actual changes.

DR. FREEMAN: You failed to go far enough in the opening statement. We posed three questions, the third of which dealt with what I was just speaking of, in other words, how does this translate to the American public in terms of their perceptions in the opening statement.

DR. TOWNSEND: Thank you.

DR. DEBETHIZY: I have a question for Mr. Peeler on the relationship between the FTC and the Surgeon General's warnings. Could you clarify that relationship for me? I was just curious about that because the questions that have been asked of me and that we have been getting into are the health implications of FTC numbers, and I was just curious about whether the FTC method is there to clarify the Surgeon General's warning, or is it related at all, or are they just two completely separate issues?

MR. PEELER: The FTC method as it was conceived and implemented was designed to provide consumers with comparative information about the relative tar and nicotine content of cigarettes. We know from the studies that we have seen that some groups of consumers look at those numbers as indicating a health benefit, which is why the Commission has asked the panel to look at the question of whether there is, for example, a dose-response relationship between the FTC tar and nicotine ratings and specific smoking-related diseases.

DR. SHIFFMAN: Let me come back to what I consider to be items of substantial consensus and maybe that will help us move on. I have not heard anyone speak against providing the consumer with more information, and so it seems to me that the appropriate education of the American smoking consumer is something we can all agree on, and that it is part of the intention of the FTC system, to give the consumer appropriate information. It seems to me that an important aspect is providing appropriate education to the consumer about the meaning of whatever information is conveyed in this labeling.

The second item on which I think we have considerable consensus is that in human smoking of particular cigarettes there is a considerable range or variability in what the consumer will actually extract from the cigarette. That was seen not only in some of the talks from past studies but also in the R.J. Reynolds study. So it seems to me the second item of substantial consensus is that no single number can completely represent the true human yield from a cigarette. Therefore, it seems to me that the direction in which we should be trying to move is to represent to the consumer the sense of that range in variability and to accompany that with appropriate educational measures so that we are providing the consumer with the kind of information on which to make informed choices, and I think that is the basis on which we ought to go forward.

DR. FREEMAN: Dr. Cohen?

DR. COHEN: Dr. Shiffman, could I ask if you would be willing to modify your view just a bit? I think that to start exactly at that point is not the right place to start because I think consumers want to know two things. They want to know if I smoke at all, how risky is it, and does that level of risk vary with the kind of cigarette I smoke. They want to know that. Now, that may be impossible to provide. That is not my field, but they do want it. We cannot finesse that issue.

DR. SHIFFMAN: I quite agree with you, and I think that part of what might go into an educational campaign would be about the meaning of these numbers or ranges in relation to health outcomes.

DR. COHEN: But it begs the question: Is there a way to provide two types of information, either in advertising or on the cigarette packages or both? The first type is the level of risk for that particular kind of cigarette or the level of harmfulness, and the second one is, can we give them a better sense of the relative magnitudes? I do not know the answer to either question, but I think that if we are going to wonder what we can do to help consumers, I think we should think long and hard about the need for those two different pieces of information.

DR. FREEMAN: At this point we are going to shift gears a little bit and get into the essence of the deliberations, and we thank the members of the tobacco industry for receiving those questions. We will go to the next phase of this discussion, which is the main phase and that is, as you remember from yesterday, we posed three questions that we were supposed to answer during these deliberations, and we are going to look at each of those three questions and get your comments on each one.

Question 1. **Does the evidence presented clearly demonstrate that changes are needed in the current FTC protocol for measuring nicotine, tar, and carbon monoxide, and if so, what changes are required?**

DR. GIOVINO: A lot has been made in this conference of the trends over time in the FTC yield in terms of tar and nicotine with a very large decline between the 1950's and 1980, roughly, and then a leveling off, and from the data that have been presented at this conference, I have to wonder, especially given Dr. Guerin's comments, what would that curve look like if consumer changes in puff frequency, puff volume, hole blocking, and vent blocking were incorporated? Dr. Guerin and Dr. Zacny have shown that the yields can be changed, given various factors, and I see that trend as a measure of yes, a standardized measure, but one that may not be as relevant now as it was 40 years ago.

So, I have to ask the panel to consider in its deliberations the issue of the usefulness of those trend data, given as was demonstrated yesterday the wide range of products now available and the different degrees of compensation that can happen with those products.

DR. TOWNSEND: May I respond to that? I believe that the trends that you saw yesterday in the chart are useful today as they always have been. One thing that I think there is consensus on within this panel is that if you change puffing conditions, what you do is shift the tar and nicotine yields up or down depending on to what level you change those puffing conditions. Even if you block the vents, you shift the tar and nicotine yields up, but in general the relative ranking does not change. If the relative ranking does not change, you are only changing the absolute values. Then that is going to have no substantive effect on the trend charts that showed nicotine and tar yield decreases over the years.

DR. GIOVINO: I have to wonder, given the situation 40 years ago when tar and nicotine levels were so high, if those behaviors would have been so common. The relative rankings may be accurate for any given year, but the range was so different 40 years ago than it is now that the actual amount of some of the compensatory behaviors may have been much less frequent 40 years ago than now.

The range in tar values and nicotine values was so much higher in the 1950's and the 1960's given the FTC yield that people may not have had to perform the compensatory behaviors and wouldn't have even had the ability to hole block because it is my understanding that there were no holes then. So, my concern is that those trend data, while representing what the FTC has presented, are not representing even what the consumer is taking out of the cigarette, let alone getting into their lungs.

DR. GUERIN: I am not sure that was ever the case anyway. In trend data, what you are looking at are the characteristics of the average cigarette, not how the cigarette was used, and that is all those data mean.

DR. GIOVINO: Exactly. I think the panel understands this, that the trend data represent what the FTC method gives. The reality is that trends over time in terms of what the consumer is taking out are quite different.

DR. BOCK: At the very earliest time that yield data were collected, the standard deviations were given, which had big meaning for the analysts but obviously did not have much meaning for people out in the street. But the variability of smoking, which is part of the fact that people in the street really need to know, the range of values for each cigarette, has not been provided by the data. The labeling might have incorporated that type of information, which would in large part, I think, answer some of the criticisms.

DR. FREEMAN: Before you go on, let me follow up on that. Are you suggesting then that might be a change in this Question 1 concern?

DR. BOCK: It would indicate that maybe there should be a change in the protocol and the way the data are collected, and there should be provision made for a range.

DR. FREEMAN: Measuring the same elements but giving the range.

DR. BOCK: With different smoking parameters.

DR. FREEMAN: That is a point of discussion. Dr. Woosley?

DR. WOOSLEY: I think in answering that first one I have to agree with Dr. Giovino that things have changed over the years, and I think that is what the FTC is actually asking us. There was this huge range of difference 30 years ago or so, and the ability for this method to predict something was great then, but now that most of the tobacco products have come down to some very homogeneous group, the variance is quite tight, and the ability of this numerical ranking to have any meaningful information or carry any meaningful information to the public is gone, in my estimation. Data yesterday were very convincing for me that numerical ranking does not really convey the exposure that occurs because of compensation. So, to me the answer to the first question is pretty clear. The current system must be changed in some way.

DR. TOWNSEND: I do not understand your comment that cigarettes today are a more homogeneous group. From the data I showed yesterday the spread in tar deliveries in 1954 was really quite narrow. Cigarettes were really quite similar then. Today there is a huge range of products available to the consumer. I see that as less homogeneous.

DR. WOOSLEY: I was referring to the potential range of intake, not the range that the tobacco industry provided us.

DR. RICKERT: One of the things that people are concerned about is the fact that consumers tend to misinterpret the information. One of the ways of coming to grips with this problem is to deal with a range of potential values rather than specific numbers. This problem was first noted, I think, back in the 1981 Surgeon General's report when at that time there was a call for publishing maximal values in addition to the values that are obtained under FTC methodology. A more recent paper in 1994 has called for the same approach, and I think serious consideration should be given to this question of range, how one might express these upper limits, and if maximum were to be used, how that maximum would be determined.

DR. GUERIN: If one examines Question 1 that we are addressing, the question says, "Is there any evidence that changes are needed in the current FTC protocol for measuring tar and nicotine and CO?" I have not necessarily seen much evidence for changes in measuring it, but a lot of reasons for changes in how we communicate it. Do we have to change the testing protocol to achieve this, or do we have to have a better way of communicating?

DR. WOOSLEY: It says, "Constituent yields," and I think the yield from that method is probably inadequate. We need data on the yield to the smoker.

DR. ZACNY: I just want to go back to something that Dr. Townsend said about 5 minutes ago and that we spent some time on yesterday when he showed charts where you increase puff volume from, I guess 35 to 55 mL, and the relative rankings would not change if puff volume were increased across the different yields. I think things change when you talk about filter vent blocking and maybe altering parameters for extensive filter vent blocking because there is a fundamental difference between lower yield cigarettes and high-yield cigarettes.

The high-yield cigarettes do not have filter vents, and so you could, by manipulating this parameter, turn a low-yield cigarette into a high-yield cigarette; the relative rankings then would not be preserved.

DR. FREEMAN: Dr. Rickert?

DR. RICKERT: I think there is one issue that we have not really looked at, and that is, there is something else that happens when you move from standardized FTC testing conditions to other testing conditions. We always consider what happens to the quantity of particulates, like tar, for example; what should be also considered is what happens to the *quality* of that tar. For example, in the Brown and Williamson documents that I received, it seemed that moving from standard conditions to behaviorally defined conditions resulted in an increase in mutagenicity of the tar fraction on a gram-per-gram basis using the salmonella assay, and so I think focusing totally on the changes in the relative ranking misses the point that the biological activity on a per-gram basis may be changing as well.

DR. FREEMAN: Dr. Henningfield?

DR. HENNINGFIELD: I would like to follow up on a point that Dr. Woosley made. I agree. My impression is that what people want to know is what gets into people, not into machines. There is only one way to do that, and that is to do what you do with any other drug: Test what gets in people, and that is the only way that you can validate the upper range. There is no way you can do that with a machine. You have to put the system in people to see what they actually get.

Also, I think you need to do that because as we have seen, with almost any system you come up with, the industry might come up with a creative way to beat that machine. Testing in humans is essential. The question for Dr. deBethizy is, when we were discussing providing a wide range of values, and there seems to be some leaning that that would be a useful thing to do, you seemed to agree that was worth considering, but that the FTC method was not up to that task. I think that is what you said. If that is what you said, why is the FTC method not up to the task?

DR. DEBETHIZY: I did not say that. What I said was that it seemed like a reasonable proposal to put on the table. I did not say anything about not providing the FTC number. I think the FTC number is a good number. It has been a standardized number we have used for a long time to provide relative ranking. If somebody is proposing that a range also be determined, with a low and a high end, then let us discuss that.

DR. SHIFFMAN: Let us, indeed, discuss that. It seems to me that the FTC assay method may be adaptable to this goal in the sense that if one looked at a different set of parameters, if one included the potential vent blocking as part of a protocol for maximum extraction or maximum yield, perhaps it would be possible to use the machine testing method to adequately describe or estimate the range of human exposures from a particular cigarette, and that could well be more informative to smokers.

DR. FREEMAN: Before we get other comments, that seems to be a recurrent point of discussion about the range being an important point to consider as a possible suggestion, and I would like to zero in on that particular point and discuss it. Is there anyone who wants to discuss that point?

DR. KOZLOWSKI: A number of the studies in the literature argue that the rankings would be preserved if you had a heavy smoke setting on the machine. I think if you consider Zacny's data and other data, the idea of tuning every cigarette up to the same maximum puff volume or maximum puff rate is probably not a good model of human smoking behavior; the higher yield cigarettes may, in fact, be undersmoked relative to the lower yield cigarettes. Zacny's data on the puff volume show clearly that the puff volumes are bigger on the ultralights than on the higher yield cigarettes, so that when you have studies that just tune everything up, and you see the ranking preserved, the fact of the matter is that if the human behavior is more appropriately modeled you may well see that some of the higher yield brands go down, the lower yield brands go up, and it would get a lot flatter than simply jacking up all the settings of the machine regardless of what the strength of that cigarette is to begin with.

DR. FREEMAN: I think perhaps the question and my own opinion as I am posing it, given a particular cigarette, would be what is the range of possible exposure of that cigarette compared to any other cigarette? The question I would like some consideration of is, is that a reasonable thing to measure; is that a reasonable approach to take as to what we should measure? Dr. Benowitz?

DR. BENOWITZ: I think that is a reasonable approach. I think Dr. Kozlowski's point of view is very well taken, but I think in practical terms it really is impossible because you would have to study large numbers of people smoking every single brand of cigarettes to be able to get individual parameters. We know what he says occurs. It seems to me that the idea of having the standard condition and an intensive smoking condition with and without hole blocking would be very useful, but what it has to be coupled with is information for consumers about how their smoking of the cigarette will influence the yields. For example, if they block, this is what is going to happen, and if they puff intensively or take a lot of puffs, then this is what is going to happen, and I think that would be the best we could do to say, "If you smoke in this way, you are going to get the maximum yields." And that way we could pick what we think would be an intensive condition and say, "If you smoke in this way, this is what your yield is going to be."

DR. FREEMAN: With a given cigarette?

DR. BENOWITZ: With a given cigarette, because I do not think it is feasible, although I would like to, either to measure puffing parameters for every brand of cigarette or even, as Dr. Henningfield suggested, to do human exposure studies if you have 900 brands of cigarettes. I do not think that would be practical. I think we should test maybe some brands of cigarettes to see how well we are doing, but I do not think it is going to be feasible for all these brands to do anything other than a standardized testing.

DR. FREEMAN: Putting that forward as a point of discussion, does anyone disagree with what Dr. Benowitz has said, that we should perhaps recommend that a given cigarette should be tested to see what its range of possible exposure would be using whatever techniques make sense; is there any disagreement with putting that forward? Dr. Hoffmann?

DR. HOFFMANN: I think that Dr. Benowitz' old studies concentrated on nicotine, but I think when we test on humans and try to see how they smoke, we should not limit it to nicotine. There are other carcinogenic toxic agents, and I think that the work done by Dr. Benowitz on nicotine is outstanding, but it is nicotine, and when we deal with cancer, at least, that is my area of expertise, there are agents that are just as important.

DR. FREEMAN: I did not understand that you were speaking only of nicotine. Were you not speaking of tar and the three things that are mentioned?

DR. BENOWITZ: Yes, in terms of the machine testing I was certainly speaking of all. In terms of human bioavailability testing, I think as Dr. Hoffmann says, if we have tools to measure tar exposure, we definitely should do that. Right now the only practical tools for large-scale studies are nicotine and CO, but when we get tar measurement tools where we can do it on hundreds of people, that should be included.

DR. TOWNSEND: If I could respond, my reaction to your proposal is that if we provide to the consumer an FTC number and a maximum deliverable number by hole blocking and a more intense puffing regimen, which I believe is your proposal, then from what I know about cigarette design those two are going to very closely parallel each other, and the ranking of cigarettes will be largely preserved. My question then is, does that provide additional and useful information to the consumer?

DR. BENOWITZ: I would like to respond to that. I do not believe that the ranking will be preserved. If you have the old-style cigarettes that are nonfilter cigarettes, no matter what you do, the ranking is going to be preserved, but if you are comparing a nonfilter cigarette and then a cigarette that has extensive ventilation and you block holes, you might see one surpass the other. I just do not believe that when you are dealing with a cigarette that has 90 percent ventilation in a standard test and people have the possibility of reducing that to zero percent ventilation, and you are comparing that to cigarettes with no ventilating filters, the ranking will be preserved.

DR. TOWNSEND: As a cigarette designer, I believe that it will be largely preserved, and I guess what I am hearing you say is that this is your suspicion, but I guess my question, is do you have data that support that, and I guess the obvious direction I am going in with this question is, should we collect data to see whether the ranking is largely preserved to convince you?

DR. FREEMAN: I think we have a question over here.

DR. HATSUKAMI: You mentioned changing the intensity of smoking. I would like to know how you determine those parameters; how do you determine the number of puffs that should be taken, the range of puffs that should be taken, or the volume that should be taken; what should that be based on?

DR. BENOWITZ: I have not looked at the current studies to see what is available, but I think you could do that on the basis of looking at observations, say in people who are smoking low-yield cigarettes and seeing what they do.

DR. HATSUKAMI: With the minimum and the maximum ranges in terms of number of puffs?

DR. BENOWITZ: I do not think a minimum is really necessary. I actually believe that we should continue to report the standard FTC method mostly because I would like to know how current cigarettes compare to cigarettes marketed 20 years ago so we could have that as sort of a minimum because in fact, you know, it is my belief, based on the evidence, that for the vast majority of cigarettes the FTC method underestimates exposure. So, we could still have that as a minimum exposure, and then we could have the test method to show what a smoker might get if they smoke in an intense way, which could then be specified.

DR. FREEMAN: Dr. Bock?

DR. BOCK: It does not make a lot of difference to me whether the ranking is changed or not. When you put down an average and a standard deviation, sophisticated people can understand whether the differences in the average are important, and a range will give that kind of information to unsophisticated people, and that is where I think the big advantage of a range is. Whether it changes the ranking, it will say that if the cigarettes are very closely ranked one above the other, it really does not matter very much which is the reality of the situation.

DR. FREEMAN: Dr. Hughes?

DR. HUGHES: You asked if there is any disagreement. I have a little bit of a disagreement, in that I am still worried about reporting numbers. I could go along with numbers if there were a disclaimer that says that 10 mg of tar does not cut your risk in half compared to 20 mg of tar. I am still very concerned that even if we give ranges that people are going to look at the averages and think that 10 gives you half the health risk of a 20, but it does not.

DR. FREEMAN: Dr. Hughes, what would you recommend in that case?

DR. HUGHES: You could go with either the nonnumerical system where you certainly had a band and put them in or numbers as long as there is a disclaimer that these are not cardinal numbers. That can be communicated fairly easily by doing that.

DR. FREEMAN: So, you favor going with numbers or not going with numbers?

DR. HUGHES: We have a long morning ahead of us; I can be persuaded either way. My only point is there must be some information to the consumer that 10 mg is not half the risk of 20. As long as that is in there, I am agreeable.

DR. FREEMAN: I think it is conceivable that whatever we decide here could also be accompanied by something in writing to explain and educate the public. I think we should assume that could be done.

DR. HUGHES: I would like to see if maybe Dr. Shiffman or Dr. Benowitz could give us a more concrete proposal here to make sure that we know what is going on because what I hear people saying, and I just want to make sure we are all saying the same thing, is that having a testing method that has a range of values, I do not know whether you want to call it the 95 percent vs. the 5 percent or something like that, some range of values based on doing different things, blocking holes and that sort of thing, but we are also talking about one thing (I was unclear), is still reporting a mean or not reporting a mean? That is what I am confused about.

DR. SHIFFMAN: You are suggesting that the current FTC system would represent a band?

DR. HUGHES: So, not a range. So, is it from the 50th to the 95th percentile?

DR. BENOWITZ: I do not think the current FTC is the 50th.

DR. DEBETHIZY: Yes, I do not think we want the current FTC method to be the bottom. I mean if you are talking about a range, the range has a low and a high, and the FTC number is in the middle. So, I think that is important. If you are going to talk about a range, you have to talk about the whole range.

DR. HUGHES: I think you have to have a range, but whether the FTC ends up in the middle I do not know. Let me suggest that I do not think that just getting an upper and a middle is fair to the consumer because there are consumers at the lower end who are getting more health benefit, if there is any, from the low-yield cigarettes than the average smoker, and I do not think it is fair to not portray that to them. So, I would like to see the full range. Everybody thinks they are the average. I would like to see it not have a mean.

DR. FREEMAN: Dr. Cohen?

DR. COHEN: I would guess that I am thinking ahead to what might happen in the marketplace, both competitively and with respect to smokers who are also consumers. I think that we have to understand that whatever analysis is done for internal purposes among specialists is one thing, but when information is presented to consumers in a form that they cannot handle, we cannot underrate the difficulty of educating them about that. It is not going to be easy to explain the idea of a range to consumers. I would ask the panel to consider a slightly different alternative, and that would be to vary the test parameters and produce a range of reasonable smoking responses on say, tar, maybe using the machine and then to pick some number like the mean plus a standard deviation, let us say, just to throw something out for discussion, because this would represent a number that a reasonable number of smokers might really encounter. In other words, that would be the tar level that a substantial number of smokers would actually encounter in smoking a cigarette, and if that were presented to consumers, yes, it would err a little bit on the high side for some consumers, but I think our duty may be to give consumers information that serves to protect a reasonable number of those who are ingesting more.

I think that if that number were provided, I do not want to call it a maximum, you would find that firms would have an incentive to modify cigarettes. They have a lot of design features they can use to modify low-yield cigarettes to be sure that the mean plus one standard deviation would be as low as possible, and I do not think we should underestimate the importance of what is done here on the design of cigarettes in the future. I do not think we should underestimate that, and I think if we give them something along the lines of what we are talking about, they have the ability to see that their cigarettes come in at as low a number as possible.

DR. FREEMAN: May I ask you, Dr. Cohen, how would you reach the mean in such a method?

DR. COHEN: I am certainly not technically competent, but in listening to the discussions and reading the papers, if the FTC testing method were adjusted to deal with such things as puff number, puff interval, and puff volume and this were done based on an observation of how smokers smoke, just as it was done when the original Cambridge Filter method was set up in the first place, then you would be able to know what the magic number would be for two-thirds of the sample or some arbitrary number, and it would be greater than the mean. I think that number would probably be a lot easier to communicate than a range, and it would have the side benefit of better informing smokers as to what their potential risk might be, and it would also provide great incentives to the industry to make cigarettes that came in at as low a number as possible.

If one of the major problems with the low-tar cigarettes is where the filter holes are and how they work and the fact that they can be covered, then if this testing protocol were followed and the mean plus one standard deviation for that cigarette the way it was smoked were a fairly large range and if the company making that cigarette did not like that large a number, it has the capability of reducing that number by putting the filter holes in such a way that they are not going to be blocked.

I would say that it is very important to consider the impact of what is done here on what they do.

DR. FREEMAN: Dr. Shiffman?

DR. SHIFFMAN: I very much share your concern that we come up with a system that is communicative and that is grasped by the smokers whom we are trying to reach. Part of what is attractive about a range is that it also communicates, to borrow a phrase, that their "mileage" will vary. My concern about any one number, no matter where you put it on the spectrum, is that it does not communicate that and implies that this is exactly what this cigarette will deliver. So, I think it is a significant challenge to health education, public education, and advertising people to design a system that communicates this idea of range and the idea that range is to some degree under the control of the smoker and his or her behavior. Part of what is attractive to me about that range is communicating exactly that, that the human yield is variable and that it is variable to some degree according to the behavior of the smoker. That is something I would like to see communicated.

DR. FREEMAN: Dr. Stitzer?

DR. STITZER: I just want to support that point. I think that we are dealing with a situation where the public is very lacking in knowledge, and the one particular thing that is not understood by smokers, I believe, is that the way they smoke their cigarette determines the yield that they get from it. I think the basis of the system we design should be to convey a very basic piece of information, and some of these ideas about ranges and so forth are important. The fact of the matter is that, with low-yield cigarettes, these ranges are going to be very wide. They are going to be completely overlapping with the higher yield brands, but that is exactly the information that we want the consumers to know.

Now, the unfortunate part is that consumers do not have any good way of knowing where they in particular fit along any range that we might present, and that is a different problem.

DR. FREEMAN: Dr. Benowitz?

DR. BENOWITZ: I would also like to support Dr. Shiffman's comments and just say that we could be specific about this, and I think we should be. For example, we can say that if you block these ventilation holes, this is what your exposure will be, and if you do not, this is what your exposure will be, and we can also request that ventilation holes be marked to make them obvious to the smoker. Make them bright red or orange or something to minimize your exposure; I am all for ultralow-yield cigarettes if people will smoke them that way. I think that is great. You have to make it possible for them to do that, and we could with labeling.

DR. FREEMAN: Dr. Henningfield?

DR. HENNINGFIELD: I also agree that the range is basic, honest, accurate information, but it is clear that it has to be coupled with education on what factors may affect your intake: how consumers can change their behavior in ways that might be helpful. But a really important point of Dr. Cohen's I think should be considered, and that is the importance of providing an incentive to the industry that may serve people. Drs. Benowitz and Kozlowski and I had this embedded in our *Journal of the American Medical Association* proposal: the notion that right now, in our estimation, virtually all cigarettes you throw into the regular category, but by providing the incentive to get that label of low, which could be a really nice selling point and may be of health benefit, you would have to work to redesign cigarettes in such a way that I think would be useful, and what you would have to do is redesign them in a way that would make sure that the upper level was lower. And that brings me again to the reason that I think we need some bioavailability testing. I agree with Dr. Benowitz, not necessarily on 900 brands, but you need to anchor it at some point to what people get, and you need an agency that can oversee that properly and also require it on demand; that is the only way you are going to prevent another Barclay cigarette type of scam, the notion that somebody comes up with a design that seems to meet the low category, and they have just done it by beating the machine. The only way you are going to check that is by seeing what people get.

DR. GUERIN: Dr. Henningfield, as a good example, the FTC test is what discovered the Barclay scheme. The FTC test has been successful in identifying those kinds of problems.

DR. SHIFFMAN: Dr. Henningfield, I take that perhaps as an additional proposal that you address a different issue than we have been talking about, which is the use of words like "light, low, ultralight" in advertising and the importance of making those accurate and not deceptive or confusing to the consumer, and that I think is something we ought to address. That the information that is presented to the public in advertising goes beyond the small numbers printed in the corner to the large "light," "ultralight," "low" printed in bold print, and I think that is something we ought to look at.

DR. HENNINGFIELD: Yes, I think those words should be banned.

DR. SHIFFMAN: I would disagree that they should be banned. They should be regulated so that they are accurate.

DR. FREEMAN: Dr. Rickert?

DR. RICKERT: I think it is obvious that many consumers choose their brands on the basis of some perceived risk to health, and it is also obvious that the FTC numbers do not and never were designed for that particular purpose. I share Dr. Hoffmann's concern in that our measure of dose is often based on nicotine, which may or may not tell us about other constituents in tobacco smoke. Specifically, at the level of molecular epidemiology, there are certain constituents that now can be tracked, and Dr. Hoffmann has mentioned NNK in urine. There is the constituent 4-amino-biphenyl, which is present in tobacco smoke and which in smokers ends up as a hemoglobin adduct. There is, also, benzo(a)pyrene, which in smokers ends up being bound to albumin. So, there are a number of traceable constituents in tobacco smoke that have known toxic or carcinogenic properties, which also then can be related to uptake in smokers and nonsmokers alike.

DR. FREEMAN: Dr. Cohen?

DR. COHEN: I would like to return to the point that Dr. Henningfield was just talking about and the point that I raised a few minutes ago. I think it is very important not to put the burden in the wrong place.

If we are going to put the burden on consumers to respond to whatever design changes industry makes and then educate them each time industry makes a clever change, as to where they put the holes or what kind of paper they use or whatever, we are fighting a losing battle. I think that the best approach here is really to allow the industry, which is able to modify its product, to modify it in order to obtain the maximum benefit to their sales from a low rating. They have an incentive to do that, and so, if the panel deems it appropriate, I would suggest that coming up with a rating system that reports to consumers a number within the range, which is not at the midpoint of the range but is tilted toward those who do compensate, is the smartest thing that can be done because that, in fact, will offer guidance to consumers who after all should not have the primary responsibility for outsmarting the designers of cigarettes, and I think that it would also provide the cigarette industry an opportunity to modify their design in order to achieve the numbers that are most beneficial for them.

DR. FREEMAN: Dr. Hoffmann?

DR. HOFFMANN: Before we got this upper limit and extreme, we should ask Dr. Guerin how far we can go. We have heard yesterday that the low-tar cigarette smoker may take up to 60 to 65 mL per puff and up to 6 or 7 puffs per minute; is that possible with our current equipment?

DR. GUERIN: Current instrumentation would have to be modified somewhat to reach some of the extremes in terms of volumes.

DR. HOFFMANN: You can do more than 50 mL?

DR. GUERIN: Right.

DR. HOFFMANN: With the machine?

DR. GUERIN: No, I said that you can, but it would require some modification.

DR. HOFFMANN: New machinery?

DR. GUERIN: To reach some of the extremes in terms of puff volumes, frequencies for a 20-port system would be too high. You can purchase systems of smaller capacity that have that flexibility.

DR. HOFFMANN: But the standard machine we have now cannot go through these extremes?

DR. GUERIN: It would not be able to go through all the extremes without some modifications.

DR. BOCK: The cost of the machine really is not something to use as a basis for this discussion. It is so small compared to the cost of labor that it is meaningless.

DR. FREEMAN: Dr. Hughes?

DR. HUGHES: We have been talking about these numbers and as scientists we like to talk about numbers, and maybe we will get to this with the third question. My major concern is conveying how much health benefit people get by these lower nicotine, lower tar cigarettes because what I saw in the 1981 Surgeon General's report and what I saw Dr. Samet present yesterday suggest to me that it is not great, and it is not very large, and I think when the normal consumer switches to a 1-mg cigarette, they think they are doing themselves a great benefit, and my concern is that the magnitude of that effect be conveyed to the consumer.

DR. FREEMAN: Dr. Rickert?

DR. RICKERT: At the present time, FTC methodology is providing us with information on tar and nicotine and CO; when we are talking about lower yield cigarettes, we tend to link tar and nicotine explicitly together, and while there is an obvious relationship between these variables, there is also extreme variation.

All one has to do is take the 933 brands that were just published recently in the FTC report and look at various plots of CO vs. nicotine or tar vs. nicotine, and you cannot help but be struck by the fact that there is a wide range of variation as far as specific nicotine level.

For example, if you look at that report and brands delivering .9 mg of nicotine, there were 54 brands with varying tar yields. So, I think, in addition to the issue of tar and nicotine, that the issue of how one communicates simultaneously changes in all three variables because you can have the situation where it could be high tar-low nicotine or low tar-high nicotine, and by constantly linking the two together, I think one is missing the point about the other two variables.

DR. FREEMAN: Yes, Dr. Stitzer?

DR. STITZER: I was going to pick up on Dr. Hughes' point because it is an important one, but I think it is very much intertwined with the whole discussion about reporting of the machine testing yields. If the smoker can visualize the fact that the actual yield from this low-yield cigarette is completely overlapping with the yield from this other high-yield cigarette, then I think that can more easily bring home the other health message, which is that switching to these cigarettes may not have any benefit whatsoever. I think that there is a dose-response problem there.

DR. FREEMAN: Dr. Benowitz?

DR. BENOWITZ: I think that it would be great if we could put something in about health risks. I think the data seem very clear that smoking any cigarette is so much greater risk than smoking none that it will be impossible to quantitate it, and I think that should be communicated. But at the same time, even if there is a small difference in exposure from high- to low-yield cigarettes, if you are talking about a huge population of smokers, it is worthwhile to encourage as many possible to get as low a yield as possible, even though it is not going to have nearly the effect of stopping smoking. It still is of some benefit. So, I think we should warn people that switching to low-yield cigarettes is not going to remove the risk of smoking, but still try to encourage that somehow people do that.

DR. DEBETHIZY: Dr. Benowitz, you are raising an important issue. It is that whatever change that gets recommended here today to the FTC, it is going to require some research and some study to make sure that some unintended things do not occur. For instance, if ranges were recommended, and put on in advertising, would that have the effect of discouraging people from switching down? As a scientist, I think it is important for us to understand the ramifications, and I am assuming that this is just the start of a process, that recommendations will be made, and that the FTC will consider those using research techniques.

DR. FREEMAN: Yes, Dr. Shiffman?

DR. SHIFFMAN: Just to proceed on the point that Dr. Hughes and Dr. Benowitz made, we have said a couple of times that the idea of educating smokers is very important. I think educating them not only about these numbers or ranges but also about the comparative benefit of not smoking at all vs. lowering the received yield is an important part, and I think it deserves some discussion, though perhaps not here, about the degree to which that can be done in this sort of labeling rating system or whether, in fact, we need other media as well. There is limited information we are going to get on a pack or in an ad, but I think there is a responsibility to educate smokers so that they do make those informed choices.

DR. FREEMAN: Dr. Woosley?

DR. WOOSLEY: I agree slightly with the representative from the tobacco industry that we have to make sure there are no adverse consequences from anything that we try to do in a meaningful way, and one of the most serious concerns I have is that we do not want to give a false impression about health risks. I think one of the most disturbing pieces of data that I saw yesterday was the indication that people who were on the ultralows had a lower cessation rate, and I am concerned that potential means that the recommendations that come out of this panel may encourage people to go to low yield instead of stopping smoking, and I think that overall will be a terribly adverse health risk or adverse effect on the overall health of the Nation.

DR. FREEMAN: Yes, Mr. Peeler?

MR. PEELER: In line with that discussion I just wanted to throw out two pieces of information for the panel's consideration. The first is from the time the ban on tar and nicotine claims in advertising was lifted, the FTC basically prohibited any health claims in the advertising. So, what you are seeing is really what consumers are inferring from the low-tar and -nicotine systems. The other thing that we have focused on and thought about in this area is the fact that the Government's position for many, many years has been that people who are concerned about their health should stop smoking. There is actually a warning on the packages right now that says that. Stopping smoking now increases your health, but it is a very difficult communications conundrum, as Dr. Shiffman has indicated, about whether you can talk about relative risk from tar and nicotine and not send an unintended message that Dr. Woosley is talking about, that this is the better way to go.

DR. FREEMAN: Yes, Dr. Kozlowski?

DR. KOZLOWSKI: I think it is pretty clear that smokers currently are turning to so-called "light" and "ultralight" brands, believing that they are doing themselves a favor with respect to their health. I think there is a real concern about health-conscious smokers who want to try to do something. They now have the impression: How could a light cigarette kill anybody; how could an ultralight cigarette kill anybody, and there is no deadly connotation to the terms "light" or "ultralight." By providing better information the hope is that some of the people who out of health concerns are turning to lower yield cigarettes will see something of the risks of that, and they may be in a fool's paradise, and they maybe should stop altogether. The pamphlet that was passed out in an earlier version about 10 years ago was titled "Tar and Nicotine Ratings May Be Hazardous to Your Health: Information for Smokers Who Aren't Ready to Quit Yet." A smoker who is smoking a 1-mg tar cigarette and enjoying it may think, "My God, I am smoking the lowest yield cigarette on the market; how could that do me any harm? I have really done something." If that smoker then sees, "I blocked the vent holes," and so on and so on, the hope is that becomes an inducement to stop. I think you expressed some reservations about use of the term "consumers," but I think it is important that continuing smokers be treated in part as consumers and be given information similar to what consumers have expected about automobiles and things like that.

DR. COHEN: Could I follow up with some numbers? I have some evidence exactly on the point that you just made, and it may be useful to the panel to hear the evidence. I apologize, again, because you couldn't read the numbers so clearly yesterday. In my survey, *83 percent* of those smoking 1- to 5-mg tar cigarettes thought that switching from a 20-mg tar cigarette to a 5-mg tar cigarette would significantly lower that person's health risks due to smoking for someone who smokes a pack a day. More than 25 percent of those smoking cigarettes with 6 or more mg of tar thought that switching from a 20-mg tar cigarette to a 16-mg tar cigarette would significantly lower that person's health risk due to smoking for someone who smokes a pack a day.

DR. DEBETHIZY: I would not be surprised at that because the Surgeon General said in 1981 that if you reduced your tar intake, you reduce risk.

It has been communicated pretty clearly that if you cannot stop or are unwilling to stop, then reducing your tar intake is a good idea.

DR. GIOVINO: I would like the Surgeon General's comments to be put on the record so that they could be stated exactly and hopefully they will be used exactly as stated. The Surgeon General said:

> The Public Health Service policy on lower tar and nicotine cigarettes must remain unchanged. The health risks of cigarette smoking can only be eliminated by quitting. For those who continue to smoke, some risk reduction may result from a switch to a lower tar and nicotine cigarette provided that no compensatory changes in style of smoking occur.

I would ask that caveat be used when these types of statements are made.

I would also remind us that while the relative risk studies on lung cancer may have controlled for number of cigarettes a day, and I am not sure of the methodology on those, they certainly have not controlled for changes in puff frequency or puff volume. So, one point I want to make is, let us make sure that we provide in any statements we make about the Surgeon General's statements the caveats that the Surgeon General's report provides, and the second point I would like to make is that the categorization of light and ultralight cigarettes in advertising and promotion is not always consistent. There are many exceptions to those rules that Ron Davis pointed out in his article in the *American Journal of Public Health*, and the current system of light and ultralight seems not totally consistent at times with the tar and nicotine ratings.

DR. FREEMAN: Dr. Headen?

DR. HEADEN: I want to go on record in support of the color-coded representation of the FTC information for the consumer and to go on record in support of a range rather than a single number. I would ask us to consider the point that Dr. Cohen made. It is important to design this information in a way that would encourage the tobacco industry to redesign cigarettes to conform to whatever standard we adopt, but I do believe that if there is a range that there will be an incentive on the part of the industry to lessen the width of that range. A cigarette brand that has a very broad range gives a very clear message to the consumer that the yield is variable, particularly when they consider the upper limit, and that there would be a high incentive for the industry to narrow the range of whatever yield there is for each of the cigarettes.

DR. FREEMAN: Thank you very much. Because we have two other major elements to consider today, and it does not mean we cannot discuss more of this, we want to go to the second question, and you can continue to raise ideas on the first question as we go along because they do overlap a bit.

Question 2. **Should constituents other than tar, nicotine, and carbon monoxide be added to the protocol?**

Dr. Henningfield?

DR. HENNINGFIELD: I do not think we have the information to decide the entire list, but we probably have some ideas of things that should be added. I would suggest that the procedure be used as the FDA uses for food labeling, which is that substances that an organization or committee with specialty in toxicology agrees are of toxicological significance be added. And with foods, under the category of other flavorings and ingredients, industries are not free of listing things that are of toxicological significance just because they call it a flavoring, as occurs with cigarettes. Rather an outside body decides what is of toxicological significance. I do not know if they are of toxicological levels, but that should not be decided by the tobacco industry, in my opinion. That should be decided by a regulatory agency with toxicology experts.

DR. FREEMAN: Dr. Benowitz?

DR. BENOWITZ: I think Dr. Henningfield's comments are well taken, but I would just like to go on record in support of the sort of labeling that Dr. Harris showed us yesterday, which I thought is very informative to consumers when you see all the cyanide and arsenic and all those things in cigarettes. I think it just helps to provide more information to a consumer about the mix of what is in their tobacco smoke. I am sure they are not going to read every bit of it, but anytime they are interested in looking and they see a list of 30 cancer-causing compounds, I think it is useful for them to know that. So, I am in favor of having that sort of listing available.

DR. FREEMAN: May I try to understand what you said, that you would not present measurements in the way that we are measuring the three elements, but you would simply list them as carcinogenic or harmful to health? How would you do this?

DR. BENOWITZ: I think you could do it either way. It would be relatively straightforward to measure those and just list how many micrograms or whatever was there, or you could just list them. I do not have a very strong feeling about it just as long as it is made clear to people what the types and the mix of toxic chemicals they are taking in their smoke.

DR. FREEMAN: What I mean is, you would treat them differently from the way we are treating tar, nicotine, and carbon monoxide?

DR. BENOWITZ: Yes, I do not think we need to provide information about standard and maximum exposures, for example. I just think if we had one number or one list it would be adequate.

DR. FREEMAN: I see. Thank you. Dr. Rickert?

DR. RICKERT: I think there should be additional communication of information. I question whether or not it should be in the form of an absolute number. For example, it could be categorized in terms of ciliatoxic agents and hydrogen cyanide, for example. It could be categorized as carcinogens and then certain carcinogens. I think, given all the discussion that we have had both yesterday and today about the potential misinterpretation of numbers, it would seem to me that to add to that confusion by a whole new set of numbers would not be serving the interests of the consumer.

DR. FREEMAN: Thank you, Dr. Rickert. Dr. Stitzer?

DR. STITZER: I am totally in favor of more information being given to the consumer, but I want to bring up priorities and to point out that cigarette packs are not very big, and personally I think it is more important to convey the information about the variability of yield in some prominent way on a cigarette package rather than using that space to list hundreds of chemicals.

Now, what I would be interested in seeing is a kind of package insert disclosure information that would be put in cigarette cartons. That might be a better format for delivering the information.

DR. FREEMAN: Dr. Petitti?

DR. PETITTI: I would like to provide support for both of the prior statements, particularly that perhaps cigarettes need to have prominently displayed the fact that they contain some list of selected carcinogens but not to portray that information in a quantitative fashion. I do not think we have the ability to decide which of the numerous carcinogens in cigarette smoke is the one or the ones that quantitatively are related to the various forms of cancer caused by cigarettes and that we would be further misleading the consumer by making them believe that, for example, a cigarette with low levels of chemical X is better for them than a cigarette with a higher level of chemical X. I do not think we will ever have the epidemiological database that will allow us to link these various carcinogens quantitatively with risk of any of the human cancers.

DR. FREEMAN: Yes, Dr. Guerin?

DR. GUERIN: If we had a list of common cigarette smoke toxins on packages, would that not discourage the industry from producing products that have undetectable quantities? Wouldn't we need some kind of a level of detection to determine when we are at basically nothing because there are advanced products that are being marketed or may be being marketed?

DR. FREEMAN: Let us go to Dr. Hughes first.

DR. HUGHES: People are interested in function. They do not care about the names. They care about what these things do. So, my proposal would be to get the word "cancer-forming" agents on there. That is the important thing, not whether it is this long name or that long name or whatever because that is the important thing that consumers need to know.

DR. FREEMAN: Yes, Dr. Townsend?

DR. TOWNSEND: Thank you, Mr. Chairman. In the U.S. market, cigarettes with comparable blends, in fact, show similar ratios of most smoke constituents per milligram of tar. What that means is, as you bring the tar level down in a cigarette, these constituents also come down more or less proportionately.

I guess the question then that leads me to is, are we providing really useful information for the consumer to use, or are we just giving them a lot of information that they are going to ignore, like I think Dr. Harris indicated that he did not read all the information on the food labeling. There is a lot of information there. Is it useful information? That is just a question I am proposing.

DR. FREEMAN: I understand. Dr. Rickert?

DR. RICKERT: I agree with what Dr. Guerin has said, in the sense that it would seem that if there are new products being developed that would have a zero yield of various carcinogens or ciliatoxic agents that must be allowed for, and I think for that, for the agent to appear on the package, there would have to be some consideration given to analytical detection limits and things of this nature. So, I do not think it should necessarily be a blanket piece of information that comes with every brand of cigarette, but there should be some differentiation based on the individual products of the cigarettes.

DR. FREEMAN: Yes, Dr. Henningfield?

DR. HENNINGFIELD: There always has to be a threshold for whether you list something, whether you are listing the lead in flour or rat droppings or whatever it is. So that is a basic concept, but I think the important thing is that an agency or panel with expertise, not the industry being regulated, make the decision. So if BHT is listed on flour or cookies, you know, we do not have to worry about how much of it is in there; I agree, that would be confusing, but another group decides if the cyanide should be listed as one of the "also contains" ingredients, for example, "also contains cyanide, formaldehyde, lead." You have somebody else decide what is of potential significance and therefore should be listed, and that is what is done with food labeling.

DR. FREEMAN: So, in principle what are you saying that we should do?

DR. HENNINGFIELD: Of course there is a threshold, but that threshold does not necessarily affect the labeling on the pack in the sense of the number because you are not putting any numbers in the same way that for potato chips you are not putting how much BHT is in there. You are listing the milligrams of things that groups decide are very important to list by milligrams like cholesterol and sodium, and then you have the list of other ingredients as Dr. Harris showed on his label, and what the thresholds are; to merit listing, another group decides that—a group with toxicology background.

DR. FREEMAN: Dr. Rickert?

DR. RICKERT: I am not really quite sure whether it is a toxicological consideration or whether it is a chemistry consideration. If you take cholesterol, for example, in order to earn a label of cholesterol-free, there has to be a certain level. I mean in the instrument you can measure this level, but it is cholesterol-free if it is less than that level. So, I think the issue, from my point of view anyway is more of a chemical issue, rather than a toxicological issue.

DR. FREEMAN: Dr. Shiffman?

DR. SHIFFMAN: I would like to come back to an issue that I think we discussed but perhaps had not gotten closure on, which is the consumer information or misinformation that is conveyed outside the formal label in the form of brand names like "light" and "ultralight," and I guess what I was hearing from several people was a proposal that the use of those terms be regulated in a manner parallel to the FDA's recent regulations of such labels on foods. That is my own view—that those labels ought to be allowed. They have the potential to provide a smoker with meaningful information, but they should be regulated so that they represent a particular number or range in the ratings and so that they have a common meaning across brands and across manufacturers. I would like to hear other people address that issue.

DR. FREEMAN: Dr. Hughes?

DR. HUGHES: I think that is a good comment, Dr. Shiffman. Where I keep seeing the break is at .5. The ones less than .5 are different from those above .5. So I would like to see the categories only be on those that are less than .5 mg of nicotine with the comparable tar.

DR. FREEMAN: I think the general question here is, should constituents other than tar, nicotine, and carbon monoxide be added to the protocol for testing? It sounds to me as though you have said that they should not be added for testing or, if testing is done, it should be done by either chemists or toxicologists but not in the same way as for the other three major substances. There is a question of whether certain substances should be listed in some way on the tobacco pack or in some other way, so the American public would know that there are harmful ingredients in tobacco other than the three elements.

Let us try to get closure on that particular point before we go on.

DR. GUERIN: I think that tar and nicotine and CO in terms of quantitative measurements are adequate. I have one question for Dr. Hoffmann. Of all of the constituents that might not necessarily correlate very well with tar, the N-nitrosamines stand out. Should we consider an N-nitrosamine measurement?

DR. HOFFMANN: When you find another HCN, benzo(*a*)pyrene, you will always get from our friends of the tobacco industry, "Yes, but this can come from air pollution." Carcinogens that derive from nicotine can come only from tobacco, and I think that should be cited. Benzo(*a*)pyrene comes from every combustion. Hydrogen cyanide comes from every combustion of a protein-containing component. Phenol comes from any combustion. The tobacco-specific nicotine-derived nitrosamines, which are strong carcinogens, come only from tobacco. I think the consumer should know that.

DR. GUERIN: To my knowledge that is the one class of chemicals that might be considered in addition, although it would be very difficult to do, relative to tar and nicotine and CO measurements.

DR. HOFFMANN: I personally do not think we confuse the smoker. I think we can let them know on the package that cigarette smoke contains toxic agents: hydrogen cyanide and known carcinogens, chloraminobiphenyls, benzo(*a*)pyrene, and the nicotine-derived nitrosamines. We should say that, though not quantitatively. Giving numbers is only confusing here.

DR. FREEMAN: Before we entertain other questions, I would like to have the committee's sense of whether you support what Dr. Hoffmann has just said, which seems to be a good summary of what we have said so far? Is there any disagreement with what Dr. Hoffmann has just said?

[NO RESPONSE]

Then we will take that as a consensus, and we will go on to consider it further in the latter part of the day.

You had another comment, Dr. Petitti?

DR. PETITTI: Just to emphasize that this information should not be quantitatively presented to the consumer because of the potential for misinformation.

DR. FREEMAN: My understanding relative to Question 2 is that there are certain elements that are proven to be harmful to human beings that are within tobacco that should be listed, though this panel is not recommending which specific compounds; that they should not be listed according to quantity; and that they should not undergo the same testing that we are recommending for tar, nicotine, and CO. I will take that as a consensus at this point.

If that is sufficient for that question, I would like to go on now to the third question that we have been asked to consider.

Question 3. Does the FTC protocol provide information useful to consumers in making decisions about their health?

Yes, Dr. Petitti?

DR. PETITTI: I think that in the context of the purpose of the FTC protocol, which is to provide information that allows consumers to choose cigarettes that reduce their risk of disease, the current FTC protocol is misleading in at least two important ways. First, it presents the consumer with a single number, thus implying that the consumer will receive exactly that exposure. Second, I think that the numbers when presented as numbers implicitly suggest that there is a ratio-scaled relationship between machine-measured yield and disease risk. I think that these numbers could be made more useful by remedying these misleading aspects of the current FTC protocol in ways that we have been discussing throughout the morning.

DR. FREEMAN: Specifically what do you recommend?

DR. PETITTI: First, present a range of numbers, thereby correcting the problem of a single number implying that the consumer will receive exactly that amount of exposure; and, second, provide some kind of graphic presentation of this information to the consumer in a way that takes away the numerical aspect of "9 is 9 times higher than 1 and 20 is 20 times higher than 1."

DR. FREEMAN: Dr. Rickert and then Dr. Hughes.

DR. RICKERT: I agree. I think the issue is, *can* the FTC protocol provide useful information rather than *does* it? In other words, are there ways that we can take this kind of information and convey it? One of the options that has been discussed and also appears in the literature is this idea of using the color of tar to communicate the range of variation that one can get in tar yields and, also, to allow individual smokers to gauge what they are receiving from the cigarette. I think a lot of us feel that if it were possible for low-yield smokers, that is those who are smoking the less-than-5-mg cigarettes, to achieve a low-yield smoke from that cigarette, there may be an accompanying health benefit to that achievement. At the present time, however, there is no means for the smoker to ascertain what the yield is. If there were some sort of graphic technique for them to visualize this process, then that may confer a health advantage to them.

DR. FREEMAN: Dr. Hughes?

DR. HUGHES: I have a question for Mr. Peeler. I was struck by the remark that talking about health benefits implies a health claim, which I understand the tobacco industry has not made with this product. Therefore my question to you is, can the FTC require such health education to come from the tobacco manufacturers when they have not made that health claim?

MR. PEELER: The numbers clearly communicate some health benefit to some portion of consumers. If we were able to determine that a significant number of consumers were being misled by that, we could require some corrective information or provide some corrective information. I think the concern has always been the one that we started out with in 1960, that as a result of that position, there basically were not any tar and nicotine numbers being made available to consumers.

In terms of our present status right now, our jurisdiction is simply to require that claims made in advertising be substantiated. Currently, there is not an FTC rule, an FTC case, or any legislation requiring the disclosure of tar and nicotine data either on labels or in advertising.

DR. HUGHES: If some surveys or several surveys showed that most consumers inferred a claim of health benefits from these cigarettes, would that be important information for the FTC to know when considering whether to force the tobacco companies to put in health information?

MR. PEELER: Consumer survey information is absolutely vital to everything the FTC does in the regulation of advertising and labeling. Therefore, the answer to the first question is yes. The next question is this point that we raised earlier: whether there would be the ability to compel disclosure of tar and nicotine information absent a health claim. You do get back to the tension between having no information out there at all and having just the accurate tar and nicotine.

DR. HUGHES: I think you are misunderstanding, because I am not talking about whether they report the numbers or not. Suppose there was a proposal that the FTC would require all cigarette advertisements that state anything about tar to have a statement that reads something like, "Switching to a low-tar cigarette is a very small health improvement compared to stopping smoking."

MR. PEELER: There is a legal analysis under the Commission's unfairness authority that could be used to require disclosure of that information, assuming the correct factual predicate could be established.

DR. HATSUKAMI: Regarding health benefits, it seems that based on Dr. Cohen's presentation there are significant numbers of people who believe that there are benefits to switching to a lower tar and nicotine cigarette, and yet some of the data do not show this relationship between tar yield and health benefits, with the exception possibly of lung cancer. Therefore, I agree with Dr. Hughes in requiring some kind of label on the package explaining that switching to a low-tar and -nicotine cigarette may or may not provide health benefits, thereby hopefully correcting an apparent misconception.

DR. FREEMAN: Dr. Benowitz?

DR. BENOWITZ: I would just like to emphasize that such language has to be stated very carefully; I believe for an individual there is very little benefit to switching. For the society of all smokers there may be benefit, and I would not want to lose that benefit. We have to walk that line of warning individuals that this is not going to help you very much, but still encourage the whole society of smokers to reduce their tar and nicotine intake. We need to find language that will serve both purposes.

DR. FREEMAN: Dr. Kozlowski?

DR. KOZLOWSKI: I would like to encourage the panel to note in the report that there is a fundamental deficiency in that the current procedures are linked to cigarette advertising. A number of presenters mentioned that currently one-third of cigarette brands are generics. There is no requirement that a cigarette brand be advertised. There is no law that says that you must advertise a cigarette, and, if it is not advertised, there is no option for any kind of brand-yield information or any kind of FTC method. I think one might see the linking of consumer information solely to advertising as a loophole in the system. I would encourage the panel to ask the FTC to try to provide some estimate of what percentage of brands are not advertised at all.

DR. FREEMAN: Mr. Peeler, can you address that question?

MR. PEELER: As I said earlier, we do not have that information today. We could certainly get that for the panel, if the panel would like it.

DR. FREEMAN: Are there a significant number of brands that are out in the market but are not being advertised?

MR. PEELER: There has been a very large increase in the number of brands that we have been reporting because of the increased number of generic brands, which are frequently not advertised.

DR. FREEMAN: And is it true that the FTC does not require that those brands undergo the same analysis?

MR. PEELER: Again, we have to go back to the beginning. The disclosure of tar and nicotine is provided for under the FTC's general authority to regulate advertising and to require substantiation of claims in advertising. At one point there was an FTC proposal to require the disclosure of tar and nicotine content in all cigarette advertising. Cigarette labeling is largely regulated by separate Federal statute called the Federal Cigarette Labeling Act. The rulemaking was suspended when the cigarette industry voluntarily agreed to put this information in all their cigarette advertising. So that is the current status of disclosure. Many companies do put that information on their packs, particularly with respect to their lower yield cigarettes. I do not have an estimate of how many packs that is.

DR. FREEMAN: Then it is conceivable that there could be cigarettes sold that do not have this labeling?

MR. PEELER: I believe it is likely that there are many cigarettes, particularly generics, that do not have these labels.

DR. FREEMAN: I think that is a very significant point. If the FTC does not regulate that, who does?

MR. PEELER: The content of the cigarette label is largely regulated by the Federal Cigarette Labeling Act, which is a Federal statute that requires a certain number of disclosures, for example, the Surgeon General's disclosure, and then basically says that, for other statements relating to smoking and health, only Congress can impose those additional statements.

DR. FREEMAN: Thank you. Dr. Hughes?

DR. HUGHES: I think we have a model with the recent food pyramid. That labeling change was accompanied by a massive educational campaign, and I do not know who did that, but it seems to me that we need a similar effort with tar and nicotine. I want my patients to know about nicotine yield much more than I want them to know about riboflavin and cholesterol and that sort of thing. My question is, why have we not had the same public education campaign around nicotine yield, spending at least as much money as we did on the food pyramid?

DR. KOZLOWSKI: To respond to that, there is a question of in whose jurisdiction does that campaign fall. I think it is not within the FTC brief in any explicit sense to do an extensive education campaign on it, and you have just heard that cigarette labeling falls under quite a different procedure.

DR. FREEMAN: Dr. Townsend?

DR. TOWNSEND: In response to Dr. Kozlowski's concern and your obvious concern about generics or unadvertised cigarettes being out there in the marketplace without any information, that really is not true. While the specific numbers are not advertised, the generic products are broken into categories of tar deliveries, the same as other brands. For example, you can find a generic sold as regular, lights or ultralights. There is information out there, even if there is no advertising that carries with it specific absolute FTC tar numbers.

DR. FREEMAN: Would you clarify this point because I am a little confused. What would be the difference on the labeling of the generic product vs. the one that is advertised?

DR. TOWNSEND: Let me take one example with the generic cigarette brand Doral. The packages are in different colors, the same as other brands, with dark green for the regular, light green for the lights, and a real light green or a white for the ultralights; and their tar category is stated on the package. That is a comparative measure of the FTC tar yield for those cigarettes even though there is no advertising that carries the FTC number with it.

DR. FREEMAN: That is how they are similar. How do they differ?

DR. TOWNSEND: What I am saying is that there is a distinction in the marketplace by virtue of what is written on the pack, that it is a light or an ultralight or a regular.

DR. FREEMAN: I understand.

DR. TOWNSEND: And by the color of the pack.

DR. FREEMAN: But other than that, the numbers are not there?

DR. TOWNSEND: Because many of these products are not advertised, the numbers in some cases are not available to consumers.

DR. FREEMAN: You have clarified my point. Dr. Benowitz?

DR. BENOWITZ: One of the central recommendations of this panel should be that cigarette labeling include these warnings. The other issue that concerns all of us is consumer information, and even though it is not a direct charge, I think we should make a strong recommendation that there be labeling about yields and the other issues we have been talking about.

DR. FREEMAN: Are you speaking also on the generic cigarettes?

DR. BENOWITZ: Yes, on all cigarettes.

DR. FREEMAN: That is your recommendation?

DR. BENOWITZ: Yes, because the FTC can regulate advertising, but what we are really talking about is labeling on the cigarette packs. If there is no vehicle for doing that now, I think we should recommend there be one.

DR. FREEMAN: Yes, Dr. Rickert?

DR. RICKERT: I would certainly support what Dr. Benowitz is saying, particularly given the amount of confusion that sometimes arises over the use of the terms "light," "ultralight," and so on. Unless these terms have been defined with some specific tar range associated with them, the use of the terms without that tar information is certainly open to the potential for misleading consumers.

DR. FREEMAN: Dr. Woosley?

DR. WOOSLEY: I agree with both of those statements wholeheartedly, but I am concerned by the reality of labeling being proscribed by legislation so that it is not to be touched by anyone but Congress. If I am interpreting that correctly, that is a terrible situation to be in. Let me just go on to say that I believe the use of the terms "light" and "ultralight" in advertising are perceived as a claim. I think there needs to be a very strong message from this committee that those are perceived claims, and they carry with it the impression of improved health, and I think that is a form of advertising.

DR. FREEMAN: Dr. Townsend, can you give the committee any sense of what percentage of cigarettes sold in America are in the generic category as opposed to the advertised category?

DR. TOWNSEND: No, I really cannot. There are some generic products or low-cost products that are advertised; most, however, are not. I cannot give you an exact percentage right now.

DR. FREEMAN: Thank you. Dr. Cohen?

DR. COHEN: Dr. Townsend, are you asserting that for cigarettes the color of the package is intended to convey the tar level of the cigarette?

DR. TOWNSEND: In practice, if you look at products that are in the market currently, in addition to having the category defined as regular, lights, or ultralights on the pack and in the advertising, in many cases the packs are different colors. If you look within one brand family, particular brands within that brand family that are in the different tar categories do have different pack colors.

DR. COHEN: Is there an intention on the part of cigarette manufacturers to convey information about tar yields by using color on packages, as well as terms such as "light" and other descriptive adjectives?

DR. TOWNSEND: There is an intention, in my opinion, by the cigarette industry in general to convey tar information to the consumer so that they can make choices. In some brands the different colors are intended to convey the different tar category in which they fall, and that category is stated explicitly in the advertising.

DR. FREEMAN: I have been informed by staff that approximately 40 percent of cigarettes sold in America are of the generic category. If that is true, then I think this is a major issue to be considered here.

DR. KOZLOWSKI: It appears that Dr. Townsend is indicating that the designations light and ultralight are in a sense being used as surrogates in a broad sense for tar and nicotine ratings and that they are carrying tar and nicotine rating information. My question is, are there industry standards or R.J. Reynolds standards for what numbers are required before a cigarette is called light or ultralight or is there variance across the industry and in what products get the label "light"?

DR. TOWNSEND: It is my understanding that the definition, of course, has changed a little bit over the years, but today the definition is really quite consistent. Cigarettes under 6 mg constitute ultralights, those from 6 to 15 are lights, and above 15 are regulars.

DR. FREEMAN: Dr. Henningfield?

DR. HENNINGFIELD: I have a recommendation and a question for Mr. Peeler. The recommendation is that, on discovering that FTC does not have the means to put on the labeling this information that we are saying is so important, I recommend that the FTC use all means at its disposal to get this information and make it readily available to consumers. My question for Mr. Peeler is, what kinds of things can you do? For example, could you put your tar report information at all points of sale, or do people just have to write for the catalog?

MR. PEELER: Let me clarify about the labeling. The place where we are preempted on cigarette labeling and where everyone is preempted on cigarette labeling is on statements relating to smoking and health, and there is a question about exactly where that is. I would think if there were a misrepresentation, for example, on a label of the tar content, and that is all that there was, that would be something on which the FTC could take action. The question of exactly how much information the FTC can affirmatively require to be disclosed absent a representation by the company is a whole other issue that we would have to look at in light of the panel's recommendations. For example, in the 1970's when the FTC required that health warnings start appearing in advertising, these requirements were based on allegations that the advertising at that point was making representations about the cigarette's healthfulness. The FTC's actions resulted in settlements between the FTC and a number of companies that provided for the health warnings in advertising, which ultimately became required by statute in 1984.

The FTC does not have the FDA-type of regulatory power over the cigarette industry. We have the power to prevent deceptive statements, and we have the power to require the disclosure of certain types of information when a failure to disclose that information would be unfair.

DR. HENNINGFIELD: Can you only regulate what appears in a magazine ad? How do we get it to the consumers who do not read the magazine ads or for the cigarettes that are not advertised?

MR. PEELER: If you are talking about information about the relationship of cigarettes to health, then the advertising and the labeling right now contain warnings, and our authority to require additional warnings or descriptions would be triggered by what representations are made.

DR. HENNINGFIELD: So you could not require that a label like the one Dr. Harris showed be put on cigarette packages?

MR. PEELER: Again, what we are here for is to hear the committee's recommendations and take those back to the five commissioners who run the agency. I think what you ought to be doing is making those recommendations that you think are right, and then it will be up to the five commissioners to sort through them in terms of what is within the FTC's authority and what is not within the FTC's authority. Clearly the focus of our concern and the reason that we are here is there has been a lot of concern that the current tar and nicotine labeling system is not serving its intended purpose, and because we are putting those numbers out every year, that is going to be the first thing that we focus on.

DR. FREEMAN: Yes, you have a comment?

MS. WILKENFELD: In the seventies and early eighties when the Commission published its number, the Office on Smoking and Health made a large chart that was available at point of purchase in pharmacies and other places where cigarettes were sold so that there was educational information at the point of sale. Whether you call that labeling or the Commission would call it advertising, I do not know. But the money ran out and that stopped.

DR. FREEMAN: I would like to just express a personal concern here. I think all of us here should be concerned with the effect of a lethal product on the American public with respect to morbidity and mortality. On the other hand, this meeting has been called by the FTC along with the Congress. My concern is that our human concerns do not become engulfed in bureaucratic problems. The 40 percent of people in America who are smoking cigarettes that you do not oversee still are smoking cigarettes and still have the same lethality for those 40 percent. I hope that although we are governed by the bureaucracy in a certain way, and you have limits, and we certainly respect that—we do have a Congress that can rule one way or another. I think we should speak to the general problem while we are giving you direction.

MR. PEELER: I would certainly agree with that.

DR. FREEMAN: Thank you. Dr. Cohen?

DR. COHEN: Consumers want information that they can use to make meaningful decisions. Assume the consumer wants to make the meaningful decision as to whether switching to a particular kind of cigarette, say a 1- to 5-mg tar cigarette, would lead to a significant reduction in health risks. Can this panel, given the state of the art, attempt to provide information that would be helpful to the consumer as to the relative risk of smoking different kinds of cigarettes? If the answer is no, then it is no, but I think that is more important information than the information currently available through tar numbers because tar numbers do not tell consumers information that is meaningful.

DR. FREEMAN: Dr. Benowitz?

DR. BENOWITZ: If you tell people that if they take in less tar, there is a small benefit, it is not one that should be denied, but I think it is misleading. I do not think we can tell people that *you* are going to reduce *your* hazard; *you* are going to live longer if *you* shift to low-yield cigarettes. So, we are caught in a bind. We want to encourage people to minimize the risk, but we cannot really tell them it is going to make a huge difference.

DR. COHEN: I think frankly that this is a subject that ought to command the attention of the panel because consumers, like it or not, are using these numbers as if they had absolute significance as numbers. The numbers mean almost nothing. The panel has to address the question of is there a way of informing consumers as to the relative risk, and perhaps the answer is to let us inform them that there is not a lot of gain; doing that, frankly, would be very useful and maybe more useful than telling them exactly what the tar differences are.

DR. FREEMAN: Dr. Rickert?

DR. RICKERT: I think the committee has thought about that to a large extent, and I think there is a consensus that what is really needed is a rather large public health education campaign to try to communicate that very information to consumers.

You are also asking for information about risk, and generally this comes from epidemiological studies, which by their very nature are extremely long and do not provide information that we can use immediately. The information that we have today has been gleaned over a number of years with respect to relative risk, and as we have seen, there is not much change.

Now, if one is going to ask what is the effect with today's cigarettes, then we are talking about a period of time that will be measured in tens of years.

Unfortunately, we have to come to grips with the problem today, and we cannot wait for tens of years to pass to obtain accurate information about today's cigarettes.

DR. FREEMAN: Dr. Hughes?

DR. HUGHES: I would like to respond very concretely to what you said, Dr. Cohen, and it is my opinion that if there is not information that you suggest about the health benefits of switching, the whole system should be junked. My concern is that we are going to say, "Yes, there should be this big public health campaign," and nothing will happen. NCI says, "We don't have money for it." FTC says, "We don't have the bureaucracy to do it." The FDA says, "We have other more important things to do," and this whole education campaign does not get done. We come up with a range of values that still has numbers on them, and people still think that they are doing themselves a big benefit, and I would rather junk the entire system than to have that happen.

The only way around it I can see is that the FTC decides that all claims of light and ultralight imply a health claim and therefore require a disclaimer. That is the only way out of it I can see, to make sure that that happens.

DR. FREEMAN: What form of disclaimer?

DR. HUGHES: I do not want to micromanage with the wording. Whether we say, "You may get a small benefit" or "You will get very little benefit compared to stopping smoking," is a tough question, and I do not think we need to decide on that wording. My point, again, is to reiterate what Dr. Cohen said, which is that the system is bankrupt unless there is some statement about the magnitude of health benefit that you will receive by switching to a low-tar and -nicotine cigarette.

DR. FREEMAN: Dr. Stitzer?

DR. STITZER: I want to return to a point I made earlier. It seems to me that we would be doing a great service if we could implement a new testing technique that involved ranges that could display and convince smokers that light cigarettes are the same or can be exactly the same as a regular cigarette. I think the data show us that all the cigarettes from .4 mg up can look exactly the same. They basically are occupying the same place in space. The range of variability is the same, and that there is no health benefit for switching to light cigarettes because of this dose variation, but there are also some data suggesting that the ultralight cigarettes, those .1 mg and below, do produce a different level of exposure.

Now, those cigarettes are not popular. They capture a very, very tiny segment of the market, but they may make a difference. We do not have the health data, but if there is a dose effect for health, those are the only cigarettes that are going to make a difference, and it seems to me that a new labeling system could potentially convey that kind of information.

DR. FREEMAN: To play devil's advocate, there seems to be a point on the other side that, if the American public becomes confused about the value of low dose vs. high dose, would it defeat the purpose of encouraging people to switch, assuming there is a benefit to low-dose cigarettes? I think I am hearing those two arguments. Yes, Dr. Giovino?

DR. GIOVINO: I think part of any disclaimer that would be given if you decided to do that would include the statement that I read earlier from the Surgeon General's report that any cigarette smoking is dangerous, that quitting is absolutely the best thing a person could do to protect his or her health, and that reducing to these brands "may." And that is exactly what the Surgeon General's report says, "May pose reduced risk, provided that no compensation occurs." I think those two caveats are absolutely essential, that quitting is better than switching and that provided no compensation there may be reduced risk.

DR. FREEMAN: Dr. Benowitz?

DR. BENOWITZ: I think there is a second function that the FTC testing does perform, and that is to mold what the tobacco companies provide. I do think that there has been a reduction in lung cancer if you compare 1950's cigarettes to modern cigarettes, and I would not want to lose that pressure to keep yields as low as possible. I think whatever we do, we do not want to lose that by saying that it does not matter at all. The other argument is if there is a 10-percent reduction of health hazard—which would be very difficult to measure by epidemiological means—if you are applying it to about 40 million smokers, that can be substantial. And I would not want to lose that for the population either.

I do not want to be misleading. I certainly appreciate Dr. Hughes' point of view, but I think we somehow should not let things slide the other way.

DR. FREEMAN: Is there any way that you can bring the two points of view together? I think this is a very important point. We need to settle it here.

DR. STITZER: There is just one other thing. The only way that this information can be relevant to the individual consumer is if there is a way for that individual to judge where he or she falls along the dose continuum. Now, that could be accomplished with a lovely sophisticated method like Dr. Rickert has described with the color coding. I do not know whether that technology is sufficiently available to incorporate into our recommendations, but it could be part of our recommendation that we try to develop a system that allows the individual smoker to know where they fall on the exposure and dose continuum.

DR. FREEMAN: Yes, Dr. Hughes?

DR. HUGHES: I disagree a little bit with you, Dr. Stitzer. Even if people could tell exactly where they were on the dose continuum, that does not solve the problem of the dose response-health benefits curve being so shallow. Also, I want to respond to your comment. I am not saying that there is no benefit, and I do not think we should say that there is no benefit because I agree the public health argument is there. But the physician in me says, "Always oversell your case," because people do not change very much. Again, I do not care what kind of disclaimer or how it is worded, but there has to be, again, something about health benefits to the consumer in all of this.

DR. FREEMAN: Dr. Shiffman?

DR. SHIFFMAN: I think the two issues we have struggled with most recently are related. While the system as now constituted has its focus on advertising and on showing a single number for an FTC measure of tar and nicotine values, in fact there are implicit claims being made both in advertising proper and in brand names, which are a form of advertising that imply a health claim. Therefore, it seems to me we ought very strongly to recommend both that the use of those terms, like "light" and "ultralight," be regulated and that when they are used, they be accompanied in fair balance by a disclosure of the sort that Dr. Hughes has suggested.

I think there is a middle ground that allows us to proceed based on what we know and based, I think, on regulatory authority that already exists.

DR. FREEMAN: Yes, Dr. Zacny?

DR. ZACNY: Based on Dr. Rickert's point about state-of-the-art epidemiological studies not being done at this time where you can say with any degree of certainty what the relationship is between nicotine dose and risk of disease with the brand of cigarettes we are dealing with now—the low-yield cigarettes and the ultralow-yield cigarettes—I disagree slightly with Dr. Hughes when he says that the relationship may be very shallow. As scientists, in any claims we make we can just say that we do not know at this time what the relationship is because it takes 10 or 20 years, but based on what we know, it would be best not to block vent holes, to take smaller puffs, etc.

DR. FREEMAN: That would be an educational campaign?

DR. ZACNY: Yes. Maybe I am wrong, but it seems that there may be a dose-response relationship between risk of lung cancer and how much smoke people take into their system, and they may realize a substantial benefit with the ultralow-yield cigarette. I do not think we know with certainty, and in the absence of that, I think the formulations that we are putting forth with bands and ranges are a good idea.

DR. FREEMAN: Dr. Kozlowski?

DR. KOZLOWSKI: I would like to draw an analogy to the FDA nutritional labeling. For a lot of the items on those labels, there is not persuasive epidemiological research to show the dose-response curves for a lot of the things that are listed as of interest. I think we do not want to be held to a higher standard. Epidemiology takes time. It has its limitations, and the basic point is there is a lot of labeling that pertains to risks that are only approximately known.

DR. FREEMAN: Dr. Benowitz?

DR. BENOWITZ: To follow up on Dr. Zacny's comments, what we really would like to know is not brands vs. risk; we would like to know actual exposure level. If we were able to measure cotinine or adducts of different compounds or whatever in smokers vs. their yields, then we would have the basis for recommending that individuals should reduce their exposure. Since there is such an overlap with the yields as marketed now, I do not think we are ever going to see a difference by yield—that does not mean that the rationale for an individual reducing their intake is not valid, and so at this point in time we may have to go forward based on scientific rationale and plausibility for reducing exposure to toxic materials.

DR. FREEMAN: Dr. Hoffmann?

DR. HOFFMANN: I think there is a misunderstanding. It has been shown in *dozens* of studies that there is a dose response with respect to cancer of the lungs and the upper respiratory tract by number of cigarettes smoked per day, length of time smoking, and groups of cigarettes. This continues for ultralow, low, and average cigarettes. There is a dose response with respect to cancer but not with respect to coronary artery disease. Any cigarette is harmful. But ultralow cigarettes have a lower risk than nonfiltered regular cigarettes when you smoke them for 10 or more years. We should not say that there is no dose response.

DR. FREEMAN: Dr. Hoffmann, just to follow up on what you said, as far as the science is concerned, you indicated that in there is no apparent dose response for coronary heart disease?

DR. HOFFMANN: We do not know from the literature any benefit with respect to coronary heart disease.

DR. STITZER: Dr. Benowitz can speak to this. Is there a dose effect based on light vs. heavy smoking for coronary disease?

DR. BENOWITZ: No, there is not. I would like to add that I agree with Dr. Hoffmann that this dose response would provide a rationale for what we are doing here today. There are data in pregnancy showing the dose response between cotinine level and the weight reduction of the newborn, and therefore that is another rationale for another disease that there is a dose-response relationship, and therefore, even though we cannot say that a particular brand is going to be less hazardous than some other brand, we can say that lowering your exposure in general will be beneficial, and then we just have to help people to do that.

DR. FREEMAN: Didn't Dr. Samet state yesterday that there is no evidence that coronary heart disease is reduced by lowering the nicotine or tar content in cigarettes?

DR. BENOWITZ: He said that there was no evidence.

DR. HOFFMANN: That may be the case, but that we have no evidence.

DR. FREEMAN: I think we should respect those data because I think more than 100,000 people die each year from cardiac death due to smoking. I do not know the exact numbers, and that is a very significant point to argue that even smoking low-nicotine, low-tar cigarettes will not protect you as far as we know from dying from coronary heart disease. Is that a fair statement, Dr. Hoffmann?

DR. HOFFMANN: No, I think we do not know.

DR. FREEMAN: Let me narrow down the point. Are you saying that there is no distinction between the low-tar and -nicotine smokers and the high with respect to death from coronary disease?

DR. HOFFMANN: There is no evidence.

DR. FREEMAN: No evidence that there is a difference?

DR. HOFFMANN: No evidence that I am aware of. We discussed it last night, and nobody came up with any, but there may be. I am not aware of it.

DR. PETITTI: Since we are relying so heavily on the 1981 Surgeon General's report, and very few data have come out since then, I would like to read the statement specifically about cardiovascular disease:

> The overall changes in the composition of cigarettes that
> occurred during the last 10 or 15 years have not produced
> a clearly demonstrated effect on cardiovascular disease, and
> some studies suggest that a decreased risk of CHD may not have
> occurred. Evidence on the association between CHD and filter
> cigarettes is somewhat conflicting. One major study showed a
> reduction of 10 to 20 percent of coronary deaths among persons
> smoking lower tar and nicotine cigarettes as compared with
> those smoking higher yield cigarettes.

That was the CPS-I study, but other surveys have shown a slightly increased risk of coronary mortality in people who smoke filter cigarettes or those who smoke nonfilter cigarettes. Recent unpublished data from the Framingham study that were ultimately published do not show a lower CHD risk among smokers of filter cigarettes. It is not that there are no data. The data that exist show no association of smoking lower yield cigarettes with reduction in coronary heart disease morbidity and mortality.

DR. FREEMAN: I think that is a very, very important point that ought to be factored into this discussion. Dr. Cohen?

DR. COHEN: I was very pleased, Dr. Hoffmann, to hear you clarify an issue for me. I heard you say that we can inform people about lung cancer, at least. Now, lung cancer is a major issue for people, and what I am wondering is, since people use tar as a surrogate for relative harmfulness, might it make some sense to restrict their usage of tar by maybe getting rid of tar and talking about cancer-causing compounds or some other component and let these numbers communicate meaningful information about something we do know something about, rather than where we do not know anything about it that is conclusive? Would it be possible, in other words, to indicate people's relative risk with respect to lung cancer for smoking these different yield cigarettes?

DR. HOFFMANN: As I see it, the public associates tar with cancer.

DR. COHEN: I think they do it more broadly and associate it with overall safety.

DR. HOFFMANN: They are not well informed. The American Cancer Society did a fantastic job, publishing this over and over again, and the public is well informed with respect to smoking and lung cancer. There has not been the same level of information communicated about coronary risk.

DR. COHEN: In your view though, is it possible to relate the differences in tar yield in cigarettes to a reduction in cancer risk? If the answer is yes, it seems to me that one of the things the panel might consider doing is trying to convey that or recommending that be conveyed.

DR. FREEMAN: Dr. Rickert?

DR. RICKERT: I would be somewhat reluctant to do that for several reasons. First of all, the information with respect to lung cancer and risk reduction is from the 1981 Surgeon General's report that relates to cigarettes that were consumed 10 to 20 years prior to that date. My other concern is in terms of "tar is tar is tar," that is, is the quality of the tar from today's ultralow-yield cigarette the same as the quality or the carcinogenic potential of tar from a cigarette from many years ago? I do not think we know that the tar of today's cigarette is the same as the tar of the cigarette many years ago that was being related to lung cancer.

DR. HOFFMANN: With respect to your first point, Dr. Rickert, there was an International Agency for Research on Cancer monograph in 1986 that presented 15 studies that all show between a 13- and 30-percent reduction. There are also reports from the World Health Organization, and there is the European study by the National Cancer Institute. It did not end with 1981.

DR. RICKERT: I am not uncomfortable with the idea that there is a risk reduction. What I am suggesting is that we really do not have enough information about the tar characteristics of today's cigarettes to directly compare them.

DR. HOFFMANN: You can do only risk biomarkers. Otherwise you cannot do it.

DR. RICKERT: I agree.

DR. FREEMAN: Yes, Dr. Hoffmann.

DR. HOFFMANN: I believe that we should do better education. I do not think that including whether it is plus or minus 3 mg or 5 mg helps the public. The public has to be much better informed.

DR. FREEMAN: It appears from what I have heard here on the question of does the FTC protocol provide information useful to consumers in making decisions about their health, that the answer seems to be not sufficiently so, and we have had an interesting discussion and debate here this morning concerning various aspects of that decision.

Things that stand out in my mind are what do the numbers mean to the public? Dr. Cohen has been eloquent in raising that issue. What is the value of projecting a range per type of cigarette to the public? What is the value of any kind of color coding to the public? What would be the value of presenting a graph to the public so a person could see by graph form what the differences in cigarettes are? We also have heard this morning, unknown to me before, that approximately 40 percent of cigarettes are not looked at by the Federal Trade Commission because they are not advertised.

MR. PEELER: They are looked at, and they are tested. The results are reported, but unless the manufacturer either voluntarily puts that information on the label or unless they advertise, those numbers aren't necessarily communicated directly to consumers.

DR. FREEMAN: Thank you for that correction. The bottom line is the public does not know those numbers.

Recommendations and Findings

DR. FREEMAN: Good afternoon, I am Dr. Harold Freeman. I am the chairman of the President's Cancer Panel. At the request of the Congress and the Federal Trade Commission, an ad hoc committee of the President's Cancer Panel has met over the last 2 days to consider the Federal Trade Commission test method for determining tar, nicotine, and carbon monoxide levels in cigarettes. Before I get into our statement, I would like to put the problem of tobacco into perspective. Tobacco use is the number one cause of preventable death in America. Cigarette smoking is responsible for more than 400,000 premature deaths every year in this country and causes one-third of cancer deaths and one-third of heart disease deaths.

Although smoking is declining among adults in the United States, it is discouraging that smoking is not declining among children, and in fact, smoking prevalence among adolescents has changed little for more than a decade.

I have with me Dr. Saul Shiffman of the Department of Psychology, University of Pittsburgh; Dr. Diana Petitti, director of the Division of Research and Evaluation, Kaiser Permanente; and Dr. William Rickert of Labstat, Inc.

This committee reviewed articles, studies, and other documents and heard presentations from a variety of experts, including tobacco industry scientists, on the subject of the FTC test method for determining tar, nicotine, and carbon monoxide levels in U.S. cigarettes. We have deliberated with the goals of answering questions and making recommendations. Our deliberations centered around the following three summary questions:

1. **Does the evidence presented clearly demonstrate that changes are needed in the current FTC protocol for measuring tar, nicotine, and carbon monoxide? If yes, what changes are required?**

2. **Should constituents other than tar, nicotine, and carbon monoxide be added to the protocol?**

3. **Does the FTC protocol provide information useful to smokers in making decisions about their health?**

I. The committee reached the following conclusions with respect to the first question.

   A. The smoking of cigarettes with lower *machine-measured* yields has a small effect in reducing the risk of cancer caused by smoking, no effect on the risk of cardiovascular diseases, and an uncertain effect on the risk of pulmonary disease. A reduction in *machine-measured* tar yield from 15 mg tar to 1 mg tar does not reduce relative risk from 15 to 1.

B. The FTC test protocol was based on cursory observations of human smoking behavior. Actual human smoking behavior is characterized by wide variations in smoking patterns, which result in wide variations in tar and nicotine exposure. Smokers who switch to lower tar and nicotine cigarettes frequently change their smoking behavior, which may negate potential health benefits.

C. Accordingly, the committee recommends the following changes to the FTC protocol:

1. This system should also measure and publish information on the range of tar, nicotine, and carbon monoxide yields that most smokers should expect from each cigarette sold in the United States.

2. This information should be clearly communicated to smokers.

3. A simple graphic representation should be provided with each pack of cigarettes sold in the United States and in all advertisements. The representation should not imply a one-to-one relationship between measurements and disease risk.

4. The system must be accompanied by public education to make smokers aware that individual exposure depends on how the cigarette is smoked and that the benefits of switching to lower yield cigarettes are small compared with quitting.

D. There should be Federal oversight of cigarette testing, but such testing should continue to be performed by the tobacco industry and at industry expense.

E. The questions involved in the purpose, methodology, and utility of the FTC protocol are complex medical and scientific issues that require the ongoing involvement of Federal health agencies, including the National Institutes of Health, Food and Drug Administration, and Centers for Disease Control and Prevention.

F. The system should be reexamined at least every 5 years to evaluate whether the protocol is maintaining its utility to the smoker.

G. When a cigarette manufacturer makes significant changes in cigarette design that affect yields, it should notify the appropriate Federal agency.

II. With regard to the second question, the committee recommends that to avoid confusing smokers, no smoke constituents other than tar, nicotine, and carbon monoxide be measured and published at the present time. Smokers should be informed of the presence of other hazardous smoke constituents with each package and with all advertisements. These constituents should be classified by toxic effects.

III. In considering the third question, the committee reached the following conclusions:

A. Information from the testing system is useless to smokers unless they have ready access to it. The information from the testing system should be made available to all smokers, including those who smoke generic brands and other brands not widely advertised.

B. Brand names and brand classifications such as "light" and "ultralight" represent health claims and should be regulated and accompanied, in fair balance, with an appropriate disclaimer.

C. The available data suggest that smokers misunderstand the FTC test data. This underscores the need for an extensive public education effort.

I would like to underscore two major points: First, the health benefits of switching to low-tar and -nicotine cigarettes are minimal compared to quitting entirely, and finally, in effect, how you smoke is much more important than what you smoke.

We have deliberated for 2 days. We believe these findings are very important to the health of the American public. We are dealing with a product that is lethal, that needs to be controlled, and we believe that these recommendations will lead to some control. I would open it up for questions to my colleagues or to myself.

PARTICIPANT: Dr. Freeman, what do you expect to be the next step in the educational process for consumers?

DR. FREEMAN: The findings from the deliberations of this committee will be reported to the Director of the National Cancer Institute, who will then formulate a report that will be passed on with the help of the President's Cancer Panel to the appropriate agencies and the Congress.

PARTICIPANT: That is a lot of reporting. Can you predict what might happen next?

DR. FREEMAN: I do not think we can predict what is going to happen in the future, but our hope is that since the FTC methodology has been in effect from 1967 and was based on findings that relate to 1936, and since in the last 25 years there has been a considerable change in our knowledge through research, as well as in the type of cigarettes that are being smoked, we now believe that these changes are very essential and should be put into effect very soon.

No one can predict because we are dealing with the FTC, possibly other agencies of the Government, and the Congress, and no one on this committee can predict how rapidly these changes may take place, but we believe they are very important.

PARTICIPANT: Are you saying that you are recommending keeping the current FTC testing method and expanding it in some way or are you talking about a whole new testing system?

DR. FREEMAN: Let me reemphasize that we are recommending the keeping of the basic parts of the FTC testing methodology with the exception that we want to expand testing to show the ranges of possible effects of the three substances that are being measured. The reason that we believe this is important is that the research has shown that people who smoke cigarettes that, for example, are labeled as having low tar can get a much higher dose from that cigarette than the label may indicate. For example, if you have a low-yield cigarette, the way you smoke it, the rapidity of the puffing, the depth of the puffing, whether you block the ventilation holes, etc., can have an extraordinary effect on the real dose to the patient. Disease, we believe, is related to the dose of carcinogens and other toxins.

PARTICIPANT: The impetus for this effort came from Congressman Waxman, a Democrat in the Congress. Now the Congress is primarily Republican. What effect do you think this is going to have on your recommendations?

DR. FREEMAN: It is conceivable that people in power who have philosophies that are different from Congressman Waxman's could present barriers to our recommendations. We are hopeful though that even with these changes that the logic of what we are saying will make sense even to people who may disagree with what we are recommending in principle. There are people, for example, who may wish to diminish the fight against tobacco, and I am sure you are referring to them. I am hopeful that even such people will listen to the logic of reporting to the American public the truth of a finding that is responsible for 400,000 deaths a year and give the public the chance of making an intelligent decision. We are not saying, "Eliminate cigarettes." We are not saying, "Stop using the methodology that has been present for 25 years." We are saying, "Give an honest report to the American public and show them the range of the risk that they are subjected to." I hope that everybody, Democrat, Republican, conservative, or liberal, will follow that logic.

PARTICIPANT: You are suggesting, in addition, putting the CO on cigarettes and also putting other ingredients?

DR. FREEMAN: One of the recommendations that I read to you indicates that we believe that in addition to putting the ranges of the tar, nicotine, and carbon monoxide that are now being measured with one number, we want to change that to a range because that is a more truthful statement. This committee is also recommending that certain key harmful substances known to be in cigarettes (we are not saying which ones should be listed) should be given as information to everyone who buys a package of cigarettes. We believe that if this is done in food, which does not apparently have the toxic effect of tobacco, then we believe it should be done in this lethal product.

PARTICIPANT: Could you explain the graphics that you would put on the package?

DR. FREEMAN: I am going to refer this question to Dr. Rickert.

DR. RICKERT: There are a number of different ways of looking at that particular problem. The graphics could involve a number of different issues; for example, it could involve a color representation of the cigarette filter. It could represent some icon that illustrates putting all of this information together. A number of different possibilities were discussed, and I do not think that the committee recommended any specific procedure. I think the feeling was that there should be some way of communicating the information to smokers without total reliance on numbers themselves.

PARTICIPANT: What would be the purpose? I do not understand the purpose of the graphics overall.

DR. RICKERT: The graphics would make several points. First of all, the point that yields to smokers depend on how the cigarette is used; that is, if you have a graphic, it gets away from the idea that there is a fixed amount of whatever the constituent happens to be. The purpose of the graphic is to illustrate the variable nature of the smoking characteristics.

DR. SHIFFMAN: If I may add, we thought it was very important to communicate to American smokers that what you get depends on how you smoke and that any system that simply gives one number is, therefore, inherently misleading. So, we envisioned a graph that would show you a band within which your particular exposure might lie and that will give smokers information on which they can make more accurate, more reasonable comparisons among brands. We think they will find that there is a good deal of overlap among brands that they now consider to be different.

PARTICIPANT: You said "light" and "ultralight." Some people say that those words represent health claims. Could you explain a little bit more about that? How does that represent a health claim, and what kind of disclaimer would be used?

DR. FREEMAN: It is the committee's belief that the public infers health claim meanings from these labels, whether they be light, ultralight or whether they be the numbers in tar and nicotine. It is anecdotal, and also studied, that people look at these numbers and these claims and translate them into what it means for their own destiny. The information gathered at this meeting indicates that smokers should not be making these predictions, first of all, and second, if the labeling by the cigarette industry of ultralight implies that you are better off according to health, if that is so, and we believe that this is so, then that represents a health claim on the part of the advertiser. If it is a health claim, it should be followed by a disclaimer saying that it is not a health claim, if it is inferred to be a health claim.

DR. SHIFFMAN: I think, again, specifically we want to be sure that the smoker understands that smoking a cigarette that is labeled as light or ultralight does not necessarily protect them from the health risks of smoking and that, in that sense, cutting down in this way may not keep people from being cut down eventually by their smoking habit. We do think that the public perceives those labels as implicit health claims.

DR. FREEMAN: It is even conceivable that a low-tar cigarette smoked in a certain way may have the same health risk as a regular cigarette, and we have pointed out in what I have already said that there is no scientific evidence that any level of tar in cigarettes protects one against death due to coronary heart disease.

PARTICIPANT: The other substances that you referred to, are you going to talk about numbers?

DR. RICKERT: I think that what the committee felt in that area was that at the present time, since there is evidence that consumers tend to misinterpret the existing numbers, that to add additional numbers may add to that confusion. At the same time there was the concern that there are additional agents, other than tar, nicotine, and carbon monoxide, that have definite implications for health. It was anticipated that these compounds would be classified in various ways, for example, "carcinogens," and then there may be a list of several carcinogens. There would be a list based on toxicological effects but not including any numerical measurement.

PARTICIPANT: Can the machinery that is currently used to test cigarettes be used?

DR. FREEMAN: We were told by an expert today that there may be some fine tuning that will be necessary to use the current equipment to do this kind of testing.

PARTICIPANT: Who would determine what that range was and how many times the machine smoked or how long the puffs?

DR. FREEMAN: This committee did not go into that kind of detail. We are talking about the principle, and the principle is that we know that human smokers smoke in different patterns. Some smokers puff many times in a minute, and some smokers may puff once a minute. Some smokers puff deeply, and there are other factors that I could mention. While we are not trying to micromanage how this should be done, the principle is that we would like the machine measurement to more closely mimic the variation that humans evidence in their patterns of smoking to give a more honest range of what a given milligram of tar really represents in range. We do not believe it is accurate at all; in fact, it is misleading to give one number when the pattern of smoking can change that number radically with respect to dose.

DR. SHIFFMAN: What the panel intended was that the range represent the range of human smoking of particular brands so that the machine would model that under different parameters, which might include things that are now not dealt with in the FTC protocol, such as the blocking of ventilation holes that are used to dilute the smoke in some brands that now list as being low yield, but in fact can become high yield when a human finger or a human lip blocks those vents.

PARTICIPANT: Can you tell us what the role of other Federal agencies is going to be?

DR. FREEMAN: I am not an expert on the bureaucracy of America. However, we did get somewhat of a description of the FTC role in our meeting here today, which is a role that I understand deals with truth in advertising as one of its major roles. And to make a personal statement here, I think that is a limited role with respect to what we are trying to accomplish for the American public.

We found out today that 40 percent of cigarettes smoked in America are generics, and these for the most part are not advertised. However, the FTC in most of its role is limited to making statements about cigarettes that are advertised. So that if nearly half the cigarettes smoked in America are not advertised, it diminishes the FTC's role. Yet, the American public needs to know about the lethal nature of all cigarettes.

Now, as far as the FDA is concerned, again, I am not an expert on what they do, but I think their role is different from the FTC and may get more into the range of health concerns, hopefully. So, I cannot give you a finite answer. Perhaps my colleagues can help me out.

DR. SHIFFMAN: I would just add that the current FTC system operates under a voluntary agreement with the tobacco industry and cigarette manufacturers, and the representatives of that industry who addressed us during this meeting expressed an interest on the part of the industry of keeping consumers and smokers informed. We expect that they would follow through on that then in taking this step to make sure that accurate, useful information is available to smokers.

PARTICIPANT: Is it your understanding that if the regulatory agencies wanted to do this, that legislation would be necessary?

DR. FREEMAN: To do exactly what?

PARTICIPANT: To carry out your recommendations?

DR. FREEMAN: It is our belief that most of what we have recommended could be carried out by the FTC without congressional change. Our worry is that 40 percent of cigarettes are not regulated in a similar manner. Our concern is about the health of the American public and that the bureaucracy that we must go through to accomplish some of these things sometimes is a barrier to that. The FTC has regulations; the FDA has regulations, but sometimes what must be done or what should be done to save lives is beyond the confines of a certain agency, and this is somewhat of a problem.

PARTICIPANT: You said that this information would be useless unless smokers had ready access to information, including smokers of generic brands. In view of what you said about the FTC's jurisdiction, how do you anticipate getting that?

DR. FREEMAN: This came up very honestly today. We have not had time to think in depth about it. This was probably a surprise, even to this committee, that that problem is so large, that 40 percent of cigarettes are of the generic type, and honestly I do not have a good answer to that question. It may be that the FDA and other agencies could help in some respects, but I will refer this question to my colleagues to see if there is an answer to that.

DR. PETITTI: I could only repeat, I think, what we heard this morning, which is that some of these changes might, in fact, require congressional action, particularly if they resulted in changes in the labeling law. We are saying that there may be the need to put things on cigarette packs in order to adequately inform the American public about the FTC protocol.

PARTICIPANT: Looking ahead to the next 5-year review, do you see any gaps in research areas that need to be addressed?

DR. FREEMAN: Yes, we do. First of all, we have this paper. Where we are now with respect to our current knowledge, of course, is based on research, not perfect research, but we know a lot more now than we knew in 1950, when Ernst Wynder and others showed that tobacco is associated with death. So, research is a critical element and at any time I think we must act on what we know, but we must always move forward to finer knowledge. For example, further research is needed to determine the extent to which smokers of lower tar and nicotine cigarettes are less likely to attempt to quit smoking. There is some preliminary evidence, for example, that low-tar smokers may have less tendency to quit smoking. This would be very bad if it turns out to be true. It needs further research.

Next, to adequately understand and evaluate the impact of what is called compensation, research is required to assess the extent to which other biomarkers are correlated with machine-measured yields of the same substance. By compensation we refer to the point that low-tar smokers frequently smoke more cigarettes apparently to get the physiological dose of nicotine, which of course is an addictive substance. Compensation needs to be studied further to see what effect it may have, and certain biomarkers may come in handy to help us. Third, the differences in smoking patterns in different ethnic groups should be studied for the implications for health education and consumer information. We know, for example, that African-Americans tend to smoke cigarettes that are higher in tar and tend to smoke mentholated cigarettes. Other examples could be given. Poor Americans tend to smoke higher tar cigarettes. Educated Americans tend to smoke lower tar cigarettes. These are all very important questions that we only have preliminary information on, and these things need to be studied much more deeply. Finally, a system should be developed to help smokers gauge where their individual smoking behavior places them on a dose continuum. What diseases you develop, whether it be cancer or anything else, is often associated with the dose that you receive, and individuals need to know what dose they are receiving. There may be other research questions, and I will open it up for Dr. Rickert and Dr. Shiffman to comment.

DR. SHIFFMAN: I would add only that in addition to refining our knowledge in these areas that there may be some very different products for smokers on the horizon. We heard some indication of those in the press, and the system would have to be very carefully considered in order to properly evaluate new kinds of products aimed at smokers.

DR. FREEMAN: I think using research in a different way, we need to better understand the way the people in power deal with tobacco in America. It is a substance that is high in the economy.

If cigarettes were invented today, they probably would be outlawed since they kill 400,000 people a year. However, it is deeply integrated into our economy. It affects policymaking. Sometimes there is a conflict, in my opinion, between making regulations and trying to balance the budget.

America in one of its Government roles is saying that tobacco kills 400,000 American people. Other parts of Government are selling it overseas and growing it in America. These are deep problems. They require further research and knowledge and action.

Are there other questions?

If not, I would like to conclude by expressing my privilege of chairing this committee. We brought together the best experts in America on the subject. Dr. Dietrich Hoffmann, for example, is one of the pioneers in the study of tobacco, and there were others, and it is a privilege to chair this committee. It is our hope that these deliberations will have an effect on the American public with respect to saving lives and preventing disease.

Thank you very much.

Overview of 1980 to 1994 Research Related to the Standard Federal Trade Commission Test Method for Cigarettes

Michael D. Mueller

INTRODUCTION   This chapter provides an overview of the major studies related to the Federal Trade Commission (FTC) test method for determining tar, nicotine, and carbon monoxide (CO) yields of cigarettes compared with yields experienced by smokers, with special reference to low-tar and low-nicotine cigarettes. Most of the studies reviewed here were published since 1980; studies published prior to 1980 were extensively reviewed in the 1981 Surgeon General's report (U.S. Department of Health and Human Services, 1981).

The apparent differences between stated yields, as measured by the FTC test method, found in cigarette advertising and on some cigarette packs and actual amounts received by smokers appear to be largely attributable to compensation behaviors related to nicotine and possibly other substances in cigarette smoke. For example, when smokers switch to low-tar and low-nicotine cigarettes, they tend to increase the volume of inhaled smoke per cigarette or increase the number of cigarettes smoked so as to maintain a steady-state level of nicotine in their blood. They may also increase the volume by changing their puffing behavior and increase yield by blocking ventilation holes in filters.

Changes in puffing patterns can substantially alter tar and nicotine yields, as reported by Rickert and colleagues (1983), who investigated the impact of varying levels of butt length, puff duration, puff interval, puff volume, and blocking of ventilation holes.

The differences in advertised tar and nicotine yields of cigarettes compared with the amounts received by smokers result largely from differences between the smoking parameters of the FTC test method and actual smoking behaviors. These differences can substantially alter the amounts of tobacco smoke constituents that smokers inhale. The FTC method was devised in 1967, and it is not clear whether these parameters were based on actual human smoking patterns and behavior. Furthermore, cigarettes have undergone substantial changes in design and content over the past 40 years. Also, much more is currently known about smoking behavior; pharmacodynamics and pharmacokinetics; and the measurement of tar, nicotine, CO, and other substances in cigarette smoke as well as in blood, plasma, urine, and expired air in smokers.

Rickert and Robinson (1981, p. 401) emphasize that

> even if compensation [changes in smoking patterns to increase
> smoke intake per cigarette] did not occur, it is likely that
> smoking machine parameters fixed about 20 [years] ago no
> longer represent the average smoker, who probably takes
> puffs of more than 45 mL every 40 s instead of a 35-mL
> puff every 58 s.

There are harmful substances in tobacco and tobacco smoke other than
tar, nicotine, and CO. These include hydrogen cyanide (HCN), acrolein, total
aldehyde, and tobacco-specific nitrosamines (TSNAs). Levels of some of these
harmful substances in low-tar and low-nicotine cigarettes probably differ
among brands and may also differ within brands when cigarettes are smoked
differently.

Smoking patterns may be influenced by factors other than nicotine
dependence. Pomerleau and Pomerleau (1984) pointed out that there is
substantial evidence that many cigarettes are smoked for reasons other than
to receive nicotine. They cite research indicating that smoking patterns are
influenced in part by environmental situations, emotions, personality, and
motivation.

Robinson and coworkers (1983) found that smoking compensation
behaviors may lead to disproportionate increases in CO and HCN when
smokers switch to low-nicotine cigarettes.

Thus, research over the past 15 years has created multiple arenas within
which scientists and policymakers may reexamine the accuracy and relevance
of the FTC testing method and, if necessary, redesign it.

PARAMETERS OF THE FTC TEST METHOD AND CURRENT SMOKING PATTERNS
The current FTC test method is based on four parameters:
puff frequency (every 60 seconds), puff volume (35 mL),
puff duration (2 seconds), and a butt length that varies with
cigarette type. Darrall (1988) noted that these parameters
were set as long ago as 1936 and were not based on observed
smoking patterns. For individual smokers, puff volume has been reported to
range from 23 mL to 60 mL; puff duration is known to vary from 0.8 seconds
to 3.0 seconds. Typically, butt length is set at 23 mm, or filter and overwrap
plus 3 mm, whichever is longer; however, the FTC reported that, for 135 of
176 brands tested, butt length was more than 30 mm (Kozlowski, 1981).

Cigarette design has undergone significant change over the past several
decades. Cigarette manufacturers can influence yields of tar, nicotine, and
other substances through changes in wrapping paper porosity; tobacco
packing density; and filter-related factors such as ventilation, particulate
matter retention, and pressure drop. Benowitz and colleagues (1983) noted
that delivery of tobacco substances also may be influenced by how fast the
paper burns because this may determine how long a cigarette is smoked.
Study results indicate substantial differences in yields when FTC test method
parameters are varied (Table 1).

Table 1
Variation of puffs and tar, nicotine, and CO yields with puff frequency

Brand Type		Tar Band	Puff Frequency (seconds)															
			50				40				30				20			
			P	T	N	CO	P	T	N	CO	P	T	N	CO	P	T	N	CO
Mini	(PI)	(M)	11	7	10	3	27	30	39	20	69	68	71	40	91	112	114	69
Reg	(PI)	(M-H)	10	14	12	11	28	31	29	26	62	60	49	38	99	100	71	65
Reg	(PI)	(M-H)	12	16	13	12	24	33	32	23	52	69	54	42	73	97	72	61
Reg	(PI)	(M-H)	12	10	4	12	29	29	23	16	57	57	37	32	110	110	72	50
Mini	(V)	(L)	3	4	12	-1	28	24	35	9	54	52	53	23	71	97	91	61
KSUM	(V)	(L)	22	35	10	18	47	55	24	43	90	154	47	67	160	300	143	188
KSEM	(V)	(L)	9	17	14	15	27	31	32	32	52	94	60	64	101	145	104	92
KSEM	(V)	(L)	8	8	6	15	30	21	19	27	69	84	48	79	118	139	96	108
KS	(V)	(L)	14	9	6	8	38	19	19	24	76	54	38	43	118	99	77	65
KS	(NV)	(L-M)	13	25	18	15	31	44	35	33	57	62	61	39	94	122	92	57
KS	(NV)	(M)	13	13	4	4	26	26	16	16	60	60	32	32	93	93	50	50
IS	(NV)	(L-M)	21	22	21	20	38	46	42	39	70	62	58	46	100	129	110	70
Percentage Increase in Machine Puffing Rate			20				50				100				200			

Note: Column numbers denote percentage increases over values obtained with a 60-second puff frequency.

Key: *P = puffs count; T = tar yield; N = nicotine yield; CO = carbon monoxide yield; Mini = minicigarette; Reg = nonfilter; KS = king size; UM = ultramild;*
EM = extra mild; IS = international size; PI = plain; V = ventilated; NV = nonventilated; M = middle tar; M-H = middle to high tar; L = low tar;
L-M = low to middle tar.

Source: Darrall, 1988.

Gori (1990a) noted that machines, unlike humans, smoke each cigarette in exactly the same way. Smokers usually inhale after taking a puff, and inhalation seems to be largely under the influence of nicotine demand. When smoking machines were invented, little was known about inhalation patterns. Today, inhalation can be measured with various biological markers, such as CO and cotinine (an indicator of nicotine intake).

In a study of eight smokers, Gust and colleagues (1983) observed that the number of puffs and the duration, volume, and time between puffs varied with each smoker. All these factors affect the amount of smoke constituents to which the smoker is exposed. Gust and colleagues also noted that smoking patterns can vary as a smoker smokes a single cigarette.

Observations of smoking behavior reveal that smoking patterns are influenced by a wide range of factors, including degree of nicotine dependence, environmental cues, stress levels, and personality variables.

A survey of 1,200 randomly selected smokers and ex-smokers in the United States and Europe showed that consumers believe that the tar yields stated on cigarette packages accurately represent what is received by the smoker (Gori, 1990b). The majority of respondents indicated a belief that the published yield is equal to the amount consumed per cigarette. However, tar intake is related to nicotine intake, and individual intake of tar varies according to the nicotine levels of cigarettes and the level of nicotine dependence of smokers.

Guyatt and coworkers (1989a, p. 192) studied the changes in puffing behavior during the smoking of a cigarette. The researchers reported

> The most important change in puffing behavior during a single cigarette is the reduction in puff volume since this directly affects smoke uptake. Most subjects showed this effect, but the proportional change was independent of the tar level of the cigarette smoked or the sex of the subject and was consistent between sessions. However, there were significant between-subject differences indicating that each individual had [an] idiosyncratic pattern. Most subjects control puff volume by varying the duration, mostly by truncating the latter part of the puff.

IMPACT OF CHANGING PARAMETERS OF THE FTC TEST METHOD ON ABSOLUTE YIELDS OF A CIGARETTE BRAND AND RELATIVE YIELDS OF DIFFERENT BRANDS

Schlotzhauer and Chortyk (1983) examined the influence of varying smoking machine parameters on yields of tar, nicotine, and other selected smoke constituents from an ultralow-tar cigarette. The smoking machine parameters were changed to reflect the deeper inhalation, more frequent puffs, and vent blocking evident among smokers of lower yield cigarettes. Specifically, volume was varied from the standard 35 mL to 45 mL and 55 mL; frequency of puffs was doubled; and puff duration was increased from 2.0 to 3.0 seconds. Only one parameter was varied at a time; yields were measured with vent holes both unblocked and completely blocked.

As shown in Tables 2 through 4, changing one parameter at a time produces substantial increases in yields, and when cigarettes were machine smoked at the average of the parameters used in Tables 2 through 4, as shown in Table 5, total particulate matter (TPM) yields were approximately doubled, and increases of 96 to 271 percent in the individual components were observed.

TAR AND NICOTINE YIELD BY THE FTC TEST METHOD AND AMOUNTS DELIVERED TO SMOKER

The issue of compensation has become a central concern in assessing intake of tar, nicotine, CO, and other constituents constituents of tobacco smoke, particularly with regard to cigarettes described as low tar and low nicotine. Various researchers have reported no correlation between cigarette brand yield and actual exposure and substantially higher relative exposures from low-delivery cigarettes than indicated by quantitative differences in stated yields (Rickert and Robinson, 1981).

The current primary measurement of the carcinogenic potential of a cigarette is its tar yield. Kozlowski and colleagues (1980a) noted that tar yield depends in part on the number of puffs per cigarette and that a major factor in tar reduction has been reduced cigarette length, which results in fewer puffs per cigarette during standard FTC testing. Increasing the number of puffs can lead to substantial increases in tar yields.

Table 2

Effect of increased puff volumes on cigarette mainstream smoke under FTC conditions of puff frequency (60 seconds) and puff duration (2 seconds)

Results	35-mL Volume	45-mL Volume	Change (±%) From FTC Values	55-mL Volume	Change (±%) From FTC Values
Cigarettes Smoked	20	20	—	20	—
Total Puffs	152	150	-1	150	-1
Puffs/Cigarette (average)	7.6	7.5	-1	7.5	-1
Total Volume Inhaled (mL)	5,320	6,750	+27	8,250	+55
TPM (mg)	86	95	+10	135	+57
TPM/Cigarette (mg)	4.3	4.7	+10	6.7	+56
TPM/Puff (μg)	566	633	+11	900	+59
Phenol/Cigarette (μg)	12	17	+41	23	+92
Glycerol/Cigarette (μg)	327	624	+91	1,000	+206
Catechol/Cigarette (μg)	28	28	0	43	+54
Hydroquinone/Cigarette (μg)	23	27	+17	41	+61
Nicotine/Cigarette (μg)	378	502	+33	713	+88
Neophytadiene/Cigarette (μg)	15	32	+113	39	+160
Palmitic Acid/Cigarette (μg)	35	63	+80	64	+83
C_{18} Acids/Cigarette (μg)	33	61	+85	55	+67

Key: TPM = total particulate matter.

Source: Schlotzhauer and Chortyk, 1983.

Table 3
Effect of increased puff frequency and increased puff duration on cigarette mainstream smoke composition

Results	60-Second Frequency	30-Second Frequency	Change (+%)	3-Second Puff Duration	Change (±%)
Cigarettes Smoked	20	20	0	20	0
Total Puffs	152	281	+85	150	-5
Puffs/Cigarette (average)	7.6	14.0	+85	7.5	-5
Total Volume Inhaled (mL)	5,320	9,835	+85	7,800	+47
TPM (mg)	86	205	+138	166	+93
TPM/Cigarette (mg)	4.3	10.2	+138	8.3	+93
TPM/Puff (μg)	566	728	+29	1,106	+93
Phenol/Cigarette (μg)	12	20	+67	13	+8
Glycerol/Cigarette (μg)	327	1,542	+371	795	+143
Catechol/Cigarette (μg)	28	66	+136	70	+150
Hydroquinone/Cigarette (μg)	23	50	+117	40	+74
Nicotine/Cigarette (μg)	378	961	+154	618	+63
Neophytadiene/Cigarette (μg)	15	29	+93	53	+253
Palmitic Acid/Cigarette (μg)	35	41	+17	39	+11
C_{18} Acids/Cigarette (μg)	33	34	+3	30	-10

Key: TPM = total particulate matter.

Source: Schlotzhauer and Chortyk, 1983.

Table 4
Effect of obstructing tipping paper ventilations on cigarette mainstream smoke composition

Results	FTC Conditions[a]	FTC With Obstructed Perforations	Change (±%)
Cigarettes Smoked	20	20	0
Total Puffs	152	131	-14
Puffs/Cigarette (average)	7.6	6.5	-14
Total Volume Inhaled (mL)	5,320	4,584	-14
TPM (mg)	86	256	+198
TPM/Cigarette (mg)	4.3	12.8	+198
TPM/Puff (μg)	566	1,969	+248
Phenol/Cigarette (μg)	12	19	+58
Glycerol/Cigarette (μg)	327	1,001	+206
Catechol/Cigarette (μg)	28	58	+107
Hydroquinone/Cigarette (μg)	23	53	+130
Nicotine/Cigarette (μg)	378	839	+122
Neophytadiene/Cigarette (μg)	15	50	+233
Palmitic Acid/Cigarette (μg)	35	85	+143
C_{18} Acids/Cigarette (μg)	33	76	+130

[a] *35-mL puff volume, 60-second puff frequency, 2-second puff duration.*

Key: TPM = total particulate matter.

Source: Schlotzhauer and Chortyk, 1983.

Table 5
Effect of combined compensatory parameters on yields of mainstream smoke components

Results	FTC Conditions	New Conditions[a]	Change (±%)
Cigarettes Smoked	20	20	0
Total Puffs	152	236	+55
Puffs/Cigarette (average)	7.6	11.8	+55
Total Volume Inhaled (mL)	5,320	11,564	+117
TPM (mg)	86	169	+97
TPM/Cigarette (mg)	4.3	8.4	+95
TPM/Puff (μg)	566	716	+27
Phenol/Cigarette (μg)	12	30	+150
Glycerol/Cigarette (μg)	327	1,212	+271
Catechol/Cigarette (μg)	28	55	+96
Hydroquinone/Cigarette (μg)	23	53	+130
Nicotine/Cigarette (μg)	378	850	+125
Neophytadiene/Cigarette (μg)	15	52	+247
Palmitic Acid/Cigarette (μg)	35	86	+142
C_{18} Acids/Cigarette (μg)	33	71	+115

[a] *Averaged, reported compensatory smoking parameters (49-mL puff, 38-second frequency, 2.5-second puff duration) set on smoking machine.*

Key: TPM = total particulate matter.

Source: Schlotzhauer and Chortyk, 1983.

In a subsequent study of four popular king size cigarettes (see Table 6), Kozlowski (1981, p. 159) found that

> the same cigarette can easily rise from a low-tar to a high-tar category [through an increase in] the number of puffs taken from it, within the range of puffs per minute consistent with human smoking behavior. Based on the standard assay, brand B has 17 percent more tar than brand C; however, based on a 10-puff estimate, their tar deliveries are identical. Those smokers who take 14 puffs per cigarette are getting 58 percent more tar than would be expected from the standard yields.

Rawbone (1984), in a study of 400 middle-tar and low-tar smokers in the United Kingdom, found that tar delivery varied significantly between middle- and low-tar cigarettes but noticeably less than expected. That is, where a 46-percent lower tar delivery was expected with the low-tar cigarettes, a 32-percent reduction was observed. Furthermore, with regard to tar delivery, 98 percent of the middle-tar cigarette smokers fell within the established bounds of 16.50 to 22.49 mg delivery, whereas only 70 percent

Table 6

Tar yields (mg) as a function of number of puffs taken by smoking machines

Brand[a]	Number of Puffs			
	6	8.7[b]	10	14
A	13	18	21	30
B	13	21	22	31
C[c]	13	18	22	31
D[c]	12	17	19	27

[a] *Four of the most popular brands of king-size filter cigarettes.*
[b] *Mean number of puffs for the standard assay for these cigarettes: A, 8.6 puffs; B, 9.3; C, 8.1; D, 8.9.*
[c] *These brands are mentholated.*

Source: Kozlowski, 1981.

of the low-tar cigarette smokers were experiencing a delivery at or below the upper limit of 10.49 mg set for low-tar cigarettes (with 30 percent experiencing a higher-than-expected tar delivery).

Rickert and colleagues (1986) machine-analyzed the nicotine, tar, and CO yields of 10 cigarette brands under 27 different conditions (the standard condition and 26 variations). Tar, nicotine, and CO yields increased with volume of smoke produced per cigarette, but yields per liter of smoke were relatively constant across the 27 conditions.

Woodward and Tunstall-Pedoe (1992) investigated the smoking patterns of 2,754 smokers (1,133 males and 1,621 females) to determine intake of smoke components by smokers of low-tar cigarettes. This study, perhaps the largest naturalistic investigation of smoking behavior ever undertaken, included smokers of low-, middle-, and high-tar cigarettes. The researchers concluded that tar yield does not accurately reflect the amount of smoke components consumed by the smoker. Specifically, tar intake increased with tar yield but much less than anticipated; expired-air CO and cotinine seemed to peak among middle-tar smokers. For women, thiocyanate increased from low- to middle-tar smokers, and for men, from middle- to high-tar smokers. The researchers found that smokers of middle-tar cigarettes may consume more of some smoke components than smokers of high-tar cigarettes. Middle-tar smokers were noted to have higher levels of expired-air CO and cotinine.

Armitage and colleagues (1988) investigated the influence of changes in tar yield when nicotine yield was maintained. Twenty-one smokers of middle-tar cigarettes were studied, with randomization to three categories: low tar and low nicotine, low tar and medium nicotine, and medium yields of tar and nicotine. With regard to nicotine uptake, there were no significant differences noted between middle-tar and nicotine-maintained cigarettes, but there were significant differences between low-tar and nicotine-maintained cigarettes. The mean total puff volume of the nicotine-maintained cigarette was significantly greater than that recorded for middle-tar cigarettes. There was no difference in mean total puff volume between low-tar cigarettes and nicotine-maintained cigarettes.

RELATIVE YIELDS OF DIFFERENT BRANDS BY THE FTC TEST METHOD AND AMOUNT OF NICOTINE ABSORBED BY SMOKERS

Ebert and colleagues (1983) undertook a study of 76 smokers to determine correlations between levels of plasma nicotine and alveolar CO and the nicotine and CO yields of cigarettes. The correlations were found to be poor (Figures 1 and 2). For the 24 smokers of low-nicotine, low-tar cigarettes, nicotine levels were statistically lower for smokers of low-nicotine cigarettes, but the levels were only slightly lower and there was great overlap in individual plasma nicotine values; there was no difference in the mean alveolar CO levels between the low-nicotine smokers and smokers of regular cigarettes.

Research by Benowitz and colleagues (1983) on 272 subjects about to enter a smoking treatment program revealed that the correlation between stated nicotine yield and actual blood cotinine levels was not significant. Furthermore, it was determined that nicotine concentration in the unburned tobacco and amount of nicotine in an unburned cigarette are not correlated positively with FTC-determined yields and that tobacco in low-yield cigarettes did not contain less nicotine than tobacco in higher yield cigarettes.

Figure 1

Relationship between plasma nicotine concentration in smokers and nicotine yield of cigarettes smoked

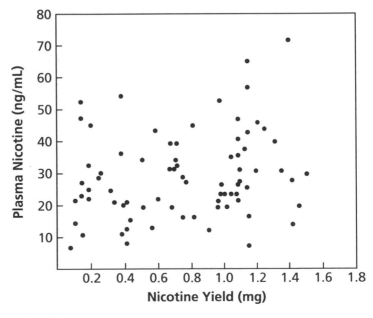

Source: Ebert et al., 1983.

Figure 2

Relationship between carbon monoxide (CO) concentration of alveolar air in smokers and CO yield of cigarettes smoked

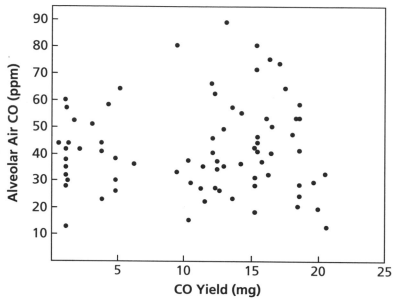

Source: Ebert et al., 1983.

Ventilation and burning characteristics are the primary determinants of machine-measured yields, and these characteristics can be controlled by smokers. Benowitz and colleagues acknowledged that blood cotinine is not a "perfect marker," but a full range of cigarettes was included in the study and there is no reason to suspect that brand is related to nicotine and cotinine metabolism.

Russell and colleagues (1986) examined blood nicotine, cotinine, and carboxyhemoglobin (COHb) levels among 392 smokers whose regular brands varied from low tar to middle tar. Tar levels were estimated from blood nicotine levels and cigarette tar yields. The authors reported

> Smokers of LT [low-tar] cigarettes had a lower intake of tar, nicotine, and CO than the smokers of higher yielding brands. On average, their estimated intake of tar was about 25 percent lower, their intake of nicotine was about 15 percent lower (17 percent and 12 percent, as measured by blood nicotine and cotinine, respectively), and their intake of CO was about 10 percent lower. These differences are substantially less than the reductions in the standard machine-smoked yields of their cigarettes (47 percent, 39 percent, and 34 percent for tar, nicotine, and CO yields, respectively), and this indicates the extent to which the LT smokers were smoking and inhaling more intensively, presumably to compensate for the lower yields. However, it is clear that

despite such compensatory changes in smoking behavior, their intake of the three major smoke components was still lower to a statistically and clinically significant degree (Russell et al., 1986, p. 83).

Maron and Fortmann (1987) examined the relationship of FTC machine-estimated nicotine yield by cigarette brand with the level of cigarette consumption and two biochemical measures of smoke exposure (expired-air CO and plasma thiocyanate) in a population of 713 smokers. These investigators found that the lower the nicotine yield, the greater the number of cigarettes smoked per day. Smokers of ultralow-nicotine cigarettes experienced smoke exposures that were not significantly different from those of smokers of higher yield brands. Only after adjustment for number of cigarettes smoked daily did nicotine yield become significantly related to expired-air CO and plasma thiocyanate. The number of cigarettes smoked per day accounted for 28 and 22 percent of the variance in observed expired-air CO and plasma thiocyanate levels, respectively, whereas nicotine yield accounted for only 1 and 2 percent of the variance, respectively. The authors concluded that machine estimates suggesting low nicotine yield underrepresent actual human consumption of harmful cigarette constituents.

In a study of 289 smokers of cigarettes in the 1-mg FTC tar class, Gori and Lynch (1983) observed that nicotine intake (measured by plasma cotinine) varied widely, from undetectable to about 800 ng/mL. The findings indicated that smokers of low-yield brands tend to take in more nicotine than posted FTC values. This observation is illustrated in Figure 3. Brand A was .9 tar and .18 nicotine, whereas brand B was .5 tar and .10 nicotine.

Coultas and colleagues (1993), working with a population of 298 mostly Hispanic smokers, studied the relationship between yields of cigarettes currently smoked and levels of salivary cotinine and expired-air CO. Spearman's correlation coefficients (Snedecor and Cochran, 1980) between the current number of cigarettes smoked and cotinine or CO were higher than correlations between the FTC nicotine data and these same markers. In multiple linear regression models, the current number of cigarettes smoked was the most important predictor of cotinine and CO levels ($p < 0.0001$), and the addition of FTC tar, nicotine, and CO to the models explained little about the variability in cotinine and CO levels.

In a large-scale study of 2,455 cigarette smokers who smoked their usual brands, Wald and colleagues (1984) observed that nicotine and CO intake was relatively constant across brands, regardless of stated yield, although tar intake appeared related to tar yield.

YIELD BY THE FTC TEST METHOD AND ABSORPTION OF NICOTINE IN SWITCHERS
As pointed out by many researchers, cigarette smoking has the hallmarks of drug-dependent behavior, with strong evidence that nicotine is the dependence-producing component (Benowitz et al., 1989). Nicotine is rapidly absorbed into the blood and quickly delivered to the brain, where

Figure 3

Observed and expected baseline plasma cotinine values as a function of FTC nicotine delivery of brands A and B

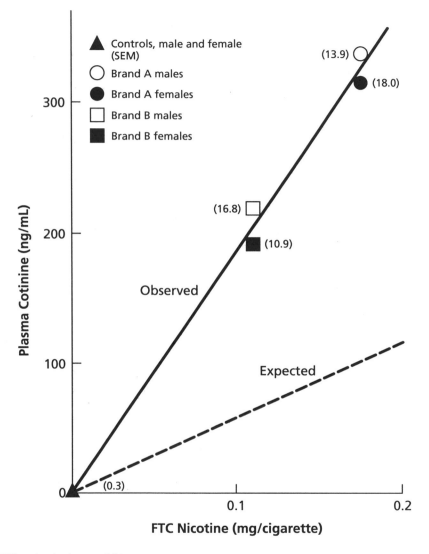

Key: *SEM = standard error of the mean.*

Source: *Gori and Lynch, 1983.*

it produces a range of mental effects on the smoker. This quick absorption and effect permit the smoker to control the nicotine level carefully; however, nicotine is rapidly eliminated from the body, which means the smoker has to deliver regular doses to the blood.

Robinson and colleagues (1982 and 1983) studied the smoking patterns of 22 cigarette smokers divided into treatment and control groups, with the treatment group switching twice to cigarettes of successively lower nicotine yields. Compensation behavior was measured noninvasively (average number of daily cigarettes, daily mouth-level nicotine exposure, butt length, expired-air CO, and saliva thiocyanate) and invasively (COHb, serum cotinine, and plasma thiocyanate). As shown in Figure 4, there were no major differences between smokers in treatment and control groups. The near-complete compensation was attributed to upward changes in smoking intensity, depth of inhalation, and cigarette consumption. In addition, there was an observed tendency of smokers of lower delivery cigarettes to smoke cigarettes down closer to the overwrap and to block ventilation holes.

In a different approach, Gritz and colleagues (1983) looked at the puffing behavior of eight smokers presented with cigarettes at two and four times

Figure 4
Average daily exposure and standardized exposure measures by period for treatment and control groups

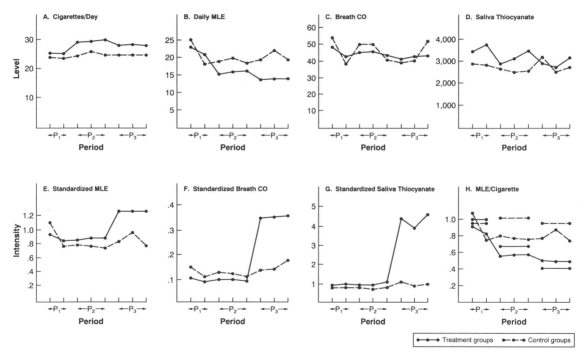

Note: *Average nominal nicotine deliveries are shown as horizontal lines in Panel H. Abbreviated variable names have been used. The increase of "standardized" exposure measure for the treatment group (Panels F and G) during period three (P_3) does not represent an increase in exposure. The exposure remains fairly constant during the entire study, as Panels C and D indicate. Panels F and G illustrate the extent of compensation necessary to maintain this constant exposure. See text for details.*

Key: *MLE = mouth-level exposure; CO = carbon monoxide.*

Source: *Robinson et al., 1982.*

their normal smoking rates. All eight smokers compensated to some degree. Despite being presented with twice the usual number of cigarettes, the smokers titrated their nicotine intake down, largely by changing their number of puffs, puff volume, and puff duration per cigarette. Gritz and coworkers disputed the view that some smokers may be compensators and others may be noncompensators, arguing that these two groups of smokers represent the opposite ends of a continuum.

Henningfield and Griffiths (1980) studied the effect of tobacco product concentration on puffing rate and total number of puffs. Tobacco concentration levels were set at 100, 50, 25, and 10 percent by means of ventilated holders (identified in Figures 5 and 6 as holders 0, 1, 2, and 4). As shown, puffs at holder 4 were about double those of holder 0. In addition, there were substantial increases in puff rate.

Compensation via alterations in puffing patterns does not explain all observed changes, however. In their investigation of puffing and inhalation patterns and yields, Nil and colleagues (1986) found that changes in puff volume account for only about one-fifth of the difference in smoke yields; no significant changes were found in inhalation patterns. On the other hand, with lower yield cigarettes, there was nearly complete compensation based on alveolar CO uptake, and the degree of increased heart rate was viewed as a nearly complete compensation for nicotine intake.

McBride and colleagues (1984) measured changes in smoking behavior and ventilation when subjects smoked cigarettes of varying nicotine yields. Nine smokers were studied, and the test order was randomized. Puff volume was noted to increase significantly during the smoking of low-nicotine cigarettes. In a study of 170 male smokers and 170 age-matched male nonsmokers, Bridges and colleagues (1986) observed that total puff volume was significantly greater for smokers of cigarettes lower in nicotine yields. As shown in Figures 7 and 8, total puff volume was significantly correlated with nicotine yield and plasma cotinine.

Researchers have observed that smokers can substantially alter tar, nicotine, and CO delivery of cigarettes by blocking the ventilation holes in the filters. In a two-part study of smokers of low-yield cigarettes, Kozlowski et al. (1982a) observed hole-blocking behavior and measured tar, nicotine, and CO levels. The investigators reported that 44 percent of 39 smokers of low-yield cigarettes blocked the ventilation holes to various degrees with their fingers or lips; 5 of 33 females left hole-blocking lipstick on the filters.

In the second part of their study, Kozlowski and colleagues (1982a) evaluated the effect of hole blocking on the tar, nicotine, and CO yields of American, British, and Canadian cigarettes of lowest or near-lowest yields. After videotaping 48 smokers, the researchers defined actual smoking behaviors and reset smoking machine parameters to reflect these real-life patterns for puff interval (44 seconds) and puff duration (2.4 seconds). Machine puff volume was set at 47 mL (2 to 13 mL below the smokers' estimated average) because this is the maximum obtainable from most

Figure 5

Mean total puffs per session (N = 4) and standard error values for each subject as a function of cigarette holder number

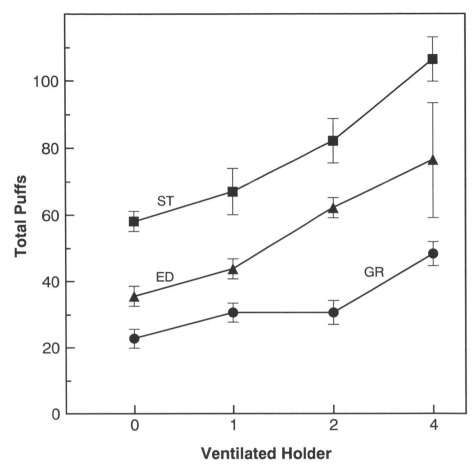

Ventilated Holder

Note: The approximate concentrations of delivered tobacco product are indicated by the holder number in which 0 = 100 percent, 1 = 75 percent, 2 = 50 percent, and 4 = 10 percent. The abbreviations ST, ED, and GR represent three paid female volunteers who participated in the study.

Source: Henningfield and Griffiths, 1980.

machines. Ventilation holes were blocked with tape. The researchers compared standard yields of cigarettes to yields resulting from the study-determined parameters and blocked ventilation holes; they observed that "tar increases from 15- to 39-fold, nicotine from 8- to 19-fold and CO from 10- to 43-fold" (Kozlowski et al., 1982a, p. 159). Five cigarette brands similar in tar yield were found to differ substantially when parameters were changed and holes blocked.

In a later study of 14 subjects, Kozlowski (1989) detected hole blocking by half the sample. Subjects blocking the ventilation holes of ultralow-yield

Figure 6

Mean number (N = 4) of cigarettes smoked by each subject during 3-hour sessions as a function of holder number (upper frame) and mean rate of puffing (puffs/minute) per cigarette (lower frame)

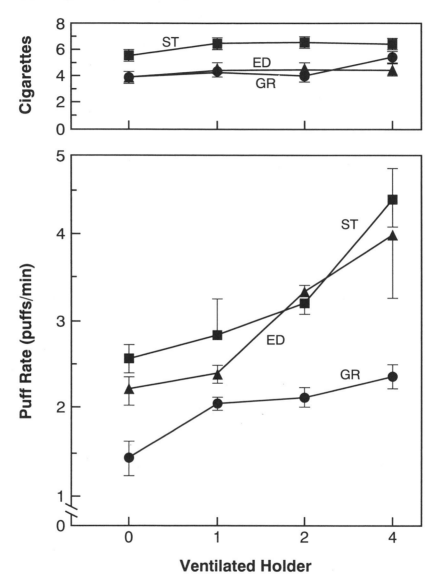

Note: *Standard error values for each subject, in both frames, are indicated by the brackets. The approximate concentrations of delivered tobacco product are indicated by the holder number in which 0 = 100 percent, 1 = 75 percent, 2 = 50 percent, and 4 = 10 percent. The abbreviations ST, ED, and GR represent three paid female volunteers who participated in the study.*

Source: *Henningfield and Griffiths, 1980.*

Figure 7

Relationship of total puff volume per cigarette with the nicotine yield of the cigarette smoked

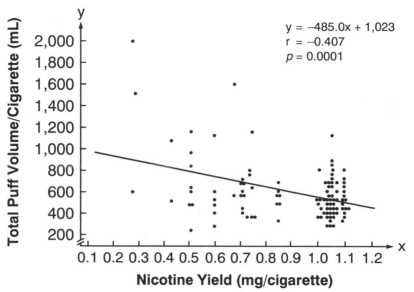

Source: Bridges et al., 1986.

Figure 8

Relationship between plasma nicotine concentration and total volume puffed per cigarette in a population smoking a single brand of cigarette (nicotine yield = 1.05 mg/cigarette)

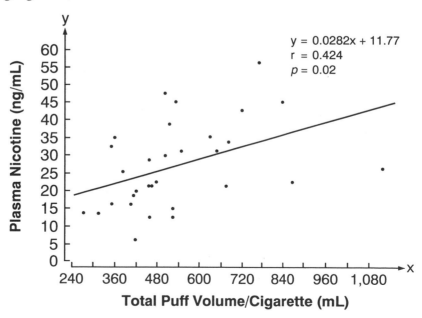

Source: Bridges et al., 1986.

cigarettes were found to have higher CO and salivary cotinine levels. Rickert and colleagues (1983) found that blocking half the ventilation holes increased the delivery of TPM by 60 percent, and full occlusion increased TPM delivery by 150 percent.

The effect of blocking on perforation ventilation (ventilation holes in the filter) and channel ventilation (longitudinal air channels around the filter) was studied by Höfer and colleagues (1991). The researchers compared results of lip smoking and holder smoking of cigarettes among 72 smokers, divided equally by ventilation type of cigarette smoked. Höfer and colleagues (1991, p. 910) found that

> under normal lip contact conditions, the CO and nicotine deliveries of the channel-ventilated cigarettes were higher than those of the perforation-ventilated cigarettes and higher than with holder smoking. With holder smoking, both types of cigarettes delivered comparable amounts of CO and nicotine (*t*-tests, n.s.).

It appeared that the nicotine boost from channel-ventilated cigarettes was twice that of perforation-ventilated cigarettes; differences in CO exposure were less well defined. The researchers judged that there was evidence of blocking in 86 percent of the channel filter cigarette smokers and in 33 percent of the perforated filter cigarette smokers.

In a novel approach to the study of hole blocking among smokers of ultralow-tar cigarettes, Kozlowski and colleagues (1988) collected 135 discarded filters from ashtrays in shopping malls. It was found that 58 percent of the filters showed some evidence of hole blocking (as measured by tar stain patterns); 19 percent showed evidence of extreme hole blocking; and 42 percent showed no signs of hole blocking. Kozlowski and colleagues (1994) extended this research to "light" cigarettes (about 9 to 12 mg tar, about 15 to 30 percent vented): Twenty-seven percent of collected filters indicated extreme blockage; 26 percent showed some blocking; and 47 percent showed no vent blocking. Although defeat of the air vents will have a relatively small effect on light rather than ultralight cigarettes, the greater sales of light cigarettes contribute to its significance for public health. In an earlier report, Kozlowski and colleagues (1980b) examined the effect of hole blocking on nicotine, tar, CO, and puffs (Table 7), noting that ventilated filters have been developed primarily as a way to make less toxic cigarettes but that smoking behavior can sabotage the benefits of these filters.

Kozlowski and colleagues (1989) demonstrated that some smokers of vented filter cigarettes are lighter smokers who appear to be seeking lower smoke doses and do not block vents, whereas others are generally heavier smokers who block vents and derive high daily doses of nicotine. Two smokers, who were vent blockers, of a 1-mg tar, 0.1-mg nicotine cigarette achieved salivary cotinine levels (303 and 385 ng/mL) consistent with smoking a high-yield cigarette.

Table 7
Effects of blocking the ventilation holes on the yields of a popular, low-yield cigarette[a]

Characteristics	Unblocked Holes	Half-Blocked Holes	Fully Blocked Holes
Constituents			
Nicotine (mg)	0.45	0.73 ± .06	0.98 ± .06[a]
Tar (mg)	4.40	7.03 ± .04	12.60 ± .20[a]
Carbon Monoxide (mg)	4.50	7.80 ± .24	17.70 ± .40[a]
Puffs	11.10	10.50 ± .20	9.20 ± .40[a]

[a] *Half-blocked vs. fully blocked comparison (t-test, 2-tailed) p < .01. Values are means ± standard deviations. Government figures for the June-July 1979 assay were used as the unblocked control; variances were not reported, but those found in similar analyses imply that all within-row comparisons would be statistically significant. All analyses in the table were performed by the same laboratory employing the same techniques.*

Source: Kozlowski et al., 1980b.

Bridges and colleagues (1990) studied 170 male smokers to determine the influence on yield of smoking topography (i.e., total smoking time per cigarette, number of puffs, interpuff interval, puff duration, volume per puff, total duration per cigarette, total volume per cigarette, flow rate). The smokers were divided into six groups according to stated nicotine yields of their cigarettes. The first four groups were most similar in age, smoking history, and alcohol and coffee consumption. There were significant negative correlations between nicotine yield and mean puff volume, total duration and volume, and flow rate. That is, as nicotine yield decreased, mean puff volume, total duration and volume, and flow rate increased significantly. These statistical relationships are shown in Figure 9. Multiple regression analysis showed that nicotine yield, alone or in combination with other factors, is a significant predictor of number of puffs or total puff volume per cigarette.

Figure 9 is of special interest because it represents smoking topography changes in a subpopulation for which nicotine yield was held constant to control for the possible confounding effects of nicotine on smoking behavior. Cumulative puff volume for a cigarette is significantly correlated with plasma nicotine, an indication that increased inhalation results in increased absorption. For the same group, the interpuff interval was negatively correlated with plasma nicotine levels (i.e., when time between puffs went down, plasma nicotine level went up).

According to Bridges and colleagues (1990, p. 31)

Smokers smoking the lowest yield cigarettes (Group 1) had significantly higher total puff volume per cigarette than did the other groups, and significantly higher mean puff volume and flow rate . . . than Groups 3 and 4. Smokers of lower yield

Figure 9
Linear relationships between nicotine yield and puffing topography measures: (A) number of puffs per cigarette, (B) total puff duration per cigarette, (C) total puff volume per cigarette

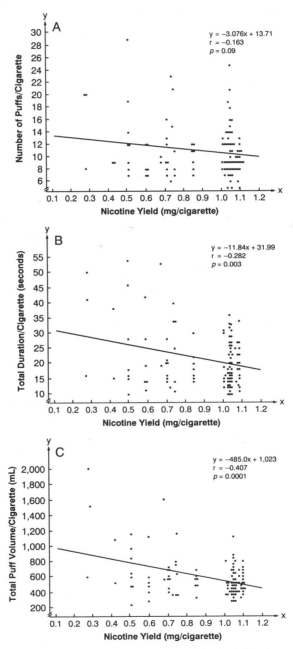

Note: The graphical representation for each of these relationships includes the equation for the inserted least-squares best fit line, the correlation coefficient (r), and the level of significance for the correlation. The data are for groups 1-4, n = 108.

Source: Bridges et al., 1990.

cigarettes also tended to have higher numbers of puffs per cigarette, decreased interpuff interval, increased duration per puff, and increased duration per cigarette, but these differences did not reach statistical significance. These results are consistent with changes in puffing topography to compensate for lower yield cigarettes.

In addition, there were significant negative correlations between nicotine yield and mean puff volume, total duration and volume, and flow rate. That is, as nicotine yield decreased, mean puff volume, total duration and volume, and flow rate increased significantly. In addition, multiple regression analysis showed that nicotine yield, alone or in combination with other factors, is a significant predictor of number of puffs or total puff volume per cigarette.

Creighton and Lewis (1978) examined changes in smoking patterns when cigarettes were varied according to nicotine delivery. Specifically, 16 smokers were monitored for 3 months. The first month, they all smoked medium-delivery cigarettes of about 1.4 mg nicotine; then the group was split for 1 month, with half smoking lower delivery cigarettes (about 1.0 mg nicotine) and half smoking higher delivery cigarettes (about 1.8 mg nicotine). During the third month, the panel of 16 smokers returned to the 1.4 mg nicotine cigarettes. Significant changes were found in smoking patterns among the 16 smokers: either the increased smoking intensity when smoking lower delivery cigarettes or decreased intensity when smoking higher delivery cigarettes. However, the researchers reported that the smokers did not equalize nicotine and TPM delivery when they switched to lower delivery cigarettes, as was the case when they switched to higher delivery cigarettes. The number of cigarettes smoked per day remained about the same throughout the study.

Russell and colleagues (1982) looked at changes in nicotine, cotinine, COHb, thiocyanate, and tar when 12 smokers switched to low-tar, low-nicotine cigarettes for 12 weeks. Plasma nicotine and cotinine were both reduced by about 30 percent and tar by 15 percent; plasma thiocyanate and COHb did not change significantly. Although mouth level of nicotine intake from low-tar, low-nicotine cigarettes was similar to the standard machine yield, the blood levels of 30 percent were substantially less than the anticipated level of 46 percent based on machine yields. There was no compensatory increase in smoke intake at the mouth level, but blood measures showed the increase in inhalation between 32.1 and 40.8 percent.

Similarly, Ashton and coworkers (1979) found that, when switched from medium- to high- or low-nicotine brands, smokers compensated for about two-thirds of the difference in standard yields. Specifically, when nicotine yield was reduced by 50 percent, nicotine intake was about 15 percent lower. Furthermore, based on machine yields, it was anticipated that the nicotine yield of low-nicotine cigarettes would be 32.6 percent that of high-nicotine cigarettes; however, in the laboratory the observed yield was 59 percent that of high-nicotine cigarettes.

Benowitz and colleagues (1986) looked at differences in tar, nicotine, and CO exposure when smokers switched from their regular brand to high-, low-, and ultralow-yield cigarettes. The researchers detected no differences in exposure among the high- and low-yield smokers. However, for smokers of ultralow-yield cigarettes, there were substantial reductions in exposure to tar (49 percent), nicotine (56 percent), and CO (36 percent). Despite these reductions, the investigators reported that the relative exposure to tar and nicotine from ultralow-yield compared with higher yield cigarettes was much greater than predicted by FTC machine-determined yields.

Kolonen and colleagues (1991) examined puffing patterns of 36 smoking students, with different smoking histories, in a natural environment. The subjects included 18 smokers of low-yield cigarettes, 10 smokers of medium-yield cigarettes, and 8 smokers who had switched from medium- to low-yield cigarettes. Subjects smoked their regular brand for the first week, a low-yield brand for the second week, and a medium-yield brand for the third week. All three groups had the highest daily puff volumes when smoking low-yield cigarettes, and the correlations between urine cotinine concentration and daily puffing in the three groups were poor. However, the urinary cotinine concentration was significantly lower for low-yield smokers compared with the switchers. The investigators concluded that cotinine excretion results in the switchers' group were in line with earlier reports showing that long-term switchers have no significant decreases in plasma and urine cotinine.

In a longer study of switching effects, Guyatt and coworkers (1989b) monitored 28 smokers who switched to cigarettes with lower tar and nicotine yields. The researchers concluded, after monitoring subjects for about 1 year, that most effects of the switch to lower yield cigarettes did not persist beyond 36 weeks. The drop in cotinine levels was only 40 percent of what was expected from stated nicotine yields; mean puff volume increased by 16 percent; and smokers seemed to achieve about 60 percent compensation when smoking lower tar cigarettes.

YIELDS BY THE FTC TEST METHOD AND OTHER CONSTITUENTS USING FTC PUFF PROFILE

Carbon monoxide yields follow somewhat surprising dynamics. For example, as Rickert and colleagues (1980) reported, efficient filters may substantially reduce tar yields of cigarettes but lead to increased delivery of CO.

In a study of reduced-draw-resistance cigarettes, Dunn (1978) found that smokers can substantially vary their inhalation patterns, leading to marked changes in the amount of smoke that reaches the lungs as measured by alveolar CO levels. Although increased levels of alveolar CO were expected with reduced draw resistance, CO levels decreased, possibly because of increased delivery of nicotine. Dunn proposed that the level of CO in exhaled air may be a good measure of depth of inhalation.

There appears to be substantial natural variation in the amount of CO inhaled by smokers, even when numbers of cigarettes smoked are approximately equal. Burling and colleagues (1985) studied 12 matched pairs of smokers, each pair smoking a similar number of cigarettes but with different levels of CO (one high-CO-level subject and one low-CO-level subject). The CO boost per cigarette was found to be significantly different for the matched pairs of smokers. The CO boost for the high-CO group was 6.9 ppm per cigarette and for the low CO group 4.4 ppm.

The study found no differences between the high-CO and low-CO groups in terms of number and duration of puffs. Given the significant differences in CO levels, the researchers speculate that the difference may reside in puff intensity, puff volume, or inhalation characteristics. These influences on CO levels are relevant to low-nicotine yields and changes in smoking behavior; Herning and colleagues (1983) reported that CO boost appears correlated to blood nicotine levels.

In an earlier study, Burling and coworkers (1983) found that a smoker's CO level is influenced by factors other than the FTC-determined CO yield of cigarettes. The researchers reported that the CO level is significantly related to interpuff interval, cigarette duration, time since last cigarette, and self-rated estimate of depth of inhalation. This research underscores the likelihood that CO levels may be determined by multiple factors, not just stated yield. However, the finding suggests that, when numbers of cigarettes are held equal, a person smoking cigarettes with a higher CO yield will likely have higher CO levels than a person smoking cigarettes of lower CO yield. Furthermore, Wald and colleagues (1984) reported that smokers of filter cigarettes have a 60-percent higher intake of CO than do those who smoke nonfilter cigarettes.

Russell and colleagues (1982), in a study of long-term switching to low-tar, low-nicotine cigarettes, observed complete compensation as measured by CO uptake, and Robinson and coworkers (1983) reported that COHb levels did not change significantly after smokers switched to cigarettes with 15- and 72-percent lower CO deliveries.

Robinson and colleagues (1984) examined exposure among 22 smokers of high-nicotine cigarettes who switched to cigarettes of similar nicotine yield but with reduced yields for tar, CO, and hydrogen cyanide. Cotinine levels remained about the same; however, although reductions of 40 to 50 percent in CO and HCN were expected, the measured reductions were 5.3 percent for expired-air CO, 12.2 percent for COHb, 2 percent for saliva thiocyanate, and 1 percent for plasma thiocyanate.

Darrall (1988) found that a 50-percent blockage of ventilation holes produced small changes in tar and nicotine yields but greater changes in CO. Nil and coworkers (1986), in a study of 117 regular smokers, reported that the CO boost of cigarettes appeared to remain steady among smokers despite controlled switching to cigarettes of higher or lower yields.

Fischer and colleagues (1989), in an investigation of six different cigarette brands (filter and nonfilter and very low to medium tar yields), found that puff volume and puff frequency, the key determinants of total volume inhaled, significantly affect the smoker's exposure to tobacco-specific nitrosamines. According to the investigators,

> The medium-tar cigarette using standard smoking conditions delivered TSNA values that were close to the calculated average intake by smokers. The calculated average TSNA intake for the low-tar cigarette, however, was about double the value determined under standard smoking conditions (Fischer et al., 1989, p. 1065).

The researchers concluded that

> since the standard smoking conditions cannot reflect the real behavior for low- and very-low-tar cigarettes, especially with respect to the total inhalation volume, risk evaluation has to consider the increase in TSNA intake with increasing total volume (Fischer et al., 1989, p. 1065).

In a subsequent study, Fischer and colleagues (1991) investigated 170 types of American, European, and Russian cigarettes. The findings revealed that the amounts of two TSNAs—NNN (*N*-nitrosonornicotine) and NNK (4-methylnitrosamino-1-[3-pyridinyl]-1-butanone)—in cigarette smoke are not correlated with tar or nicotine delivery and the amounts of TSNAs in mainstream smoke are related to the amount of preformed nitrosamine in the tobacco.

In an investigation of compensation behaviors among smokers switching to lower delivery cigarettes, Robinson and coworkers (1983) noted disproportionate increases in HCN levels. The researchers concluded that machine-determined "standardized" deliveries do not reflect potential exposure to HCN.

Rickert and Robinson (1981), in a study of delivery by low-hazard and high-hazard brands and actual levels, found that differences in HCN and CO yields of the two different delivery types varied much more widely than actual levels of COHb and plasma thiocyanate obtained from smokers of each. High-hazard cigarette smokers had nearly four times the HCN of low-hazard cigarette smokers; however, the actual levels differed by only 20 percent. These differences were not statistically significant, possibly due to small sample size (n = 31).

Rickert and colleagues (1983) looked at variations in smoking patterns and reported that HCN delivery is influenced by blocking of ventilation holes and, to a lesser degree, by puff duration, puff volume, and butt length. Blocking half the ventilation holes increased HCN yield by 70 percent; covering all the holes produced a 250-percent increase in yield. These investigators determined that HCN yield for the cigarette brand investigated ranged from 5 to 241 μg, depending on variations in smoking parameters, although the mean HCN yield was 39 μg. For 115 Canadian cigarettes, the average HCN yield varied from 2 to 233 μg. This impact of smoking pattern on HCN yield was cited by Rickert and colleagues as a possible explanation for the poor correlation between HCN yield and levels of plasma thiocyanate and saliva thiocyanate.

Rickert and colleagues (1980) indicated that aldehydes, gas-phase constituents of tobacco smoke, are known to be ciliatoxic and may not be removed to a substantial degree from cigarette smoke by filters. Acrolein, a toxin restricted in occupational and industrial settings, also may contribute to the chemical toxicity of tobacco smoke. In a study of 102 brands of Canadian cigarettes, Rickert and colleagues found that tar level was a poor predictor of total aldehydes and acrolein delivery. The effect of changes in smoking patterns on phenol, glycerol, catechol, hydroquinone, palmitic acid, and neophytadiene are shown in Tables 2 through 5 (Schlotzhauer and Chortyk, 1983).

PROPOSALS TO CHANGE THE FTC TEST METHOD   At least three proposals have been published for changes in the FTC cigarette test method. Kozlowski and colleagues (1982b) made a proposal addressing the issue of the variability in human smoking behavior. These investigators suggested a three-level (i.e., light, average, and heavy) machine regimen linked to a color-matching technique to help smokers gauge the extent of puffing on a given cigarette—the darker the stain, the greater the exposure, with the tar stains keyed to a range of tar doses. Rickert and colleagues (1986) proposed an estimate based on average yields of tar, nicotine, and carbon monoxide per liter of smoke. Henningfield and coworkers (1994) proposed that multiple tests be used: an average smoking test and a heavy smoking test. The heavy smoking test would include vent-blocking conditions for those cigarettes incorporating ventilation holes and if it is possible for those holes to be blocked by the smoker's lips or fingers.

REFERENCES

Armitage, A.K., Alexander, J., Hopkins, R., Ward, C. Evaluation of low to middle tar/medium nicotine cigarette designed to maintain nicotine delivery to the smoker. *Psychopharmacology* 96(4): 447-453, 1988.

Ashton, H., Stepney, R., Thompson, J.W. Self-titration by cigarette smokers. *British Medical Journal* 2(6186): 357-360, 1979.

Benowitz, N.L., Hall, S.M., Herning, R.I., Jacob, P. III, Jones, R.T., Osman, A.L. Smokers of low-yield cigarettes do not consume less nicotine. *New England Journal of Medicine* 309(3): 139-142, 1983.

Benowitz, N.L., Jacob, P. III, Yu, L., Talcott, R., Hall, S., Jones, R.T. Reduced tar, nicotine, and carbon monoxide exposure while smoking ultralow- but not low-yield cigarettes. *Journal of the American Medical Association* 256(2): 241-246, 1986.

Benowitz, N.L., Porchet, H., Jacob, P. III. Nicotine dependence and tolerance in man: Pharmacokinetic and pharmacodynamic investigations. *Progress in Brain Research* 79: 279-287, 1989.

Bridges, R.B., Combs, J.G., Humble, J.W., Turbek, J.A., Rehm, S.R., Haley, N.J. Puffing topography as a determinant of smoke exposure. *Pharmacology, Biochemistry and Behavior* 37: 29-39, 1990.

Bridges, R.B., Humble, J.W., Turbek, J.A., Rehm, S.R. Smoking history, cigarette yield and smoking behavior as determinants of smoke exposure. *European Journal of Respiratory Disease* 146(Suppl): 129-137, 1986.

Burling, T.A., Lovett, S.B., Richter, W.T., Frederiksen, L.W. Alveolar carbon monoxide: The relative contributions of daily cigarette rate, cigarette brand, and smoking topography. *Addictive Behaviors* 8(1): 23-26, 1983.

Burling, T.A., Stitzer, M.L., Bigelow, G.E., Mead, A.M. Smoking topography and carbon monoxide levels in smokers. *Addictive Behaviors* 10: 319-323, 1985.

Coultas, D.B., Stidley, C.A., Samet, J.M. Cigarette yields of tar and nicotine and markers of exposure to tobacco smoke. *American Review of Respiratory Disease* 148: 435-440, 1993.

Creighton, D.E., Lewis, P.H. The effect of different cigarettes on human smoking patterns. In: *Smoking Behavior. Physiological and Psychological Influences*, R.E. Thornton (Editor). Edinburgh: Churchill Livingstone, 1978. pp. 289-300.

Darrall, K.G. Smoking machine parameters and cigarette smoke yields. *Science of the Total Environment* 74: 263-278, 1988.

Dunn, P.J. The effects of a reduced draw resistance cigarette on human smoking parameters and alveolar carbon monoxide levels. In: *Smoking Behavior. Physiological and Psychological Influences*, R.E. Thornton (Editor). Edinburgh: Churchill Livingstone, 1978. pp. 203-207.

Ebert, R.V., McNabb, M.E., McCusker, K.T., Snow, S.L. Amount of nicotine and carbon monoxide inhaled by smokers of low-tar, low-nicotine cigarettes. *Journal of the American Medical Association* 250(20): 2840-2842, 1983.

Fischer, S., Spiegelhalder, B., Preussmann, R. Influence of smoking parameters on the delivery of tobacco-specific nitrosamines in cigarette smoke—A contribution to relative risk evaluation. *Carcinogenesis* 10(6): 1059-1066, 1989.

Fischer, S., Spiegelhalder, B., Preussmann, R. Tobacco-specific nitrosamines in commercial cigarettes: Possibilities for reducing exposure. *IARC Scientific Publications* (105): 489-492, 1991.

Gori, G.B. Cigarette classification as a consumer message. *Regulatory Toxicology and Pharmacology* 12(3 Pt 1): 253-262, 1990a.

Gori, G.B. Consumer perception of cigarette yields: Is the message relevant? *Regulatory Toxicology and Pharmacology* 12(1): 64-68, 1990b.

Gori, G.B., Lynch, C.J. Smoker intake from cigarettes in the 1-mg Federal Trade Commission tar class. *Regulatory Toxicology and Pharmacology* 3(2): 110-120, 1983.

Gritz, E.R., Rose, J.E., Jarvik, M.E. Regulation of tobacco smoke intake with paced cigarette presentation. *Pharmacology, Biochemistry and Behavior* 18: 457-462, 1983.

Gust, S.W., Pickens, R.W., Pechacek, T.F. Relation of puff volume to other topographical measures of smoking. *Addictive Behaviors* 8: 115-119, 1983.

Guyatt, A.R., Kirkham, A., Mariner, D.C., Baldry, A.G., Cumming, G. Long-term effects of switching to cigarettes with lower tar and nicotine yields. *Psychopharmacology* 99: 80-86, 1989b.

Guyatt, A.R., Kirkham, A.J.T., Baldry, A.G., Dixon, M., Cumming, G. How does puffing behavior alter during the smoking of a single cigarette? *Pharmacology, Biochemistry and Behavior* 33(1): 189-195, 1989a.

Henningfield, J.E., Griffiths, R.R. Effects of ventilated cigarette holders on cigarette smoking by humans. *Psychopharmacology* 68(2): 115-119, 1980.

Henningfield, J.E., Kozlowski, L.T., Benowitz, N.L. A proposal to develop meaningful labeling for cigarettes. *Journal of the American Medical Association* 272(4): 312-314, 1994.

Herning, R.I., Jones, R.T., Benowitz, N.L., Mines, A.H. How a cigarette is smoked determines blood nicotine level. *Clinical Pharmacology and Therapeutics* 33: 84-90, 1983.

Höfer, I., Nil, R., Bättig, K. Ultralow-yield cigarettes and type of ventilation: The role of ventilation blocking. *Pharmacology, Biochemistry and Behavior* 40(4): 907-914, 1991.

Kolonen, S., Tuomisto, J., Puustinen, P., Airaksinen, M.M. Smoking behavior in low-yield cigarette smokers and switchers in the natural environment. *Pharmacology, Biochemistry and Behavior* 40(1): 177-180, 1991.

Kozlowski, L.T. Tar and nicotine delivery of cigarettes: What a difference a puff makes. *Journal of the American Medical Association* 254(2): 158-159, 1981.

Kozlowski, L.T. Evidence for limits on the acceptability of lowest tar cigarettes. *American Journal of Public Health* 79(2): 198-199, 1989.

Kozlowski, L.T., Frecker, R.C., Khouw, V., Pope, M.A. The misuse of "less-hazardous" cigarettes and its detection: Hole-blocking of ventilated filters. *American Journal of Public Health* 70(11): 1202-1203, 1980b.

Kozlowski, L.T., Heatherton, T.F., Frecker, R.C., Nolte, H.E. Self-selected blocking of vents on low-yield cigarettes. *Pharmacology, Biochemistry and Behavior* 33(4): 815-819, 1989.

Kozlowski, L.T., Pillitteri, J.L., Sweeney, C.T. Misuse of "light" cigarettes by means of vent blocking. *Journal of Substance Abuse* 6: 333-336, 1994.

Kozlowski, L.T., Pope, M.A., Lux, J.E. Prevalence of the misuse of ultra-low-tar cigarettes by blocking filter vents. *American Journal of Public Health* 78(6): 694-695, 1988.

Kozlowski, L.T., Rickert, W.S., Pope, M.A., Robinson, J.C. A color-matching technique for monitoring tar/nicotine yields to smokers. *American Journal of Public Health* 72(6): 597-599, 1982b.

Kozlowski, L.T., Rickert, W.S., Pope, M.A., Robinson, J.C., Frecker, R.C. Estimating the yield to smokers of tar, nicotine, and carbon monoxide from the "lowest yield" ventilated filter cigarettes. *British Journal of Addiction* 77(2): 159-165, 1982a.

Kozlowski, L.T., Rickert, W.S., Robinson, J.C., Grunberg, N.E. Have tar and nicotine yields of cigarettes changed? *Science* 209(4464): 1550-1551, 1980a.

Maron, D.J., Fortmann, S.P. Nicotine yield and measures of cigarette smoke exposure in a large population: Are lower-yield cigarettes safer? *American Journal of Public Health* 77(5): 546-549, 1987.

McBride, M.J., Guyatt, A.R., Kirkham, A.J., Cumming, G. Assessment of smoking behavior and ventilation with cigarettes of differing nicotine yields. *Clinical Science* 67: 619-631, 1984.

Nil, R., Buzzi, R., Bättig, K. Effects of different cigarette smoke yields on puffing and inhalation: Is the measurement of inhalation volumes relevant for smoke absorption? *Pharmacology, Biochemistry and Behavior* 24: 587-595, 1986.

Pomerleau, O.F., Pomerleau, C.S. Neuroregulators and the reinforcement of smoking: Towards a biobehavioral explanation. *Neuroscience and Biobehavioral Reviews* 8(4): 503-513, 1984.

Rawbone, R.G. Switching to low-tar cigarettes: Are the tar league tables relevant? *Thorax* 39(9): 657-662, 1984.

Rickert, W.S., Collishaw, N.E., Bray, D.F., Robinson, J.C. Estimates of maximum or average cigarette tar, nicotine, and carbon monoxide yields can be obtained from yields under standard conditions. *Preventive Medicine* 15(1): 82-91, 1986.

Rickert, W.S., Robinson, J.C. Estimating the hazards of less hazardous cigarettes. II. Study of cigarette yields of nicotine, carbon monoxide, and hydrogen cyanide in relation to levels of cotinine, carboxyhemoglobin, and thiocyanate in smokers. *Journal of Toxicology and Environmental Health* 7: 391-403, 1981.

Rickert, W.S., Robinson, J.C., Collishaw, N.E., Bray, D.F. Estimating the hazards of "less hazardous" cigarettes. III. A study of the effect of various smoking conditions on yields of hydrogen cyanide and cigarette tar. *Journal of Toxicology and Environmental Health* 12(1): 39-54, 1983.

Rickert, W.S., Robinson, J.C., Young, J.C. Estimating the hazards of "less hazardous" cigarettes. I. Tar, nicotine, carbon monoxide, acrolein, hydrogen cyanide, and total aldehyde deliveries of Canadian cigarettes. *Journal of Toxicology and Environmental Health* 6(2): 351-365, 1980.

Robinson, J.C., Young, J.C., Rickert, W.S. A comparative study of the amount of smoke absorbed from low-yield ("less hazardous") cigarettes. Part 1. Non-invasive measures. *British Journal of Addiction* 77(4): 383-397, 1982.

Robinson, J.C., Young, J.C., Rickert, W.S. Maintain levels of nicotine but reduce other smoke constituents: A formula for "less-hazardous" cigarettes? *Preventive Medicine* 13(5): 437-445, 1984.

Robinson, J.C., Young, J.C., Rickert, W.S., Fey, G., Kozlowski, L.T. A comparative study of the amount of smoke absorbed from low-yield ("less hazardous") cigarettes. Part 2. Invasive measures. *British Journal of Addiction* 78(1): 79-87, 1983.

Russell, M.A.H., Jarvis, M.J., Feyerabend, C., Saloojee, Y. Reduction of tar, nicotine, and carbon monoxide intake in low-tar smokers. *Journal of Epidemiology and Community Health* 40(1): 80-85, 1986.

Russell, M.A.H., Sutton, S.R., Iyer, R., Feyerabend, C., Vesey, C.J. Long-term switching to low-tar low-nicotine cigarettes. *British Journal of Addiction* 77(2): 145-158, 1982.

Schlotzhauer, W.S., Chortyk, O.T. Effects of varied smoking machine parameters on deliveries of total particulate matter and selected smoke constituents from an ultra-low-tar cigarette. *Journal of Analytical Toxicology* 7(2): 92-95, 1983.

Snedecor, G.W., Cochran, W.G. Correlation. In: *Statistical Methods,* G.W. Snedecor and W.G. Cochran (Editors). Ames, IA: Iowa State University Press, 1980.

U.S. Department of Health and Human Services. *The Health Consequences of Smoking: The Changing Cigarette. A Report of the Surgeon General.* DHHS Publication No. (PHS)81-50156. Rockville, MD: U.S. Department of Health and Human Services, Public Health Service, Office on Smoking and Health, 1981.

Wald, N.J., Boreham, J., Bailey, A. Relative intakes of tar, nicotine, and carbon monoxide from cigarettes of different yields. *Thorax* 39(5): 361-364, 1984.

Woodward, M., Tunstall-Pedoe, H. Do smokers of lower tar cigarettes consume lower amounts of smoke components? Results from the Scottish Health Study. *British Journal of Addiction* 87(6): 921-928, 1992.